# GENETICS
## IN THE CLINIC

*Clinical, Ethical, and Social Implications
for Primary Care*

# GENETICS
## IN THE CLINIC
### Clinical, Ethical, and Social Implications for Primary Care

MARY B. MAHOWALD, Ph.D.
Professor
Department of Obstetrics and Gynecology
  and MacLean Center for Clinical
  Medical Ethics
Committee on Genetics
University of Chicago
Chicago, Illinois

ANGELA S. SCHEUERLE, M.D.
Medical Director
Texas Birth Defects Research Center
Texas Department of Health
Austin, Texas

VICTOR A. McKUSICK, M.D.
Professor of Medical Genetics
Institute of Genetic Medicine
Johns Hopkins University
Baltimore, Maryland

TIMOTHY J. ASPINWALL, J.D.
Nossaman, Guthner, Knox, Elliott, LLP
Sacramento, California

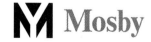 Mosby

*A Harcourt Health Sciences Company*

St. Louis   London   Philadelphia   Sydney   Toronto

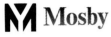

**Mosby**

*A Harcourt Health Sciences Company*

*Editor:* Liz Fathman
*Editorial Assistant:* Paige Mosher Wilke
*Project Manager:* Carol Sullivan Weis
*Designer:* Mark A. Oberkrom

Mosby, Inc.
*A Harcourt Health Sciences Company*
11830 Westline Industrial Drive
St. Louis, Missouri 63146

Printed in the United States of America

**Library of Congress Cataloging in Publication Data**

Genetics in the clinic: clinical, ethical, and social implications for primary care/Mary B. Mahowald . . . [et al.].
    p. ; cm.
    Includes bibliographical references and index.
    ISBN 0-323-01203-5
    1. Medical genetics. 2. Primary care (Medicine) I. Mahowald, Mary Briody.
    [DNLM: 1. Genetics, Medical. 2. Primary Health Care. QZ 50 G32827 2001]
RB155 .G3894 2001
616'.042—dc21

00-135004

01  02  03  04  05  TG/FF  9 8 7 6 5 4 3 2 1

# Editors

**VICTOR A. McKUSICK, M.D.**
Professor of Medical Genetics
Institute of Genetic Medicine
Johns Hopkins University
Baltimore, Maryland

**ANGELA S. SCHEUERLE, M.D.**
Medical Director
Texas Birth Defects Research Center
Texas Department of Health
Austin, Texas

**MARY B. MAHOWALD, Ph.D.**
Professor
Department of Obstetrics and Gynecology
  and MacLean Center for Clinical
  Medical Ethics
Committee on Genetics
University of Chicago
Chicago, Illinois

**TIMOTHY J. ASPINWALL, J.D.**
Nossaman, Guthner, Knox, Elliott, LLP
Sacramento, California

# Contributors

**JAMES E. BOWMAN, M.D., FASCP, FCAP**
Professor Emeritus
Department of Pathology
University of Chicago
Chicago, Illinois

**DAN W. BROCK, Ph.D.**
Professor
Department of Philosophy and Biomedical
  Ethics;
Director, Center for Biomedical Ethics
Brown University
Providence, Rhode Island

**C. THOMAS CASKEY, M.D.**
President and Chief Executive Officer
Cogene Biotech Ventures, LP
Houston, Texas

**SHELLY A. CUMMINGS, B.S., M.S.**
Assistant Director and Genetic Counselor
Cancer Risk Clinic
Section of Hematology/Oncology
Department of Medicine
University of Chicago
Chicago, Illinois

**CATHLEEN M. HARRIS, M.D., M.P.H.**
Assistant Medical Director
Phoenix Perinatal Associates
Phoenix, Arizona

**LYNN A. JANSEN, R.N., Ph.D.**
Assistant Professor and Assistant Director
  of the Bioethics Institute
New York Medical College
Valhalla, New York;
Senior Medical Ethicist
The John J. Conley Department of Ethics
  Saint Vincents Hospital
New York, New York

**JASON H.T. KARLAWISH, M.D.**
Assistant Professor of Medicine
Department of Medicine
University of Pennsylvania
Philadelphia, Pennsylvania

**JOHN D. LANTOS, M.D.**
Associate Professor and Section Chief,
  General Pediatrics
Department of Pediatrics and Medicine;
Co-Director
MacLean Center for Clinical Medical
  Ethics
University of Chicago
Chicago, Illinois

**MICHAEL J. MALINOWSKI, J.D.**
Associate Professor of Law
Widener University School of Law
Wilmington, Delaware

**MARGARET R. MOON, M.D.**
Vice President
Ethics and Clinical Programs
Doctors Community Healthcare
  Corporation
Scottsdale, Arizona

**ROBERT J. MOSS, M.D.**
Clinical Assistant Professor
Department of Family Practice
University of Illinois
Chicago, Illinois;
Director of Geriatrics
Department of Family Practice
Lutheran General Hospital
Park Ridge, Illinois

**OLUFUNMILAYO I. OLOPADE, M.B., B.S., FACP**
Associate Professor
Department of Medicine;
Director, Cancer Risk Clinic
University of Chicago
Chicago, Illinois

**WILLIAM H. PERANTEAU, B.A.**
University of Pennsylvania
School of Medicine
Philadelphia, Pennsylvania

**LAINIE FRIEDMAN ROSS, M.D., Ph.D.**
Assistant Professor
Departments of Pediatrics and Medicine;
Assistant Director
MacLean Center for Clinical Medical
  Ethics
University of Chicago
Chicago, Illinois

**ANITA SILVERS, Ph.D.**
Professor
Department of Philosophy
San Francisco State University;
Community Member
Medical Ethics Committee
San Francisco General Hospital
San Francisco, California

**MARION S. VERP, M.D.**
Associate Professor
Departments of Obstetrics and Gynecology
  and Human Genetics
University of Chicago
Chicago, Illinois

*To James V. Neel, Ph.D., M.D. (1915-2000), pioneer in the application of genetics in the clinic and perceptive student of the implications of genetics for society, and*


*to Beth Fine Kaplan, M.S., C.G.C. (1956-1998), who prepared others to make those applications as knowledgeably, sensitively, and effectively as possible.*

# Acknowledgments

This book is the culmination of a 3-year project supported by the U. S. Department of Energy (DOE) entitled "Implications of the 'Geneticization' of Healthcare for Primary Care Practitioners" (DE-FG02-95ER61990). I wish to thank the DOE's Ethical, Legal, and Social Issues (ELSI) Program and Office of Biological and Environmental Research for that support. I am also grateful to my co-investigators in the project: Christine Cassel, John Lantos, Mira Lessick, Robert Moss, Lainie Friedman Ross, Greg Sachs, and Marion Verp. Practitioners who worked with each of the co-investigators were Laurel Anderson, Cathleen Harris, Jason Karlawish, Sheila Malm, Margaret Moon, and Darrel Waggoner. Dana Levinson and Timothy Aspinwall coordinated the project in its early and later phases, respectively. National advisors or consultants who contributed by presentations on specific topics were Lori Andrews, James Bowman, Dan Brock, Tom Caskey, Sherman Elias, Wolfgang Epstein, Beth Fine, Stephen French, Jeff Leiden, Noralane Lindor, Abby Lippman, Victor McKusick, Carole Ober, Julie Gage Palmer, Colleen Scanlon, Anita Silvers, and Joe Leigh Simpson. Although not formally involved in the project, Shelly Cummings and Olufunmilayo Olapade extended its scope to include cancer genetics. I am thankful to all these individuals for helping to bring this book to fruition.

Others helped immensely in the editing and publication process. At the University of Chicago, our department librarian, Gail Isenberg, her assistant Samina Ahmed, and our tech staff facilitated the process through their computer expertise. Tim Jacobs spent long hours preparing electronic and hard copies of the manuscript, and Beatrix Merigold enabled me to review and return the page proofs with considerable efficiency.

At Harcourt Health Sciences, Liz Fathman is the kind of editor I would like my friends to find, and I feel similarly about Paige Mosher, editorial assistant, and Carol Weis, Project Manager. Mark Oberkrom designed an unusually attractive cover, and Joanne Worley-Pellegrini made my involvement in the marketing process as easy as it could be.

Finally, I wish to acknowledge support groups with whom I am affiliated at the University of Chicago, including the Department of Obstetrics and Gynecology, the MacLean Center for Clinical Medical Ethics, and the Committee on Genetics. To all the individuals in all these settings who have supported the work on this book, I am most grateful.

MARY B. MAHOWALD

# Foreword

## THE FUTURE OF MEDICAL GENETICS

The announcement of the completion of the Human Genome sequence in 2000 alters the landscape for medical care with particular opportunities emerging for heritable diseases. Medical genetics is a rapidly expanding element of practice in specialties such as obstetrics, pediatrics, and internal medicine. Carrier testing for common recessive diseases, such as sickle cell anemia, cystic fibrosis, or Tay Sachs, should be available to all couples. All pregnant women over age 40 should be counseled for prenatal diagnostic options related to risk of Down syndrome. All newborns should receive genetic screening of treatable metabolic disorders such as galactosemia or phenylketonuria. Adults with late-onset genetic disorders should be diagnosed as early as possible to maximize lifestyle and management opportunities.

The clinical importance of genetic diagnostics and therapeutics has increased with the mapping and sequencing of the Human Genome and now focuses on gene functions in disease and health. The pace at which genes are associated with specific diseases will undoubtedly accelerate as new tools, such as DNA expression chips and bioinformatics, are applied to disease problems. Medical applications of human genetics thus deserve careful consideration. In applying this knowledge, primary care physicians must consider individual, family, and societal attitudes and evaluate the medical risks and benefits of new genetic practices as acceptable standards of care.

Genome science will provide an increasing list of therapeutic targets. Some estimate that 8000 to 10,000 of our 100,000 genes will emerge as targets of therapy. New genetic information will also accelerate the development of improved drugs and protein replacement through gene therapy. Seen simply as new techniques, the genetically engineered treatments pose no major new issues for individual patient care because, ideally, medicine embraces the most efficacious and safe treatment. Accordingly, we should view these new therapies with positive expectations and the realization that new therapeutic strategies require focus on safety.

A major therapeutic concept that will benefit through collaboration between genome science and human genetics is the use of vaccines. Vaccines have long provided an accepted strategy for prevention of infectious disease. Prevention of childhood diseases and, recently, adult viral illnesses has had enormous impact on improved health. For example, infantile paralysis is virtually eradicated, and mother-to-child liver cancer transmission is greatly reduced in China because of polio and hepatitis B vaccines. We anticipate additional vaccines against agents such as human papillomavirus (HPV, cervical cancer), human immunodeficiency virus (HIV, AIDS), malaria, and *mycobacterium tuberculosis* (TB). The 20 bacterial genomes fully sequenced and annotated for gene functions facilitate identification of vaccine gene targets.

With the new technology, individuals at risk for genetic disease will be identified and treated before they become patients through presymptomatic therapy. This is the new medical paradigm forecast by human genetics and genome science. The most compelling example of this paradigm is the use of cholesterol-lowering drugs to prevent cardiac and cerebrovascular occlusion. Lipid, lipoprotein, and genetic diagnostic markers can reliably identify individuals at risk for vascular occlusion. With these drugs' proven efficacy and safety and multiple options for patient identification, genetic testing may be utilized on a national level to identify at-risk persons, who can receive presymptomatic therapy for this most common fatal disease in the United States. The risk/benefit ratio is clearly favorable for this initiative. Nonetheless, since individuals of normal health will be treated for extended periods, use of presymptomatic therapy raises the threshold for drug safety to a level nearly equivalent to that required for vaccines. Genetic risk of the disease must be weighed against the risk and cost of chronic therapy.

We are experiencing a renaissance in medical diagnostics made possible by the Human Genome Project and disease-related DNA testing. Current clinical diagnostic tests measure pathological changes in select patients through automated blood chemical measurements, Papanicolaou testing (Pap smears), and cranial magnetic resonance imaging (MRI). DNA testing not only identifies individuals at risk but also raises the capacity of detecting disease risk in relatives. The challenges include poor patient understanding of disease risk, concern about the privacy of family information, and discrimination in regard to insurance and employment. All of these areas demand education not only of patients but also of primary care physicians. A national educational framework of general principles for DNA diagnostic applications must be developed. Such education will need to be continually refocused as effective therapy options emerge for specific diseases such as cancer, diabetes, and vascular occlusion.

The first widespread DNA-based diagnostics will probably occur in treatment of cancer, where both germline and somatic gene mutations contribute to disease predisposition and progression. Economic and rapid DNA systems are in development but not widely accepted or available. For the near future, the medical community will depend on specialty reference laboratories, and medical genetics programs will serve a critical role in providing this service. The absence of DNA test kits with U.S. Food and Drug Administration (FDA) approval will challenge reimbursement decisions on whether to provide this new and highly specific testing. Examples already exist for fluorescence in situ hybridization (FISH) and DNA sequence diagnosis. New therapeutics, such as Her-2 neu antibodies (herceptin) for breast cancer, will accelerate these decisions and policies.

Implementation of new DNA diagnostic systems, matched to appropriate therapy, deserves special consideration. Such tailoring of medical therapy to each patient's individual genetic makeup has created the field of *pharmacogenetics*. Some scientists speculate that pharmacogenetics will improve the matching of patients to specific drug responsiveness and will allow drug selection to minimize side effects. Proposals in this area will need to withstand the traditional assessment of risk/benefit considerations, outcome research, and cost-effectiveness.

Specialty-trained medical geneticists and genetic counselors have been touchstones of quality genetics care. Typically, these providers focus on the individual and family for diagnosis, education, and presentation of appropriate care options. Their number is limited, however, and their care is currently focused in pediatrics, obstetrics, and oncology. Specialists in genetics are needed for the education of primary care physicians, who will be the responsible for providing established medical genetics practice. Clearly, the day-to-day genetic health providers of the future will be primary care clinicians.

C. THOMAS CASKEY, M.D.
President and Chief Executive Officer
Cogene Biotech Ventures, LP
Houston, Texas

# Contents

# GENETICS
## IN THE CLINIC
*Clinical, Ethical, and Social Implications
for Primary Care*

# INTRODUCTION

# Geneticization in the Clinic

*Mary B. Mahowald*

In 1991, Abby Lippman coined a term that has since been used to characterize the impact of advances in genetics on the population at large. *Geneticization,* she wrote, is "an ongoing process by which differences between individuals are reduced to their DNA codes, with most disorders, behaviors and physiological variations defined, at least in part, as genetic in origin."[1] This ongoing process has significant implications for primary caregivers, even those whose practice required little knowledge of genetics in the past. Despite the rapid advances in genetics, the majority of health caregivers go about their daily tasks with little attention to the impact these developments have on patient care. Gradually, as members of diverse specialties recognize the relevance of genetics to diagnosis and treatment of their patients, attention to genetics is increasing. The goal of this book is to accelerate and facilitate the integration of genetics into routine primary care practice.

Greater understanding of genetics and its social and ethical implications is important for primary caregivers for several reasons. First, there is ample evidence of their deficiency of training in and knowledge of genetics and its implications. For example, when physicians from ten states who were not geneticists or academics were questioned about genetic information judged relevant to their practice by a panel of their peers, they answered more than 25% of the questions incorrectly.[2] Second, the usefulness of genetic diagnosis and possibilities for prevention or treatment have extended beyond prenatal and early childhood care where they have concentrated for decades. Genetics is now relevant to clinical encounters with patients of any age and either sex, whether well or ill. Third, the clinical relevance of genetics is no longer limited to single-gene disorders of relatively rare occurrence but applies to a huge array of common complex disorders that physicians who are not geneticists confront routinely. To the extent that all disease has a genetic component, this far-reaching relevance is undeniable.

Many clinicians, however, seem resistant to learning about and incorporating genetics into their practice. For example, a national conference entitled "The New Genetics in Primary Care," organized through support from the National Institutes of Health in 1997, mainly attracted specialists who were already well trained in genetics, along with some specialists in ethics. Although some of these individuals probably served as conduits of their knowledge of genetics and ethics to primary caregivers, it is doubtful that this transmission occurred on the scale warranted by relevant advances. In recent years, education about genetics and ethics expanded in medical school training, nursing education, postgraduate training, and continuing education programs, and ties between genetics and ethics are increasingly addressed in all of these programs. The National Board of Medical Examiners now lists "Genetics" as a separate category for questions on the licensing examination for all U.S. physicians. Nonetheless, huge gaps remain between the preparedness of most general practitioners for dealing with implications of genetics and their preparedness in other areas of clinical medicine.

As primary caregivers learn more about genetics to optimize their care of particular patients, they also need to recognize situations in which their patients should be referred to genetics experts for counseling about specific conditions. Referrals to specialists are a long-standing requirement of good generalist practice. As genetic information proliferates, this practice is even more necessary because those who optimally treat "the whole person" cannot themselves acquire expertise in genetics that is comparable to those who concentrate exclusively on genetics or its subspecialties. Knowing how and when to refer, however, assumes a basic knowledge of genetics.

Many clinicians have been relatively disinterested in genetics because curative or definitely preventive measures are usually unavailable when a positive genetic diagnosis is obtained. This inability to affect outcome probably serves as a disincentive to primary care practitioners. In the absence of treatment modalities after positive prenatal genetic testing, the legal option of terminating the pregnancy may be unavailable, morally objectionable, costly, and psychologically onerous. Although elective abortions are medically induced, they are neither experientially nor morally equivalent to the medical treatment that clinicians are accustomed to offering to restore health, prevent disease, or sustain life. Abortions after prenatal diagnosis may be particularly troubling for clinicians and patients because they are usually performed late in pregnancy with the specific goal of ending particular fetal lives.

Predictive tests for late-onset and multifactorial disorders present new challenges to traditional diagnosis and treatment. In addition to the discomfort clinicians may feel about lack of effective treatment modalities, communicating either negative or positive results may be complicated by the remaining uncertainty about whether a given individual will actually contract the disease to which he or she is susceptible. In the absence of symptoms, for example, the clinician is unable to tell a patient who tests positive for breast cancer or prostate cancer that she or he will in fact have the disease sometime in the future. Also, a negative result does not eliminate the possibility of disease onset. In other words, good news does not preclude a bad outcome and vice versa.

In a health care system that rewards procedures more than talking with patients, the communication skills and time required for effective counseling about genetics are scarce commodities. Primary care practitioners are given little incentive to provide information about genetics and genetic testing. Although medical geneticists and genetic counselors may provide genetic information and counsel patients about its implications, primary caregivers remain responsible for obtaining adequate informed consent for genetic tests and procedures undertaken in their practice. Moreover, to the extent that genetic information affects them, family members of particular patients may also require information and counseling. Thus issues of confidentiality become much more complicated for primary caregivers because of the problems of disclosure raised by the unique impact of genetic information on other family members. Similar issues are raised with regard to the potential right of insurance companies and employers to such information.

Although genetic counseling is a young profession, its emphasis on nondirectiveness has been central to its practice and to the education of its members throughout its history. This emphasis has been reinforced by the desire to avoid eugenic applications or interpretations of genetic counseling and by the fact that most genetic counseling has taken place in the context of reproductive decision making, where the law and social mores support the right of individuals to make decisions consistent with their own moral values. However, nondirectiveness stands in contrast to the explicit priority given by primary caregivers to their patients' health. Typically, patients expect and desire directiveness with regard to that goal. To the extent that genetic tests or interventions are conducive to their patients' health, general practitioners should probably remain directive. To the extent that this is not the case, physicians may need to learn how to counsel patients nondirectively.

To facilitate directive and nondirective uses of genetic information by primary caregivers, Part I of this book reviews the underlying principles of genetics and their implications for diagnosis and management of genetic disease. Victor McKusick, who was trained in internal medicine but is most widely known for his monumental and continually updated catalog of human genetic conditions, *Mendelian Inheritance in Man,* introduces this section with a review of the background, progress, and promise of the Human Genome Project. Angela Scheuerle, a clinical geneticist trained in pediatrics, follows with chapters on genetic testing and possibilities for treatment of genetic disease. Because cancer in its various manifestations across different age groups is a common concern of primary caregivers, a chapter is included on cancer genetics by Marion Verp, an obstetrician and geneticist; Shelly Cummings, a genetic counselor at a cancer risk clinic; and Olufunmilayo Olopade, a medical oncologist. This section concludes with a chapter on clinical aspects of prenatal testing and interventions by obstetricians Cathleen Harris and Marion Verp.

Part II examines topics of relevance to clinicians who practice in a primary care setting. Dan Brock, a philosopher, examines how concepts of health and disease are influenced by knowledge of genetics. James Bowman, co-author of *Genetic Variation and Disorders in Peoples of African Origin,*[3] considers cultural and ethnic differences in genetic testing; I discuss issues of gender justice in genetics; and Anita Silvers, co-author of *Disability, Difference, Discrimination,*[4] addresses issues that are relevant to care of persons with disabilities and their families. Shelly Cummings draws on her experience to discuss how the skills of genetic counseling are applicable to the primary care setting, and Lynn Jansen, a nurse and a political scientist, examines the role that nurses may play in the provision of genetic services.

Part III deals with ethical and social issues raised by advances in genetics for specific groups of practitioners. Obstetricians Cathleen Harris and Marion Verp address ethical issues for those who provide prenatal care. Pediatricians Margaret Moon and Lainie Friedman Ross consider diagnostic and presymptomatic genetic testing of children; Ross also discusses the problem of consent to genetic testing of pediatric patients. Internist Jason Karlawish and medical student William Peranteau examine whether general internists should offer genetic screening to their patients, and family physician Robert Moss, in collaboration with Shelly Cummings and me, addresses presymptomatic and predictive genetic testing as "a family affair."

Part IV considers policy topics that primary care providers face because of the role they play in safeguarding the confidentiality of medical information. John Lantos, a pediatrician, and Timothy Aspinwall, a lawyer, track the impact on primary caregivers of an unregulated market in genetic testing and interventions. Aspinwall also examines the impact of reportable or discoverable genetic information on insurance coverage and employment of primary care patients. Michael Malinowski, lawyer and author of a recent text on biotechnology,[5] addresses some of the ethical and legal challenges raised for practitioners through the commercialization of genetic tests.

The final section is a glossary of terms used in genetics and a selective bibliography of articles, books, policy statements, and electronic resources on clinical, ethical, and social implications of advances in genetics. Recognizing the busyness of today's primary caregivers, our hope is to facilitate optimal care for patients by assisting them in meeting the challenge these advances pose.

## REFERENCES

1. Lippman A: Prenatal genetic testing and screening, *Am J Law Med* 17:15-50, 1991.
2. Holtzman NA, Watson MS, editors: *Promoting safe and effective genetic testing in the United States,* Baltimore, 1998, Johns Hopkins University Press.
3. Bowman JE, Murray RF: *Genetic variation and disorders in peoples of African origin,* Baltimore, 1990, Johns Hopkins University Press.
4. Silvers A, Wasserman D, Mahowald MB: *Disability, difference, discrimination: perspectives on justice in bioethics and public policy,* New York, 1998, Rowman & Littlefield.
5. Malinowski MJ: *Biotechnology: law, business, and regulation,* New York, 1999, Aspen.

# PART I

# CLINICAL APPLICATIONS OF GENETICS

# CHAPTER 1

# Mapping the Human Genome: Retrospective, Perspective, and Prospective

*Victor A. McKusick*

## HISTORY

In human genetics, 1956 was a watershed year. In Copenhagen at the First World Congress of Human Genetics, the correct chromosome number in humans was announced: a diploid number of 46 (not 48 as previously thought). It was not merely getting the count right that was significant; it was also the demonstrated ability to study human chromosomes with relative facility, leading to discovery of aberrations causing birth defects, such as Down syndrome, and cancers, such as chronic myeloid leukemia, during the subsequent 5 to 6 years. Medical genetics as a clinical discipline now had its organ, as cardiology has the heart and neurology has the nervous system.

Developments in the laboratory were accompanied by the growth of medical genetics as a clinical discipline. One of the newest and fastest-growing areas of medical specialization, it became the twenty-fifth member of the American Board of Medical Specialists in 1991 and thus gained recognition as a separate medical specialty, equal with pediatrics or surgery. However, the application of genetic medicine is not limited to this relatively small group of practitioners, any more than distribution of antibiotics is limited to those board-certified in infectious disease. All physicians should be prepared to counsel concerning the genetic problems of families and individuals who come under their care. Genetic counselors or medical geneticists can do only a small portion—the more complex portion—of genetic counseling.

A genetic counselor should have the fullest possible understanding of the human genome and how variations in it can lead to disease and other deviant phenotypes. With increasing knowledge, focus on gene structure shifts to a focus on gene function. Focus on the basic etiology of genetic disease becomes a focus on pathogenesis. The psychosocial aspects of genetic counseling are also important and require improving, but those aspects have limited value if less than accurate and comprehensive information is available for the counselors to transmit.

### Chromosome Structure

The karyotype is a low-resolution optical microscope view of the human chromosomes. The following are visible in this view:

1. Twenty-four types of chromosomes (the 22 autosomes and the X and Y chromosome)
2. An estimated 70,000 genes (range of estimates, 50,000 to 100,000) carried by the chromosomes
3. An estimated 3 billion nucleotides in the haploid genome (one chromosome from each pair)

Each chromosome constitutes a single molecule of deoxyribonucleic acid (DNA) packaged so tightly that if unwound, each cell's complement would stretch to 5 feet in length. (A small 25th chromosome is located in the mitochondria in the cytoplasm. It has already been sequenced completely with mapping of its genes and identification of disorders caused by mutations in those genes.)

By 1968, approximately 68 genes were known to be located on the X chromosome because of the characteristic pedigree pattern of traits, such as colorblindness and hemophilia, but it was not until that year that a gene was assigned to a specific autosome: Duffy blood group locus to chromosome 1 by linkage to a normal morphologic variant of chromosome 1. In the 1970s, human-rodent somatic cell hybridization became a method for mapping genes to chromosomes. In the 1980s, molecular genetics came to the further aid of gene mapping. It provided the following:

1. Gene probes that made it possible to search directly for the gene in somatic cell hybrids, eliminating the need for the gene to be active in the hybrid
2. Probes for reliable mapping of single-copy genes by in situ hybridization
3. Polymorphic DNA markers for linkage studies in families

In the 1990s, the methods of molecular genetics were used to break down the entire genome into overlapping segments (e.g., yeast artificial chromosomes [YACs]), which could be used for mapping cloned genes and as the basis for sequencing. (A "clone" is simply a genetically identical copy. To speak of a gene as having been cloned means that the gene has been identified and that multiple copies of the gene have been made through manipulation, usually in an experimental organism such as bacteria or yeast.) "Radiation hybrids" similarly dissect the genome into multiple segments of varying lengths that can be used for mapping gene clones to specific segments and therefore to specific chromosomal sites.

## HUMAN GENOME PROJECT

**Genome** is a hybrid word created by elision from genes and chromosomes. **Human genome** denotes the complete complement of genes and chromosomes in the nucleus of each human cell. The Human Genome Project (HGP) was first formally proposed in 1985 as a multinational effort to identify all the genes on the human chromosomes. Robert Sinsheimer, Walter Gilbert, Renato Dulbecco, and others further suggested undertaking the project to determine the sequence of the four kinds of nucleotide bases (abbreviated A, T, C, and G) in the DNA of both the coding and the noncoding parts of all the chromosomes. In an influential editorial in 1986, Dulbecco suggested that major understanding of human cancer could result from complete sequencing. No mention of gene mapping was made by Dulbecco or the others in the field. Gene mapping is fundamentally a cartographic project; it aims to map all the genes on the chromosomes and also to determine the ultimate map: the nucleotide sequence of the DNA. Thus the HGP is an enterprise for complete mapping of the human genome. By 1986, more than 800 genes were mapped to specific chromosomes and most genes to specific chromosomal regions.

The HGP was debated, discussed, and planned during a 5-year gestational period. In the United States, the project was initiated October 1, 1990 and predicted to take 15 years for completion. On this schedule, the last gene and the last nucleotide should be identified by midnight September 30, 2005. At the 5-year mark, Francis Collins, director of the HGP in the National Institutes of Health (NIH), said the project is "ahead of schedule and under budget." Projections then suggested that the enterprise may reach its goal by April 25, 2003, which is the 50th anniversary of the landmark paper by Watson and Crick (1953), or that it will at least be finished by February 2, 2004, which is the 60th anniversary of the report by Avery, MacLeod, and McCarty that DNA is the genetic material. A completion date of 2006 would be satisfactory, since this would be the 50th anniversary of the report of the correct chromosome number in the human. Going from a correct count of the chromosomes to a complete chemical description in 50 years would be a great achievement. A first draft of the complete sequence was jointly announced on June 26, 2000, by publicly funded laboratories and a commercial laboratory.

## Retrospective

In late 1986 the National Academy of Sciences (USA) called for a committee to examine whether the HGP could and should be undertaken. In its report in early 1988, the committee concluded that the project should be undertaken and proposed that it could be completed within 15 years at an expense of approximately $200 million a year. Their recommendation was map first, sequence later. The logic behind this suggestion was that physical and genetic maps of the genome would be required as substrate and scaffolding for efficient sequencing and the intervening time would allow the sequencing technology to evolve to maximal efficiency.

The HGP is not confined to North America. As plans were made in the United States, similar plans were made in Europe and Japan, and important contributions have come from other countries, each with its own programs. Coordination of the HGP among countries has been the role of the Human Genome Organization (HUGO), which Norton Zinder, one of its founding council, referred to as a "UN for the human genome." HUGO was constituted in Montreux, Switzerland, in September 1988 at a meeting of 32 scientists from 19 countries. HUGO is not an agency for funding of the research but rather a coordinating agency. HUGO played a role in integrating the physical and genetic mapping of chromosomes through workshops and is involved with international aspects of intellectual property rights; patenting; ethical, legal, and social issues; genome databases and other research resources; the human genome diversity project; and conduct of international genome conferences.

HUGO programs are particularly significant in Europe where multiple nations have individually funded human genome projects. In the United States, coordination in the public sector has been provided mainly by two funding agencies that work collaboratively: roughly one third of federal funding is through the Department of Energy and two thirds is funded through the National Institutes of Health (NIH). In keeping with the expansion of the project and the recognized impact of the work, the National Center for Human Genome Research (NCHGR) became the National Human Genome Research Institute (NHGRI) in 1997.

## Perspective

In the United States, James Watson was the first director of the NIH genome program; Francis Collins has been director since 1993. Progress in the first 5½ years was aided greatly by several technical advances not yet known when the HGP was proposed in 1985 and 1986. Three of these technical advances are PCR (1985-1986), which is known by most, at least by name, since the O.J. Simpson trial; YACs for cloning large segments of DNA (1987); and microsatellite DNA markers (1989), which are a much improved tool for genetic linkage studies in families because of high-order polymorphism (normal variation).

The HGP involves creation of genetic and physical maps and the ultimate definition of the nucleotide sequence. A genetic map is in essence a statistical model that represents one gene's distance from another based on observation of how frequently those two genes are inherited together. More commonly, "markers" were developed against which to observe gene inheritance. These markers are identifiable pieces of DNA, or short intervals of sequence, that themselves do not function as genes but which are standard enough to use as tools. During the first 5 years, genetic reference maps have been constructed with DNA markers at close intervals, useful for linkage mapping of traits and disorders in families or for defining somatic deletions in cancers. Physical maps of overlapping DNA segments, such as those cloned in YACs, have also been created. These are called physical maps because they consist of tangible, testable pieces of DNA that can serve as substrate for sequencing and locating genes through hybridization.

In addition to the genetic map of DNA markers and the physical map of chromosomal segments, an important step in the HGP is the development of expressed sequence tags (ESTs). This approach involves isolating parts of genes by working back from the messenger RNA through the complementary DNA (cDNA) formed using reverse transcriptase; these parts of genes are called ESTs. The ESTs represent the business part of the genome. Many thousands of ESTs have been mapped, covering all the chromosomes. This array is referred to as the *transcript map;* it is a map of the elements of the genome (genes) that are transcribed into messenger RNA for translation into specific proteins.

## Map-Based Gene Discovery

From the first, a main justification for the HGP was its potential for identifying the basic genetic defects, not only in cancer but also in hereditary disorders such as muscular dystrophy and Huntington disease, and its potential for defining the basis for genetic susceptibility to multifactorial disorders such as diabetes, hypertension, and mental illness. In the early stages of gene mapping, clinical application was limited to use of the linkage principle to diagnose a disorder prenatally or presymptomatically or in the carrier state. For example, in 1983 Huntington disease was linked to DNA markers at the end of the short arm of chromosome 4. Although the gene itself had not been cloned, linkage to those markers could be used for diagnosing the disorder before onset of clinical disease under favorable circumstances (i.e., if DNA was available from both affected and unaffected relatives and the markers showed proper variation among the family members).

Originally, genes were located indirectly by identifying the gene product, a protein typically active in metabolism, and then tracking down the responsible gene. In 1986, *positional cloning* (initially known as reverse genetics because the protein need not be found first) allowed map-based gene discovery. In simple terms, positional cloning involves finding DNA markers that flank the region where the disorder maps and "walking in on the gene." This is roughly analogous to locating a small town along a highway in Texas by starting at one state border driving in the correct direction. Once the gene involved in a given disorder is isolated by positional cloning and specific disease-causing point mutations are identified in the gene, specific DNA tests for the disorder become possible. For example, in 1993, 10 years after Huntington disease was mapped to the short arm of chromosome 4, the gene was finally cloned; the unusual type of mutation (an expansion of a 3-nucleotide CAG repeat) was found; and specific DNA tests were designed for diagnostic, presymptomatic, prenatal, and even preimplantation diagnosis.

Map-based gene discovery has become a leading paradigm in biomedical research. By this approach, many disorders have by now been characterized at a basic level. All specialties of medicine use map-based gene discovery to study their most puzzling diseases.

## Sequence-Based Gene Discovery

The complete sequence of the human genome is necessary for finding all the genes, as well as for learning what the noncoding parts of the genome represent.

An exciting aspect of the HGP is the nonhuman genome project (i.e., work involving model organisms in parallel with the work in the human) and the work in various databases containing genomic information on humans and other organisms. These two areas are related and have great potential for advancing the understanding of the human genome.

Homology, an ancient and highly useful concept in biology, recognizes that organisms that share a common evolutionary ancestor likely have similarities in their genes. Important genes are likely to have changed very little over the course of evolution. The National Academy of Sciences (USA) committee recommended that the genomes of model organisms be mapped and sequenced in parallel with the mapping of human genomes. Comparative gene mapping in mouse and human has been going on since the early 1970s. Interestingly, if two genes are on the same chromosome (syntenic) and not far apart in the mouse, chances are they share a chromosome in humans. Mapping and sequencing in organisms such as the mouse, a genus of flies *(Drosophila)*, baker's yeast, and bacteria, in which genetic information is more extensive or can be acquired more readily than in the human, are proving highly useful to human genome analysis. The complete genome sequence has been determined for several bacteria, *Saccharomyces cerevisiae,* (baker's yeast), *C. elegans* (roundworm), and *Drosophila.* In these organisms, sequence information has been used to identify all the genes, with guesses as to their function—an exciting preview of what will be possible with a knowledge of the full human sequence. The sequence in these other organisms is a Rosetta stone for deciphering the human genome.

The scientific and technological revolutions in molecular genetics and information of the last half century converge in the HGP and make it possible. Computerized databases of several types have been created for the information coming out of the HGP. Examples are GenBank (and its equivalent and coordinated databases in Europe and Japan) for DNA sequences, Genome Database (GDB) for genetic maps and related information, and the *Online Mendelian Inheritance in Man (OMIM),* a full-text catalog of human genes and genetic disorders. These databases are available on the Internet to all scientists involved in the HGP. In part, the easy availability of this growing body of knowledge has propelled the project ahead of schedule.

Database searching is becoming a leading method for biological research. Algorithms are being developed for recognizing genes in the midst of DNA sequence and motifs in the deduced amino acid sequence of the gene product that are clues to gene function. Identifying genes in the human sequence and determining their function also rely heavily on the search for similar sequences in other organisms where function may not be known or can be obtained more easily than in the human. This is research not *in vitro* or *in vivo,* but *in silico.* Database searching is the *in silico* equivalent of the "zoo-blot" used in the "wet lab" to establish homology and evolutionary conservations by hybridization of DNA.

## Prospective

The 1986 human gene map and the diagram of the vascular system from the anatomy of Vesalius (1534) are both anatomical diagrams. The ability to study the chromosomes microscopically, to map genes on chromosomes, and to dissect the anatomy of the human genome in molecular detail has provided medicine and biology with a neo-Vesalian basis (to quote Charles Scriver). Vesalius' anatomy represented important information for medicine and was the basis of Harvey's physiology of 1628 and Morgagni's pathology of 1761. A century from now, historians are likely to point to the HGP as having provided a similar infrastructure for phenomenal advances in biology and medicine that occurred earlier in the twenty-first century.

What are likely to be the long-term effects of the HGP on medicine, biology, and society? In general, the HGP increases the gap between what we know how to diagnose and what we know how to treat. (Huntington disease is an example.) The output from the HGP increases the risk of widening the gap between what we *think* we know and what we *really* know. For example, associations may be found between certain characteristics, such as behavioral traits, cognitive ability, and criminality, and particular genomic constitution. Some of these associations may turn out to be spurious, and others, even though they are statistically significant, may be blown out of proper proportion to the detriment of individuals and population groups. There is also risk that the gap will be widened between what science really knows and what the public thinks is known and between our ability to know and our wisdom in using that knowledge.

There are also the hazards of reductionism and genetic determinism, or the idea that when we know the last nucleotide in the genome sequence, we will know everything it means to be human, as well as the notion that there is a direct and inevitable one-to-one relationship between a particular genomic constitution and a particular phenotype. When the HGP is finished, the complete inventory of genes and the full sequence will represent an immensely valuable source book for biology and medicine. We will not know, however, the function of all the genes in isolation, let alone in concert; we will not know how they are regulated; we will not know the worldwide variation in the genes among the some 6 billion persons who will inhabit this globe by that time; and we will not know the complex relationship between variation in genome constitution and variation in phenotype. These matters will require study far into the future. "As the radius of knowledge gets longer, the circumference of the unknown expands." There will be plenty to do.

## SUMMARY

The scientific and technical infrastructure provided to biology and medicine by the HGP should be highly useful in unraveling molecular mechanisms of differentiation, development, and cognition. How is it determined that only certain genes are expressed in a kidney tubule cell, for example, and, in the main, a different set of genes is expressed in a cartilage cell? What controls and regulates the orderly and coordinated succession of gene expression that determines the development of an organ or other body part? Why are we self-aware, and what is memory? Completion of the HGP is only the end of the beginning.

Medicine can be expected to become powerfully more predictive and preventive than it is now. The HGP can provide the technology and background information for determining susceptibility to disorders that may develop later in life, to diagnose disorders in fetuses as early as preimplantation, and to identify the carrier status for disorders that can become manifest in our children. At the same time, diagnosis and treatment, the traditional turf of medicine, will become more specific and effective. In the future we will look back on our current cancer management as we do today on the treatment of infectious disease in the preantibiotic age. Medicine will become more "scientific." The potential contribution of the HGP to diagnosis and therapy are already recognized by pharmaceutical firms and biotech companies that have invested heavily in genome research. Advances in genomics have also stirred controversy over the appropriateness of patents on DNA.

Biological research will become DNA-focused (sequence-based) to a large extent. It will be more integrated and multidimensional as it seeks to discover how all the genes act and interact and how interplay with environment affects both. Studies of gene structure, regulation, and expression will extend through the following dimensions:

- Across species
- Across the 6 billion or more inhabitants of this globe
- Across stages of development and aging
- Across organs, tissues, and cell types
- Across subcellular compartments

All of these dimensions for each gene are related in a complex network to those of all the other genes with which it or its product(s) interacts. It is likely that the global, "big picture" approach taken by the HGP will extend to much of biological research in the future, with an increase in the size of laboratory groups and with collaborating groups from multiple laboratories.

# RELATED READINGS

1. Collins FS: Ahead of schedule and under budget: the Genome Project passes its fifth birthday (review), *Proc Natl Acad Sci USA* 92:10821-10823, 1995.

2. Guyer NS, Collins FS: How is the Human Genome Project doing, and what have we learned so far? (review), *Proc Natl Acad Sci USA* 92:10841-10848, 1995.

3. McKusick VA: Mapping and sequencing the human genome, *N Engl J Med* 320:910-915, 1989.

4. Lander ES: The new genomics: global views of biology, *Science* 274:536-539, 1996.

# CHAPTER 2

# Diagnosis of Genetic Disease

*Angela E. Scheuerle*

Genetic conditions and other birth defects occur at a surprisingly high rate. It is estimated that 2% to 3% of newborns have a significant congenital anomaly.[1] Birth defects are the leading cause of infant mortality in the United States, accounting for approximately 21% of infant deaths.[2] Also, anomalies are found in children previously thought to be normal; for example, a 5-year-old girl undergoing evaluation after a urinary tract infection is found to have a horseshoe kidney, a congenital anomaly not found at birth because there was no indication for testing. Also, there are biochemical genetic conditions that do not manifest until after the newborn period; newborn screening for phenylketonuria (PKU) is performed in all states because PKU is not clinically apparent in the nursery and presymptomatic treatment can alleviate its symptoms. Therefore in older cohorts of children the prevalence of genetic disease and other birth defects may be much higher than a single-digit percentage.

Medicine's ability to treat congenital anomalies and genetic disease has improved greatly in just a few generations. Children who might have died early from tetralogy of Fallot or cystic fibrosis (CF) now receive treatment that prolongs their life span—even so far as to allow them to have children of their own. This increased survival means that the management of children with complex disease has moved out of the neonatal intensive care unit into the primary care arena. Even the general internist may be approached for care by a patient with sickle cell disease or CF. Some practitioners enjoy the intricacy of managing such patients and concentrate their practice in that direction; however, all primary care offices seeing 75 to 100 patients per day can expect to see a child with Down syndrome and an ear infection, a parent concerned about developmental delay, or a woman with high cholesterol. On a more basic level, when a diagnostic "zebra" rears its head, all practitioners need to be able to answer patient and family questions, initiate testing, and proceed with appropriate consultation or referral. Thus it is no longer sufficient simply to diagnose and treat the condition; appropriate risk counseling and presymptomatic diagnosis for at-risk relatives also should be considered.

It is possible to separate genetic diseases and birth defects (Figure 2-1). Genetic diseases are caused by some aberration of DNA. For some genetic diseases there is a distinct family history, but for many others the patient in the office will be the first member of the

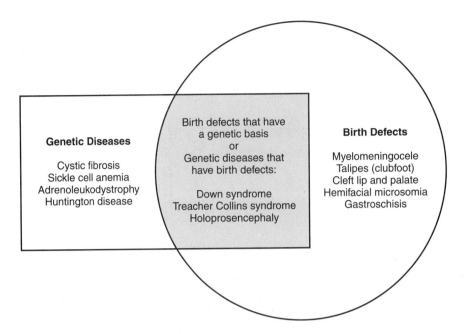

FIGURE 2-1  The interrelationship between genetic diseases and birth defects.

family to be diagnosed. Some birth defects are genetic; for example, the presence of duodenal atresia in a child with Down syndrome is a birth defect with a genetic basis. Holoprosencephaly is now recognized about 40% of the time to be caused by a mutation in a single gene.[3] On the other hand, the cause for many structural birth defects, such as cleft lip and spina bifida, has not been defined; these are typically said to arise because the correct combination of factors was present. Significant diseases of adults—atherosclerosis, breast and colon cancer, Alzheimer disease—have a genetic component. Although many genetic diseases are not as acutely striking as the birth of a child with a meningomyelocele, the implications for family health and risk are similar. Therefore the categories of "genetic diseases" and "birth defects" overlap but are not equivalent.

Genetics as a practice can be intimidating because of a plethora of eponymous conditions and the reliance on subtle differences in physical appearance. Just describing genetics gives one pause. Management of infectious disease becomes comfortable by sheer repetition, and the treatment of broken bones is blatantly obvious. Genetic conditions are too numerous to memorize (one Internet site just celebrated its 10,000th entry[4]) and are notorious for not providing enough diagnostic clues. Nevertheless, the skills necessary to make genetic diagnoses are not significantly different from those used for strep throat or femur fracture: history, physical examination, and appropriate laboratory testing. The remainder of this chapter emphasizes the aspects of each step that are particularly relevant to genetic medicine.

Throughout this chapter and the remainder of the book, multiple genetic syndromes are mentioned as examples for diagnostic tests or counseling issues. Some may be unfamiliar to many readers. The bibliography at the end of the book can provide resources for further investigation of these conditions.

# HISTORY AND PHYSICAL EXAMINATION

In general, "genetic medicine" is no more complex than standard clinical or hospital practice. It does, however, require (1) a thorough family history and (2) a heightened awareness of genetic disease. The second of these is probably self-evident; however, some issues surrounding information sources and referrals should be reviewed. Since history comes before physical examination and diagnosis, the family history is discussed first.

A thorough family history includes information about the health status, causes of death, and pregnancy outcomes of the patient and the most genetically related relatives. It is not sufficient to know just the ages and causes of death of the patient's parents. The health problems of the patient's siblings and children can give clues to disease. Additionally, the identification of a family member with multiple pregnancy losses or apparent infertility can be important.

Another helpful tool is family photographs. The physician can ask to see pictures of the family if there are suspicions that other members of the family may have the same condition as the patient. Many people carry pictures of their family, or the physician can suggest that the patient bring a family photo album to the next clinic visit. Advanced technology of copy machines and computer scanners allows good-quality reproductions of family photos to keep in the patient's chart.

Record keeping of the family history is best done using the "genogram" or the family tree, which is a symbolic representation of the family that allows delineation of each person (Figure 2-2). The great practical advantage is that it is faster than writing the information in long hand. Learning the symbols takes some practice, like typing or using medical abbreviations, but once the skill is mastered, it is possible to record a complex family history in a short time. In addition, patterns of disease can emerge as the record is being made. What might take time to decipher in notes may be obvious in pictures.

The flow of information collection may differ, depending on the age of the patient (Figures 2-3 and 2-4). For children, it might be patient, parents, siblings, aunts/uncles, and grandparents. For adults, information could be collected as patient, children, siblings, parents, aunts/uncles, and grandparents. The order is not as important as gathering complete information. It is imperative to remember siblings of both children and adults and children of adult patients.

Some information requires specific questions. It is important to ask about pregnancies and pregnancy outcomes for the patient, patient's parents, and when appropriate, patient's siblings. This information is as important for male patients as it is for females because genetic disease and chromosome translocations can be transmitted by and can affect men as well as women. If the patient reports an elective pregnancy termination in self or partner, it is necessary to determine whether this was for medical or social reasons. If an elective termination was done for medical reasons, the diagnosis should be noted. Asking the questions in that manner is acceptable to patients because it allows the collection of medical information without dwelling on social reasons for elective termination or invading patient privacy.

Learning about early infant or childhood deaths is important because genetic disease and birth defects are the primary cause of infant mortality. Interestingly, one must inquire separately about infant deaths. Children who die before a year of age are only rarely thought

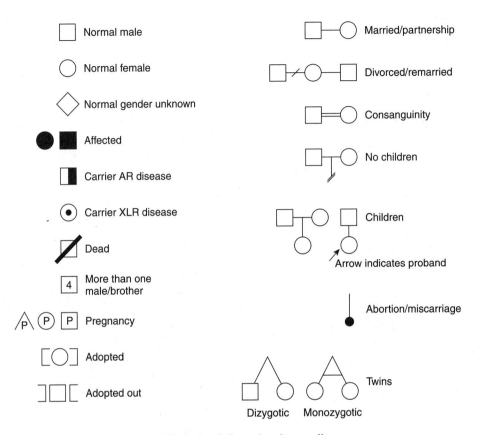

FIGURE 2-2 Symbols used to draw pedigrees.

of as siblings, particularly if there was no reciprocal relationship established between that infant and the patient. Likewise, a child who dies after birth does not fall into the category of stillbirth or miscarriage and may not be mentioned by the patient when that question is asked.

Questions that should be asked in a family history to elicit information regarding the diagnosis of genetic disease are listed in the box.

## AWARENESS OF GENETIC DISEASE

A thorough family history may raise suspicions of a genetic condition in the family. Repeated occurrences of the same or similar conditions may be an easy clue to diagnosis. In large part, diagnosing a genetic condition is a function of awareness, just as with any type of disease. Unfortunately, genetic conditions have long been thought of more as Grand Rounds cases than as serious possibilities in a differential diagnosis. The "genetic revolution" in medicine is likely to change that.

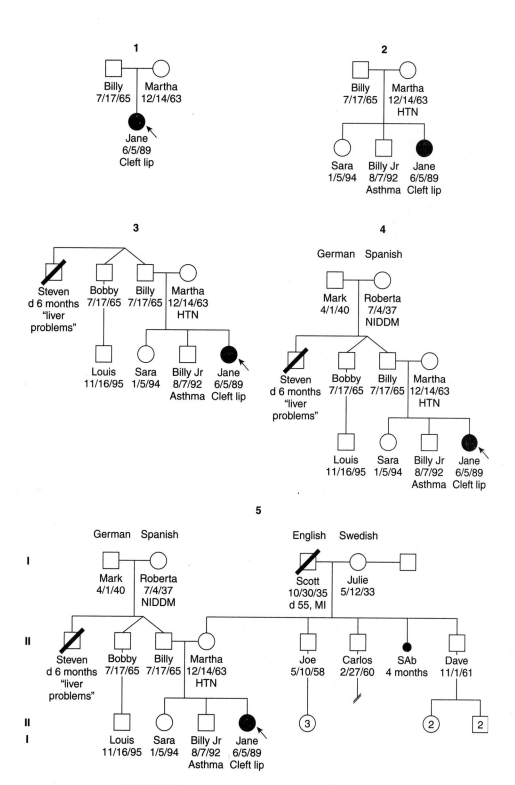

FIGURE 2-3 Steps in collecting the pedigree of a child.

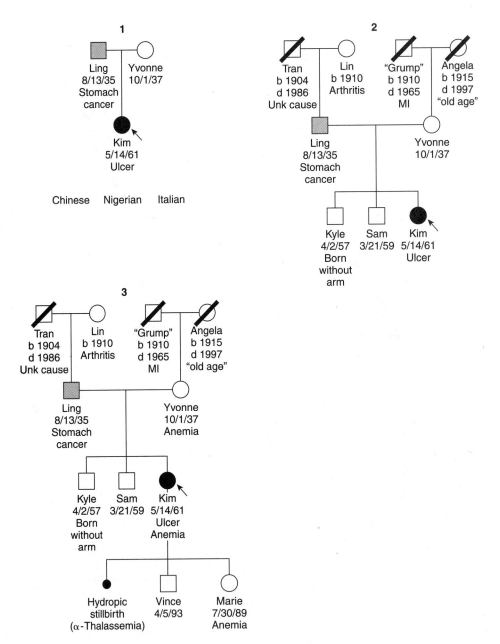

FIGURE 2-4   Steps in collecting the pedigree of an adult.

## QUESTIONS TO ASK WHEN OBTAINING A FAMILY HISTORY

**General**

1. Current or past history relevant to the condition of the proband
2. Information about relatives: names, birthdates, any health or developmental problems, causes of death, surgeries, and so on
3. Ask specifically about miscarriages, stillbirths, and children who died in infancy
4. Racial and ethnic background
5. Family origin: as in England, Taiwan, Guatemala
6. Record family names. Family names can indicate consanguinity and ethnicity. Do not assume that a person has the father's last name. Do not assume that the child of a single mother has her name.

**Specific**

1. "Who do you look like in the family?" Remember that others in the family might be affected, too.
2. "Is there anyone in the family with birth defects, mental retardation, or learning problems?"
3. "Are you aware of any miscarriages or stillbirths in you mother/sisters/daughters?"
4. "Are there any early infant deaths or children who died before 1 year of age?"
5. "Are you and your spouse related?" "Do you share distant cousins or great-grandparents?" The physician should ask politely and preface this with "I ask everyone this question." There are cultures, including some in the United States, in which it is not taboo for one's spouse to be a cousin. Persons in these cultures will not be offended by the question and will probably know their family history well. People who are not related will not be offended. If the patient refuses to answer, the physician should consider incest.
6. "Are you interested in having more children?" This can be awkward to ask immediately after the birth of an affected child; the physician can defer if necessary. However, it is good to know the answer to this question because it can help the physician determine how important recurrence risk information is for this family.

In general, a genetic disease should be considered whenever there is an indicative family history, developmental delay/mental retardation, intrauterine growth retardation, or a physical malformation (including some cancers). These broad categories frequently generate referral to genetic clinics and should prompt appropriate investigation. Recognition of less striking physical characteristics in genetic conditions may also lead to a diagnosis. Some characteristics are obvious and common, such as the features of Down syndrome, and others are less familiar, such as the facies of Noonan syndrome. Recognizing these features is a matter of sheer practice, but the gestalt of "unusual appearance" is a place to begin. (The phrase "funny looking kid," or FLK, is now out of favor. It is considered inappropriate and unkind by parents of the children and the physicians who care for them.)

On a practical level, how does a physician "keep up" with advances in genetics, particularly when it is difficult to stay current in one's own specialty? Ironically, one way is the general media. Genetic discoveries attract attention of the mass media, so newspapers and television news magazines abound with information. However, the physician must be careful about the details. In general, if announcements about a disease affect one's specialty, a quick search of the medical literature or one of the weekly online services is likely to yield more adequate and accurate data.

Annual meetings of various medical specialties sometimes offer workshops or symposia dedicated to genetics, as do continuing medical education (CME) and board review courses. When possible, these are given by medical geneticists recruited for the purpose. Taking advantage of these opportunities increases the opportunity to obtain advice from those who concentrate in the field.

The specialty of medical genetics has existed since 1993, and as of 1999 there were 1006 physicians certified by the American Board of Medical Genetics (ABMG). Although some medical geneticists operate private practices or consulting services, the majority work within academic medical centers. As with any medical consultant, a geneticist can see a patient by referral from any other physician, from other sources such as teachers and from parents. A majority of medical geneticists have also been trained in another specialty and will see patients from conception to old age. Local practice directories can identify geneticists in a particular city or insurance plan; Internet sites allow physicians to search more wide-reaching directories.

Because of its complexity, genetic diagnosis and counseling is not offered over the Internet; however, websites provide updated information about genetic disease or give background information helpful in patient management. A list of these sites is included in the bibliography at the end of the book, along with several dysmorphology books that are good additions to a clinic library.

## LABORATORY TESTING

Three common types of genetic tests are cytogenetics, molecular testing, and biochemical analysis. All of these should be available to any physician through local medical center laboratories or in laboratories around the country. For some tests there may be only one laboratory available in the United States (for a few tests, there is only one in the world!). Other tests are so common they are advertised on billboards.

### Cytogenetics

The analysis of chromosomes (a karyotype) is a fundamental genetic test. Cells from any nucleated, replicating body tissue (i.e., not red blood cells, nerve, or muscle) can be used for this test. The most common tissues used are leukocytes and fetal cells in amniotic fluid. These cells are grown in culture and arrested at metaphase, when the chromosomes are condensed and visible by light microscopy. The cells are dropped onto a slide, which breaks the cell membranes and spreads the chromosomes for better examination. Giemsa stain is used to mark the chromosomes and aid in analysis. The chromosome spreads are then photographed or computer scanned, and the chromosomes are arranged in a karyotype. The Giemsa stain creates striping or "banding" patterns on the chromosomes that are consistent from person to person. This banding facilitates evaluation. Chromosomes are numbered from largest to smallest, 1 to 22, and the sex chromosomes are designated by letter X or Y. Each chromosome is divided into two "arms" designated p (the short arm) and q (the long arm) (a mnemonic for which is "pint" and "quart"—pints are smaller than quarts).

Banding patterns are consistent within a species. Thus it is possible to compare a patient's karyotype against a human standard to determine whether there are abnormalities. Each chromosome is a single molecule of DNA that has been very tightly compacted. On average, each chromosome contains 1000 genes. Each chromosome band can contain 100 genes. So even a small change (one just barely visible by light microscopy) may have devastating results.

Normal human karyotypes contain 46 chromosomes with an XX or an XY sex chromosome complement. Thus a female karyotype is designated 46,XX and a male karyotype is designated 46,XY (Figure 2-5). A few small changes are seen with reasonable frequency in normal individuals and are thus considered "normal variants." Otherwise, any alteration from this baseline is considered abnormal; the term is *aneuploidy* (*an,* not; *eu,* true/normal; *ploid,* number/complement). There can be aneuploidies that are additions or subtractions of a single chromosome, as in Down syndrome (47,XX,+21) or Turner syndrome (45,X). Complete duplication of the entire chromosome complement in triploidy (69,XXY) and

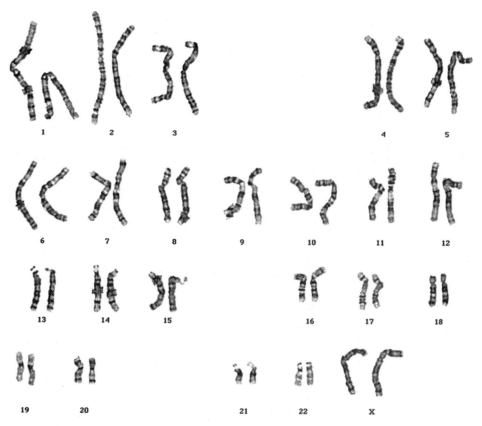

FIGURE 2-5   Karyotype of a normal female—46,XX.

(Courtesy Lisa Shaffer, MD, Baylor College of Medicine, Houston, Texas.)

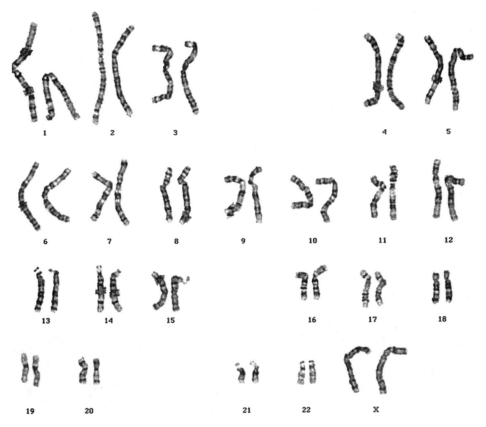

FIGURE 2-6   Karyotype of a male with Wolf-Hirschhorn syndrome—46,XY, del (4) (p14). Arrow shows where cytogenetic material is missing. Note difference in length of the two chromosomes 4. (Courtesy Lisa Shaffer, MD, Baylor College of Medicine, Houston, Texas.)

tetraploidy (92,XXYY). Missing or additional pieces of chromosomes also cause clinical syndromes. The most widely known of these syndromes is cri du chat, which is caused by a missing piece of the fifth chromosome (5p−), and Wolf-Hirschhorn syndrome (4p−) (Figure 2-6).

Microscopic and molecular techniques have progressed so that it is possible to find small duplications and deletions in chromosome structure. The corresponding clinical diagnoses are known as "microdeletion syndromes"; some are thought to be common. Another name for them is "contiguous gene deletion syndromes" because numerous genes are involved. Velo-cardiofacial/DiGeorge syndrome results from a small deletion of chromosome 22q; Williams syndrome results from a deletion of chromosome 7q; and Prader-Willi/Angelman syndromes result from a deletion of chromosome 15q. Where there is one thing in genetics, there is usually the opposite as well. Charcot-Marie-Tooth disease type I is the corresponding "microduplication syndrome" that results from a duplication of 17p.

The technique of fluorescence in situ hybridization (FISH) facilitates diagnosis of the microdeletion and microduplication syndromes. Technically a molecular test, it is used by cytogenetic laboratories and should be ordered through them. FISH is included as appropriate on their result reports. A DNA "probe" is manufactured in the laboratory. This probe is a short strand of DNA that corresponds to the genomic region of interest. A fluorescent tag is attached to this probe, and this tagged probe is applied to the patient's chromosomes. If the probe has a place to attach, it will do so; if not, it is washed off. Microscopic (or computerized) examination with the appropriate color filters shows colored spots (signals) that correspond to the fluorescent tag. The standard procedure is to use one color for control probes and another color for the test probes. So, for example, a normal chromosome number 22 would show a green control spot and a yellow test spot. The results are easy to interpret, although somewhat counterintuitive since the test is looking for deletions. The *absence* of the fluorescent tag indicates an abnormal result. The absence of a colored test spot means that the probe had nowhere to attach, indicating that the region of interest has been deleted.

Cytogenetic analysis of malignant tissue has become a mainstay of oncology. There is a high rate of cytogenetic abnormality in malignant cells. Some patterns of aneuploidy or chromosome rearrangement have been recognized, and the karyotype of a cancer can give information about diagnosis and prognosis. This is true for leukemias, lymphomas, and other solid tumors. Cancer cytogenetics is a specialized field of cytogenetics and should be performed at a laboratory familiar with the nuances.

A standard chromosome test can take from 48 hours to 2 weeks, depending on the laboratory procedures and tissue type. Skin and amniocentesis samples typically take more time because it takes longer for the cells to grow and divide. (Some laboratories use newer computer technology for karyotyping; others rely on microphotography. There are benefits and problems with each type of procedure.) It is possible to have a "stat" karyotype result. Some FISH probes can be done in a few hours, and complete karyotypes can be finished in as few as 48 hours. However, it is necessary to notify the laboratory in advance because the "stat" cell cultures must be handled differently from the routine ones. Additional requested tests, such as high-resolution banding and FISH testing, may require more time and be more expensive; however, advanced technology is beginning to decrease time and cost for some specific tests. Cytogenetic testing is a "send out" test for essentially all hospitals, and the laboratory used may be dictated by the patient's insurance carrier or the hospital's university affiliation.

Blood samples for cytogenetic testing should be sent in a *sodium* heparin tube that may have a green or a dark-blue top. (Most green-topped tubes have lithium heparin. Lithium interferes with cytogenetic techniques and should be avoided.) Tissue samples can be sent in a sterile container in tissue medium or sterile saline. Samples preserved in formalin or embedded in paraffin will not work because the cells are dead. The samples may be refrigerated for short-term storage (24 to 48 hours) but can be sent at room temperature. They should not be frozen. The sample must be viable for the test to work since the test relies on the presence of dividing cells.

The following information is important to know when ordering cytogenetic testing:

- Cost for routine, high-resolution, oncology, and "stat" karyotyping
- Collection and transport instructions
- Samples accepted: blood, solid tissue, amniotic fluid, chorionic villus, hair, urine, and so on
- Cost for and availability of FISH testing
- Turnaround time for each specimen type
- Whether the laboratory will report preliminary results

- How reporting is done—by mail, fax, e-mail, or telephone
- Availability of the laboratory director if there are questions
- The laboratory's quality control procedures—will they repeat tests for free?
- The laboratory's false-negative and false-positive rates

## Molecular Testing

DNA testing, or molecular testing, looks directly at changes in the DNA to diagnose disease. There are numerous techniques, and some are individualized for particular diseases. A full discussion is outside the scope of this work and can be found in any good genetics text. This overview is divided into tests that look directly at the gene in question and tests that are indirect.

The most obvious way to diagnose a known genetic disease is to look at the gene. A causative mutation found in that gene is a definitive diagnosis. These tests require that the gene be known and that the mutation be identifiable by standard technique. Sickle cell anemia meets these requirements. The mutation in sickle cell anemia is known and is the same in essentially all persons with the condition. The standard DNA test compares the normal sequence to the known mutant sequence using the *allele specific oligonucleotide* (ASO) technique. The same type of test is used for CF, although the increased number of mutations in CF limits the sensitivity of the test.

Direct mutation testing also is used with the *triplet repeat expansion* diseases. Throughout the genome there are sections of DNA that have repeated patterns of bases. These can be pairs, CGCGCGCGCG, triplets, CAGCAGCAGCAG, quadruplets, CCAACCAACCAA, and so on. There are also complex repeats, but thus far these have not been associated with disease. It is normal to have these repeats in baseline sizes; however, when there are errors in DNA replication, the repeats can "expand," which disrupts the transcription of the gene.

Disease has been associated with expansion of the triplet repeats in approximately a dozen conditions, including Huntington disease and fragile X syndrome. All of these conditions involve neurological abnormality, and most are degenerative in nature. There is some direct correlation between the size of the repeat and the severity of the disease; however, it is not possible to predict an exact disease course based on the DNA test. Using DNA technology, it is possible to measure the number of repeats in these genes. The general techniques are applicable to all the triplet repeat diseases but must be tailored to the particular segment of DNA and to the expected size of the expansion. The results are reported in repeat sizes relative to normal for the gene in question.

The most common type of indirect DNA testing is the *linkage analysis*. The type of test is used when the gene is unknown, when the mutation is difficult to test with consistent results, or when the number of possible mutations exceeds the number that can be easily tested. Linkage testing looks at *polymorphisms* (benign changes in DNA sequence) and analyzes how they are transmitted through the family. Polymorphisms do *not* cause disease, rather they are serendipitous tools supplied by nature that are exploited for testing purposes. Analyzing the inheritance of polymorphisms around or within a gene allows indirect examination of the gene's inheritance.

Linkage testing requires samples from other members of the family, at least one of whom must be affected with the condition. Linkage is not diagnostic for the first affected family member; however, after the birth (or diagnosis) of the first affected family member, the information can be used for diagnosis in the next baby or other relatives. Since gene locations are usually known before the genes themselves, most DNA tests began as linkage analyses. CF, Huntington disease, and Duchenne muscular dystrophy can now be diagnosed by direct mutation analysis; these were previously tested using linkage analysis.

Blood for DNA analysis is most commonly collected in a purple-top tube with EDTA. Tissue samples can be sent in any form. Since DNA analysis does not depend on viability of the tissue, anything with nuclei is a reasonable sample, assuming the laboratory is prepared to handle it. DNA has been extracted from preserved tissue, but it is technically more difficult. The longer the sample has been preserved, the less likely intact DNA will be extracted. The samples may be refrigerated. For long-term storage, freezing or liquid nitrogen may be used.

DNA testing requires a few days to 2 weeks, depending on the test being performed. Some laboratories "batch" samples for better handling. For example, a laboratory that handles large volumes of CF testing may begin processing on Monday to generate reports on Friday. A sample arriving on Tuesday will not be processed until the next week. Most DNA testing is labor intensive and requires a time-consuming series of procedures (PCR amplification, gel electrophoresis, and so on). Molecular diagnostic laboratories are available nationwide, but most tests will be sent to a laboratory from the clinic or hospital. The laboratory used may be dictated by the hospital's university affiliation or the patient's insurance.

The following information should be solicited from a laboratory performing DNA or molecular testing:

- For what diseases do they test?
- What samples are required for a particular test; how many family members must participate?
- What is the cost for the various tests?
- What discounts are available for the same test in multiple family members?
- What samples are accepted: blood, solid tissue, amniotic fluid, chorionic villus, hair, urine?
- What is the turnaround time?
- Will the laboratory report preliminary results?
- How is reporting done: a report in the mail, fax, e-mail, or a telephone call?
- Is the laboratory director available if there are questions?
- What are the laboratory's quality control procedures—will they repeat tests for free?
- What are the laboratory's false-negative and false-positive rates?

Another type of molecular testing does not involve DNA. For a handful of conditions, even if the gene is known, it is easier to test the affected protein than it is to test DNA. This is largely true for abnormalities of connective tissue, such as collagen IA (osteogenesis imperfecta), elastin (Ehlers-Danlos syndrome), and fibrillin (Marfan syndrome). Although these tests are offered as fee-for-service diagnostic tests, they may be done in only one or two laboratories in the United States. For all of these tests, the sample required is solid tissue containing the protein in question, usually a skin punch biopsy.

**Biochemical Testing**

Inborn errors of metabolism result from defects in metabolic enzymes and can be detected using standard laboratory techniques. Biochemical analysis for metabolic disease may be the most understandable type of "genetic testing" because it is similar to other, more standard, medical testing. Also, most physicians are familiar with newborn screening for PKU, which involves biochemical testing.

Defective metabolic enzymes can be found indirectly by screening their metabolites; an increase in the level of one biochemical can indicate a dysfunction of enzyme for which it is a substrate. There may be a corresponding decrease in the concentrations of the enzyme's products (Figure 2-7). The compounds (substrates and products) routinely measured are amino acids and organic acids, although other panels may include mucopolysaccharides and cholesterol metabolites. Rather than evaluate them one at a time, they can be tested in batch panels of amino acids or organic acids and are commonly ordered that way. While it is possible to do either of these tests on blood or urine, the most useful combination of tests is serum (or plasma) amino acids and urine organic acids.

Organic acids are measured by gas chromatography/mass spectroscopy against a calibrated standard. Amino acids may be measured this way or with specific reactants. If a laboratory uses a single technique for all samples, thus allowing for standardization, there is no distinct advantage of one method over another. Blood samples are submitted in a red-topped serum separator tube or in a test tube that will separate plasma (different laboratories are calibrated for different samples). Urine can be submitted in any sterile container and may be refrigerated or frozen.

An abnormality found by amino or organic acid screening may then be confirmed by direct enzyme testing in some cases, although not in all. Some enzymes remain unidentified. Direct testing is specialized and is likely to require particular samples. For example, some tests require fresh liver biopsy, whereas others can be done on leukocytes. Rather than memorize a list of test samples, which is too long to include here, the best plan is to contact the laboratory directly and learn their preferred samples and handling methods.

The turnaround time for biochemical testing depends largely on the frequency that a particular test is done. "Stat" testing is generally available when there is a diagnostic emergency, and the turnaround time can be less than 24 hours. As mentioned with the other tests, it is best to let the laboratory know in advance that a sample will be sent for "stat" turnaround.

Other information to know from a biochemical genetics laboratory includes the following:

- What diseases do they test for, and how often do they run a particular test?
- Are results reported quantitatively (more informative) or qualitatively?
- What samples are required for a particular test?
- What is the cost for the various tests?

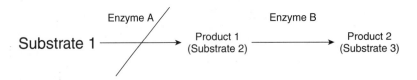

FIGURE 2-7   Basis of biochemical testing. Malfunction of enzyme A leads to an accumulation of substrate 1 and a relative decrease in the concentration of product 1 and product 2.

- What discounts are available for the same test in multiple family members?
- What samples are accepted: blood, solid tissue, amniotic fluid, chorionic villus, hair, urine?
- What is the turnaround time?
- Will the laboratory report preliminary results?
- How is reporting done?
- Is the laboratory director available to answer questions?
- What are the laboratory's quality control procedures—will they repeat tests for free?
- What are the laboratory's false-negative and false-positive rates?

## SUMMARY

Genetic disease is becoming relatively more prominent because of the progressive control of death from infectious disease and accidents. With improved survival techniques, children who would have died in infancy are living into childhood and coming to the attention of medical specialists other than neonatologists. Additionally, persons with conditions that were previously lethal are reaching adulthood and bearing children who are likewise affected. As a result, physicians in all branches of medicine must become familiar with at least the subset of genetic conditions that affect their practice.

A few simple techniques are useful for evaluating genetic disease. First, a complete family history, with full information about all family members, may reveal other affected persons. Reviewing photographs of relatives can be enlightening. Second, maintaining a high level of suspicion for genetic disease is imperative for generating a complete differential diagnosis, including the "zebras." If genetic disease is suspected or clinically diagnosed, several laboratory tests are available for confirmation.

Information about genetic disease is increasingly common, in both the popular media and the medical literature. While any physician can be expected to recognize the need for genetic diagnosis (for practical purposes, no different from recognizing infectious or rheumatologic conditions), helpful tests and websites are easily available, as are consultants in medical genetics.

## REFERENCES

1. Accardo PJ, Capute AJ: Mental retardation. In Oski FA, DeAngelis CD, Feigin RD, et al, editors: *Principles and practice of pediatrics,* Philadelphia, 1994, Lippincott.
2. Sever L, Lynberg MC, Edmunds LD: The impact of congenital malformations on public health, *Teratology* 48(6):547-549, 1993.
3. Belloni E, Muenke M, Roessler E, et al: Identification of Sonic hedgehog as a candidate gene responsible for holoprosencephaly, *Nat Genet* 14:353-356, 1996.
4. *Online Mendelian inheritance in man,* http://www.ncbi.nlm.nih.gov/htbin-post/Omim.

# CHAPTER 3

# Management of Genetic Disease

*Angela E. Scheuerle*

The concept of genetic diagnostics is somewhat new and foreign in medicine, and the treatment of genetic diseases can seem like futuristic science fiction—thoroughly laced with complex manipulation and "technobabble." However, diagnosis of genetic disorders involves the comfortable methods of history and physical diagnosis, and with the exception of some still experimental therapies, treatment of genetic disease and birth defects employs standard techniques that mirror those used in more common conditions. Giving insulin to a patient with type I diabetes and factor VIII to a patient with hemophilia A are equivalent treatments. Restricting eggs because of an allergy and restricting phenylalanine because of mental retardation require the same processes. Yes, the treatments must be tailored to the conditions, but that is true for every patient who comes through the clinic door.

This chapter briefly explores some ways to manage genetic disease. Many of these treatment concepts will be familiar to most physicians, even though this particular viewpoint may be new. As new treatments become available, they will fit most likely into one of these categories. It is also probable that every physician will recognize each of these situations within his or her own patient population.

## MANIPULATING DISRUPTED ANATOMY: SURGERY AND TECHNOLOGY

A child born with a neural tube defect, congenital heart defect, or autosomal dominant ectrodactyly has the immediate attention of two medical specialties, one of which is surgery. In some cases, the surgeon will have been consulted before the child's birth. These birth defects and many others are managed partly by surgical means. Other treatments may include the use of prostheses and orthoses; occupational, physical, or speech therapy; or specialized education programs. In some cases, entire clinics have evolved to provide multispecialty care for a particular defect or set of conditions. A "craniofacial clinic" may include a plastic surgeon, geneticist, otolaryngologist, pediatrician, social worker, neurosurgeon, ophthalmologist, psychologist, speech pathologist, dentist, prosthodontist, and nutritionist. The Shriners' Hospital system offers this type of coordinated care for children with physical birth defects.

Some common surgeries might be considered surgical management of a birth defect, for example, radial keratotomy for treatment of myopia, cochlear implants to reverse deafness, or laser treatment of hyperpigmentation. Some surgeries are more controversial. The "normalization" of the face of a child with Down syndrome, including tongue reduction and elimination of epicanthal folds, is thought by some to improve the socialization of such children; thus they will not be treated so differently because they look more "normal." Others argue that a "normal"-looking person with mental retardation is less likely to be treated with patience and extra help than one who is obviously dysmorphic.

Surgery or physical therapies can also address late manifestations of genetic disease. For example, a boy with Duchenne muscular dystrophy may stay out of a wheelchair an extra year or two with some surgical management or specialized exercises.[1] Splenectomy in some red cell dyscrasias may improve anemia.[2] And, as Steven Hawking has shown, aggressive use of computer technology may enable a patient with amyotrophic lateral sclerosis to function at an amazingly high level even after his body has effectively "shut down."

## MEDICAL TREATMENT OF SYMPTOMS

The cornerstone of many medical treatments is not to cure a condition as much as it is to alleviate the symptoms of disease. This is also true for the treatment of many chronic conditions, for example, a drug given to a patient with congestive heart failure is not expected to return the heart to normal, only to maximize the function of the ailing heart. Some genetic conditions can thus be managed with otherwise common medications. For example, retinoic acid derivatives are useful in managing some forms of ichthyosis,[3] and patients with Marfan syndrome who are at risk for aortic dilation and dissection can be given beta blockers to decrease pressure on a fragile aorta.[4] The pharmacological action of the drugs has not changed; their usefulness has expanded.

It is important to remember also that a person with a known genetic disease remains susceptible to all the same conditions prevalent in the general population; a child with achondroplasia can get chickenpox and a woman with spina bifida can become pregnant. While some patients may need special monitoring, there is no reason to assume that normal therapies and management will be inadequate. Sometimes having a genetic disease can place a patient at even greater risk for a common problem. Persons with Down syndrome are at high risk of hypothyroidism. The standard treatment is thyroxin supplementation but the suspicion for testing must be high. Children and adults with albinism must be cautioned strongly against sun exposure because of their increased susceptibility to sunburn and skin cancer.

## DIETARY RESTRICTIONS

Manipulation of diet is rampant in today's society. There are those who avoid fat, sugar, gluten, monosodium glutamate, lactose, eggs, all processed food, or red meat, while others "load" themselves with vitamin C, protein, carbohydrates, zinc, selenium, or androstenedione. All physicians are familiar with the patient who chooses a diet to be smarter, slimmer, more muscular, less hyperactive, or more athletic. Placebo affect aside, there may be some benefit to a controlled diet. Among official recommendations are five fruits/vegetables a day, the recommended daily allowance (RDA) of vitamins and minerals, and the "food pyramid" found on many grocery store items. Whatever the goal of dietary intake for an individual person, we are at least comfortable with the idea that to some extent we are what we eat.

Dietary restriction is perhaps one of the more familiar concepts in treatment of genetic disease, since it is the cardinal management for the "newborn screening" conditions. In phenylketonuria (PKU), for example, the body is unable to catabolize the phenylalanine so it accumulates and becomes a neurotoxin. The obvious treatment is to restrict phenylalanine in the diet. However, this is easier said than done, since phenylalanine, an amino acid, is present is virtually all foods that have protein, including pediatric staples such as peanut butter and ice cream, so the diet is very limited. Some phenylalanine is needed for normal growth, and it is an essential amino acid—the body does not produce it. Thus dietary management becomes a balancing act between not enough and too much. In general, the approach is to restrict all protein, then provide a supplemental formula that contains all the amino acids except phenylalanine. Because this treatment is effective, women with PKU are now living into adulthood and bearing children. During pregnancy the diet must be even further restricted because phenylalanine concentrates in the fetus and acts as a teratogen.

The same dietary procedure applies to other inborn errors of metabolism such as maple syrup urine disease (MSUD) and galactosemia. Conceptually, this is not different than managing a diabetic or low-fat diet, but it is much more detailed. Previously, it was thought that the specialized diets could be discontinued after childhood. Now it is recognized that the diets should be maintained throughout life.

Some genetic conditions manifest only in the presence of a particular substance. These conditions define a new branch of science called *pharmacogenetics.* Two easy examples are malignant hyperthermia and glucose-6-phosphate dehydrogenase (G6PD) deficiency. Overall, management is aimed at avoiding those things that precipitate symptoms. Malignant hyperthermia is an autosomal dominant condition that manifests when an affected person is given halide anesthetics. Such administration results in high fevers, which can be detrimental or even fatal.[5] G6PD deficiency causes hemolytic anemia only when the affected person is exposed to particular oxidants. This condition is also called "favism" because ingestion of fava beans can precipitate attacks. Many medications must also be avoided in these patients.[6]

Pharmacogenetics may eventually allow physicians to tailor treatments to individual patients. For example, the propensity for deafness as a sequela of aminoglycoside treatment has a genetic basis—mutation in the mitochondrial DNA in the ear.[7] A patient identified as having the genetic susceptibility could be treated with a different class of antibiotics or at least be more closely monitored for toxicity. It is reasonable to assume that side effects of other drugs may have a genetic component.

## DEPLETION OF AN EXCESSIVE SUBSTANCE

Physicians who train in Florida only learn about lead poisoning as an academic exercise because lead-based paint, which causes problems in the North and Midwest, is not used in

Florida. The diagnosis of plumbism (such as from inhaling fumes of leaded gasoline) was usually reserved for Grand Rounds. In the northern and Midwestern states, however, EDTA infusion for the treatment of lead intoxication is routine. Although avoidance is still the gold standard, chelation therapy with EDTA is the treatment of choice for lead intoxication, and it serves as an example for the next set of genetic diseases—those in which excessive storage of a substance must be depleted. Lead intoxication differs from genetic diseases since it is an acute problem needing a single course of treatment. Comparable genetic conditions must be treated throughout a lifetime, so the toxic/therapeutic ratio of the medications becomes more important.

Wilson disease is characterized by an accumulation of copper in the liver, which is caused by reduced incorporation of copper into ceruloplasmin and reduced biliary excretion of copper. Since 1956, the standard of treatment has been oral administration of D-penicillamine, which increases urinary excretion of copper. Zinc salts, which appear to block intestinal absorption of copper, have also been successful. Unlike the affect of EDTA on lead, reduction in liver copper is slow, and the benefits of therapy may not be visible for months. A copper chelating agent, ammonium tetrathiomolybdate (TTM), is useful for rapid "decoppering" but is too toxic to use in lifelong management. TTM may be useful while a patient waits for a liver transplant or in acute decompensation from copper accumulation.[8]

A more prevalent condition involves accumulation of iron. Bloodletting as a medical panacea has long been abandoned, but it remains the primary treatment for hemochromatosis, a common autosomal recessive disease. In hemochromatosis there is an excess storage of iron, which can deposit in solid organs and cause cirrhosis, diabetes, and ultimately heart failure. Phlebotomy can mobilize the iron, decreasing secondary damage, and is standard treatment. Because women lose iron with the menstrual cycle, they are somewhat protected from the complications, at least until menopause. Unfortunately, this may mean that premenopausal women are underdiagnosed because their symptoms are not as severe.[9]

## REPLACEMENT OF A MISSING GENE PRODUCT

The two examples of "routine" genetic diseases used earlier were insulin-deficiency diabetes and hemophilia. Since the etiology of type I diabetes remains obscure and is only partially genetic, this section expands instead on hemophilia A and Smith-Lemli-Opitz syndrome; both are treated by replacement of a missing gene product.

Hemophilia A (factor VIII deficiency) is familiar to all physicians because it is a common condition with definable genetics and an historic impact on the royal families of Europe. The unfortunate consequences of acquired immunodeficiency syndrome (AIDS) brought hemophilia to the attention of the medical and lay communities. Patients with hemophilia are susceptible to AIDS and other viral diseases because of the manner in which they are treated. Administration of exogenous factor VIII controls the symptoms of hemophilia by supplying the missing link in the clotting cascade. Since factor VIII is a circulating protein found in the serum, it functions equally well whether manufactured in the liver or delivered by intramuscular injection. Before recombinant DNA technology, factor VIII was concentrated from the blood of many donors, thus exposing the patient to potential infection from many people. Hemophilia is now treated with recombinant factor VIII manufactured and excreted by bacteria, eliminating exposure to human immunodeficiency virus (HIV), hepatitis, and all other viruses and increasing the purity of the protein itself.

A more recently discovered condition, Smith-Lemli-Opitz syndrome (SLOS), is also treated with an exogenous compound. SLOS has been recognized for years as a dysmorphology syndrome with mental retardation. In 1994 Tint et al[10] demonstrated that these patients had a defect in cholesterol biosynthesis, which was suspected because of very low serum cholesterols in numerous patients. In the field of medical genetics, this was the first malformation syndrome to be linked to a biochemical defect. The reason cholesterol deficiency causes dysmorphology is unknown but conceptually it follows, since cholesterol functions in formation of cell membranes. Although it seemed simplistic, some patients began treatment with bile salts and oral cholesterol in various forms (e.g., pure cholesterol or egg yolk). The dysmorphic features have not been affected by the cholesterol intake, but other changes have been noticed.[11] Kelley[12] presented a most vivid description of what cholesterol treatment can do for a patient with SLOS:

> . . . *the impact on the families of some SLOS children and adults has been profound when their cholesterol deficiency syndrome was treated. Growth improves, older children learn to walk, and adults speak for the first time in years. Equally important is how much better the children feel. Sometimes after just days or weeks of cholesterol treatment, head banging stops, agitation passes to calm, and older children and adults verbalize how much better they feel.*

## ORGAN AND TISSUE TRANSPLANTATION

Some organs can be removed without life-threatening consequence to the human organism. This is not an unusual treatment approach for many conditions, including genetic ones. Cancerous organs, inflamed appendices, and impacted wisdom teeth are all treated by removing the involved tissue. Splenectomy for management of spherocytosis was mentioned previously, and there are other parallels in oculotomy for retinoblastoma, nephrectomy for polycystic kidney disease, and the removal of extra digits in polydactyly.

When the offending organ cannot be removed without a threat to life, an alternative treatment is organ transplantation. Although transplantation is laced with ethical, political, and biological problems, exchanging a dysfunctional organ with a functional one seems a straightforward way of managing disease, particularly when disease pathogenesis involves an isolated organ. Technically, genetic diseases involve the entire body, since the defective gene is present in all cells; however, when the gene is active in only one organ, replacement of that tissue may affect a "cure" of the genetic disease. Currently the most common transplantations are liver and bone marrow.

Bone marrow transplantation, preceded by ablation therapy of the patient's own marrow, has been used in severe cases of hemoglobinopathy, particularly sickle cell disease. Because bone marrow transplantation has its own risks, it is not a standard therapy for hemoglobinopathy, and patients must meet some severity criteria: frequency of pain, occurrence of stroke, young age, and so on. Nothing is done to the donor marrow, but it must not be autologous—it must be from someone who is not affected with a hemoglobinopathy. When the transplant is successful, the patient no longer manifests the genetic disease in the relevant tissue.

For some metabolic diseases, liver transplantation is an effective treatment. Hepatorenal tyrosinemia, which is caused by a deficiency of fumarylacetoacetate hydrolase, is one example. Symptoms include liver failure, cirrhosis, hepatocellular carcinoma, renal Fanconi syndrome, glomerulosclerosis, and peripheral neuropathy. Although there are renal symptoms, hepatic transplant is curative because the liver is the site of enzyme production.[13] This is also true for ornithine transcarbamylase deficiency, which results in hyperammonemia and subsequent brain damage.

Ideally, organ transplantation in genetic disease should occur before the onset of irreversible sequelae such as encephalopathy. Unfortunately, the current scarcity of replacement organs makes early transplant difficult; patients must be "sick enough" to receive a new organ. As such, genetic patients are caught in a quandary, since the best time for them to receive transplant is before other damage occurs, but without that damage, they may not rank high enough on the transplant list.

## GENE THERAPY

Gene therapy is the transfer of genetic material (DNA or RNA) for the purpose of treating or curing a genetic disease. Organ transplantation was discussed as a treatment of genetic disease. Transplantation is a type of gene therapy, but it is undirected—all of the genes in the organ have been replaced. New therapies aim to replace just the defective gene. In theory, this sounds simple enough, and the goal is indeed for it to be simple. (There is a scene in the fourth *Star Trek* movie in which the twenty-third-century physician gives a tablet to a twentieth-century dialysis patient who is later seen proclaiming, "The doctor gave me a pill and I grew a new kidney!") In practice, the studies have been disappointing. In the early 1990s, a review of existing gene therapy research showed that it had not lived up to expectations. Researchers essentially retreated and regrouped, moving more carefully and in many new directions. The literature in this area is extensive and rapidly changing. Two treatment strategies, ex vivo and in vivo gene therapy, are addressed here, as well as a few of the vectors that may be used.

### Treatment Strategies

The ex vivo strategy involves genetic engineering of a patient's tissue while it is outside the body. Some of the affected tissue would be removed from the patient, a new functional gene would be inserted into the tissue, and the tissue would be reimplanted in the patient. The easiest tissue to manipulate in this way is blood, so the earliest successful gene therapy protocols involved hematopoietic precursors. If the patient's own marrow is used, so that the transplant is autologous tissue that has undergone gene insertion, the immunological consequences of transplant are eliminated. Bone marrow transplantation has been used in treatment of adenosine deaminase deficiency (a form of severe combined immunodeficiency) and is being experimented with in a number of other conditions. Ex vivo therapy has also been attempted in familial hypercholesterolemia using hepatocytes, taking advantage of the liver's high cell turnover.[14] The advantages to the ex vivo strategy are that the cells exposed to the new DNA/RNA are precisely controlled, a high concentration of vector can be used, and the transfer conditions can be optimized.

In vivo gene therapy is likely to have more applications than ex vivo gene therapy, since it requires less manipulation of patient tissue. In this context, a new gene programmed to be active in the relevant tissue is introduced directly into the patient. Gene therapy research in cystic fibrosis (CF), for example, has involved inhaling genetically engineered viruses that deposit a working CF transmembrane conductance regulator (CFTR) gene directly into the alveoli of the patients. Other research involves parenteral routes. This approach to gene therapy better mirrors standard medical practice in which medications are given directly to the patient. In vivo the vector can be delivered to sites that may not be available by the ex vivo method. Disadvantages of the in vivo method include difficulty controlling the exposure conditions and the potential contamination of tissues other than the target organ by the new genetic material. Diseases for which in vivo gene therapy has been attempted include malignant melanoma and CF.

### Vectors

Just as the malaria parasite is transferred via the mosquito, genetic materials need a vector. Although technology continues to advance, naked DNA and RNA usually cannot be injected into a cell; something has to put it there. The most commonly used vector in genetic engineering and gene therapy is the virus. There are known, common viruses whose wild-type function includes insertion of viral DNA into the human genome. These retroviruses, including HIV and human T-lymphotropic virus (HTLV), have as their genome a single strand of RNA. Within a host cell, the viral RNA is reverse transcribed into DNA and that DNA is inserted into the host genome. Using genetic engineering, the viral genome is manipulated so that the pathogenicity is lost, but the ability to transfer genetic material remains and a therapeutic gene is substituted for the viral genes. The patient's tissue can then be "infected" with the engineered retrovirus, which will insert a functional copy of the therapeutic gene into the patient's genome. This vector offers the high efficiency of genetic material transfer and good long-term expression. Unfortunately, this method requires dividing cells (so it is not useful in nerve or muscle tissue), and the size of the DNA insert is limited. The greatest danger is the potential for mutation during or as a consequence of insertion.[14]

Larger genes can be transferred using adenoviruses, which are a second type of viral vector. The adenovirus can be manipulated like the retrovirus to carry new, functional genetic material without the pathogenicity. In this case, the genetic material is double-stranded DNA, and it does not insert into the host DNA but exists in the cell as an episome. The efficiency of DNA transfer is high, and there is a broad range of target cells due to the many types of adenovirus available. Since the DNA of the host genome is not disrupted, there is no danger of insertional mutagenesis and the target cells do not need to be dividing. The disadvantages to adenovirus vectors are that many patients mount an immune response to them, making their repeated use in one patient very limited, and the virus can be cytopathic. Also, since the DNA lies free in the cell, it can be lost so expression of the therapeutic gene is transient.[14]

Other viral vectors that are under experiment include the adeno-associated viruses, herpesviruses, vaccinia, and influenza viruses. Liposomes, a nonviral vector, coat DNA in a lipid layer to facilitate movement through cell membranes. The lipid layer can be impregnated with a particular ligand, which will bind receptors on a target cell and thus limit the potential contamination of nontarget tissues.[14]

Insertion of naked DNA directly into the target tissue is a relatively new way to solve the transfer problem. Used for several years in plant research, the gene gun is gaining popularity in human research. Dispersion of the new genetic material is limited by the "power" of the injection. Currently, the experimental usefulness is in relatively superficial tissues such as skin and skeletal muscle. More widespread use has been made of the gene gun in vaccinations in which the injected DNA stimulates an immune response by the host. Conceptually similar to common vaccines, this application broadens the field to include vaccination against some types of cancers and currently resistant microorganisms.

### Treatment Goals

The goal of gene therapy is to replace a nonworking gene with a functional one; however, there are many nuances to this goal. To treat a recessive condition caused by loss of gene function, gene therapy could replace the missing DNA or at least provide a functional copy of the gene in the most critical tissue. Gene therapy for CF and muscular dystrophy fall into this category. Most dominant diseases would not be successfully treated in this manner because they do not typically involve loss of function. Diseases for which the amount of gene expression would have to be regulated are also difficult to treat in this manner—not enough is understood about gene regulation at this time.

Gene therapies can focus on expression of a substance that is toxic to a particular type of cell, which is the mainstay of cancer therapy. The substance may be directly toxic, or it may introduce into the malignancy a susceptibility to some other drug. For example, one patient had a large, malignant brain tumor into which a gene was inserted for thymidine kinase, which is an enzyme that makes ganciclovir highly toxic to mammalian cells. The patient was then given ganciclovir, which was benign to all the cells in the patient's body except the cells in the tumor. After gene therapy, the patient showed a normal brain without evidence of tumor.

Other gene therapy goals could include blocking translation or inactivation of a harmful mRNA or disrupting the function of a deleterious protein. There are many potential levels at which gene therapy could work; understanding them has just begun. As previous genetic research has shown, each new discovery shows increased rather than decreased complexity. This increasing complexity can be daunting at first, until new ways are learned to take advantage of the biochemistry.

## SUMMARY

Perhaps the most exciting aspect of medical treatment is that it is always changing. The "genetic revolution" is changing medicine the way that sulfa drugs did in the 1940s. More defined diseases will be added to each of the categories discussed, and more categories most likely will be discovered. As discussed briefly in these early chapters, diagnosis and treatment of genetic disease are becoming ubiquitous to medical practice. All physicians see patients who will be affected by new genetic technology, whether they have a genetic condition or are treated by a genetic manipulation. The remainder of this book focuses on how practitioners can incorporate this new knowledge into practice without losing perspective.

## REFERENCES

1. Smith SE, Green NE, Cole RJ, et al: Prolongation of ambulation in children with Duchenne muscular dystrophy by lower limb tenotomy, *J Pediatr Orthop* 13(3): 336-340, 1993.

2. Schwartz SI: Role of splenectomy in hematologic disorders, *World J Surg* 20(9):1156-1159, 1996.

3. Shwayder T: Ichthyosis in a nutshell, *Pediatr Rev* 20(1):5-12, 1999.

4. Mange EJ, Mange AP: *Basic human genetics,* ed 2, Sunderlin, Mass, 1999, Sinauer Associates.

5. Kalow W, Grand DM: Pharmacogenetics. In Scriver CR, Beaudet AL, Sly WS, et al, editors: *The metabolic and molecular bases of disease,* ed 7, New York, 1995, McGraw-Hill.

6. Luzzatto L, Mehta A: Glucose 6-phosphate dehydrogenase deficiency. In Scriver CR, Beaudet AL, Sly WS, et al, editors: *The metabolic and molecular bases of disease,* ed 7, New York, 1995, McGraw-Hill.

7. Fischel-Ghodsian N, Prezant TR, Chaltraw WE, et al: Mitochondrial gene mutation is a significant predisposing factor in aminoglycoside ototoxicity, *Am J Otolaryngol* 18(3):173-178, 1997.

8. Danks DM: Disorders of copper transport. In Scriver CR, Beaudet AL, Sly WS, et al, editors: *The metabolic and molecular bases of disease,* ed 7, New York, 1995, McGraw-Hill.

9. Botwell TH, Charlton RW, Motulsky AG: Hemochromatosis. In Scriver CR, Beaudet AL, Sly WS, et al, editors: *The metabolic and molecular bases of disease,* ed 7, New York, 1995, McGraw-Hill.

10. Tint GS, Irons M, Elias ER, et al: Defective cholesterol biosynthesis associated with the Smith-Lemli-Opitz syndrome, *N Engl J Med* 330:107-113, 1994.

11. *Online Mendelian inheritance in man,* http://www.ncbi.nlm.nih.gov/htbin-post/Omim.

12. Kelley RI: RSH/Smith-Lemli-Opitz syndrome: mutations and metabolic morphogenesis, *Am J Human Genet* 63(2):332-336, 1998 (editorial).

13. Mitchell GA, Lambert M, Tanguay RM: Hypertyrosinemia. In Scriver CR, Beaudet Al, Sly WS, et al, editors: *The metabolic and molecular bases of disease,* ed 7, New York, 1995, McGraw-Hill.

14. Gelehrter TD, Collins FS, Ginsburg D: *Principles of medical genetics,* ed 2, Baltimore, 1998, Williams & Wilkins.

# CHAPTER 4

# Cancer Genetics in the Clinic

*Marion S. Verp*

*Shelly A. Cummings*

*Olufunmilayo I. Olopade*

In the past it was believed that the etiology of cancer would be found through the identification of toxic environmental agents; however, recently it has become apparent that most cancers develop as a result of a combination of genetic and environmental factors. In some cases, genetic predisposition to a particular type of cancer is the strongest risk factor for an individual. Therefore properly obtaining and interpreting a family history of cancer is important in evaluating a patient's risks and implementing strategies to reduce that risk.

Several genes responsible for inherited predisposition to cancer have been identified, and new cancer susceptibility genes continue to emerge (Table 4-1). Clinical tests are now available to identify carriers of some of these genes, and additional tests will become available in the future.

This chapter reviews the basic principles governing genetic cancer susceptibility, describes the more common familial syndromes and tests, and suggests appropriate scenarios for counseling and screening. In the future it will certainly be the purview of general practitioners to identify their patients who are at increased risk of cancer by virtue of their family history and who can benefit from genetic counseling and testing.

## GENETIC COUNSELING

Genetic counseling is primarily a communication process. The role of the counselor, whether generalist or geneticist, is to assess the counselee's risk for the disorder in question, to determine the options (e.g., genetic testing of appropriate individuals), and to help the counselee develop a strategy for dealing with the risk that is appropriate for their belief system. Because of the complexity of the testing and the importance of the results to the counselee's physical, mental, and social well-being, appropriate caution must be exercised in offering and interpreting presymptomatic tests.

## TABLE 4-1

## Selected Syndromes of Cancer Predisposition

| Syndrome | Mode of Inheritance | Gene | Neoplasms |
|---|---|---|---|
| Hereditary breast/ovarian | Dominant | BRCA1 | Breast, ovarian, prostate, colorectal |
| | | BRCA2 | Breast, ovarian, prostate, colorectal, melanoma, fallopian tube |
| Prostate | Dominant | HPC1, PCAP, HPCX | Prostate |
| Li-Fraumeni | Dominant | TP53 | Soft tissue sarcoma, osteosarcoma, breast, leukemia, brain, adrenocortical |
| Cowden disease (multiple hamartoma) | Dominant | PTEN | Breast, thyroid, hamartoma of skin; oral, thyroid, facial papules, intestinal polyps |
| Peutz-Jeghers | Dominant | STK11 | Breast, uterine, ovarian, testicular, gastrointestinal |
| HNPCC | Dominant | MLH1, MSH2, MSH6, PMS1, PMS2 | Colon, endometrial, ovarian, gastrointestinal, breast |
| FAP | Dominant | APC | Colon, sebaceous cysts, lipomas, desmoid tumors, facial bone osteomas |
| MEN I | Dominant | MEN1 | Pancreatic islet cell tumors, pituitary, parathyroid adenoma |
| MEN IIa | Dominant | RET | Medullary thyroid, pheochromocytoma, hyperplasia of parathyroid |

*HNPCC,* Hereditary nonpolyposis colorectal cancer; *FAP,* familial adenomatous polyposis; *MEN,* multiple endocrine neoplasia.

TABLE 4-1

## Selected Syndromes of Cancer Predisposition—cont'd

| Syndrome | Mode of Inheritance | Gene | Neoplasms |
|---|---|---|---|
| MEN IIb | Dominant | RET | Medullary thyroid, pheochromocytoma, mucosal neuromas |
| FAMMM | Dominant | CDKN2(MLM), CDK4 | Malignant melanoma, dysplastic nevi |
| Neurofibromatosis 1 | Dominant | NF1 | Neurofibrosarcoma, pheochromocytoma, optic glioma |
| Neurofibromatosis 2 | Dominant | NF2 | Bilateral acoustic neuroma, other nervous system |
| Hippel-Lindau disease | Dominant | VHL | Neural system hemangioblastoma, pheochromocytoma, renal cell, pancreatic |
| Retinoblastoma | Dominant | RB1 | Retinoblastoma, osteosarcoma |
| Wilms' tumor | Dominant | WT1 | Nephroblastoma, rhabdomyosarcoma, hepatoblastoma, neuroblastoma |
| Fanconi anemia | Recessive | FACC | Leukemia, esophageal, skin, hepatoma |
| Ataxia-telangiectasia | Recessive | ATM | Leukemia, lymphoma, ovarian, gastric, brain, breast |
| Bloom syndrome | Recessive | BLM | Leukemia, tongue, esophageal, Wilms' tumor, colon |
| Xeroderma pigmentosa | Recessive | XPA, XPC, XPD, XPF | Skin, melanoma, leukemia |

*FAMMM,* Familial atypical mole malignant melanoma.

Respect for the autonomy of the individual and the need for confidentiality must be kept in the forefront. Although there may be agreement between counselor and counselee on the desirability of prevention and early diagnosis in general, the extent to which counselees are willing to adopt various medical and surgical interventions varies enormously. Therefore the counselor's role is to present and encourage risk reduction strategies while being mindful of the different social, economic, cultural, and personal circumstances that will determine those strategies the patient wishes to adopt. In general, the goal of genetic counseling is to avoid the imposition of the practitioner's personal preferences when medical options are not fully proved. For multiple reasons, including the assumption of benefit from some regular screening and early detection options, cancer genetic counseling may be more directive than reproductive counseling.

In many families of average size, a two- or three-generation pedigree reveals two or more cases of cancer. The physician must decide whether a family may have a specific gene strongly associated with cancer or whether the family shows a clustering of unrelated cancer cases. In the former case, it may be appropriate to offer testing for the specific gene; in the latter, counseling regarding environmental risk factors or mere reassurance may be most appropriate.

To distinguish these possibilities, the physician must take a detailed family history. The following guidelines are useful:

- Query the patient about all first-degree relatives (parents, children, siblings), then second-degree relatives (grandparents, grandchildren, aunts, uncles, nieces, and nephews), and third-degree relatives (first cousins).
- Ask the patient to recall each relative and whether that individual has had cancer or not.
- Record the type of cancer and age of onset for each affected relative.
- Note the ethnic/racial background of the family.
- Inquire about consanguinity.
- Note relatives who have had bilateral cancers, multiple cancers, cancer before age 50, and cancer of the same type as others in the family.

The extensive characterization of familial cancers (breast, ovarian, prostate, renal, and so on) has led to specific screening strategies for each. Although genetic testing is not available yet for some forms of cancer, early detection by other screening measures has been suggested for at-risk relatives. A positive family history is one of the most common risk factors for cancer and is used as a guide to assess level of risk. In general, risk varies from moderately increased when one first-degree relative has cancer to more highly increased when a first-degree relative is diagnosed at an age less than 50 years or when there are two first-degree relatives with the same type of cancer.

An error sometimes made by patients and physicians is assuming that breast cancer susceptibility can only be transmitted through the maternal side of the family. Obtaining historical information from both sides of the family is equally important in determining whether one is dealing with a familial cancer syndrome. The next section has descriptions of some of the well-characterized familial cancer syndromes and a suggested approach to each.

### Breast/Ovarian Cancer

The strongest risk factors for breast cancer are age, family history, and personal history of breast cancer. Most (90% to 95%) breast cancers are sporadic and are not associated with inheritance of a highly penetrant gene. Three out of four breast malignancies occur in women over age 50; those that occur at younger ages have a much higher chance of being the result of a genetic predisposition.

Young women are unlikely to receive breast cancer screening as part of their routine health care. Therefore it is important to recognize those who are at high risk by virtue of their family history. Daughters of any patient with breast cancer occurring before age 50 would be included in this group.

## ASSESSING FAMILIAL BREAST CANCER RISK

Several models are available for estimating a patient's risk for breast cancer. The most readily available is the Gail model, which was initially derived from 2852 cases and 3146 matched controls in the Breast Cancer Detection and Demonstration Project[1,2,3]; the model has since been modified. A number of variables are used to calculate risk ratios: ethnic background, current age, age at first live birth, age at menarche, number of first-degree relatives with breast cancer, number of prior breast biopsies, and whether atypical hyperplasia or lobular neoplasia was diagnosed. A computerized program is available through the National Institutes of Health (NIH) to calculate individual risk. This program, however, does not include a detailed family history analysis and therefore may underestimate or overestimate risks for some women. The Claus model, derived from the Cancer and Steroid Hormone Study, estimates age-specific risks for breast cancer based exclusively on the numbers and age of affected first-degree and some second-degree relatives.[4] This model may provide more accurate prediction of risk for women with a strong family history of breast cancer. Several features of familial breast cancer help clinicians recognize persons who are at high risk because of inheritance of a breast cancer susceptibility gene. One feature is the early age of onset. Relative risk is more than fivefold in close relatives of breast cancer patients who were diagnosed younger than 40 years of age. On the other hand, relative risk is less than twofold in relatives of patients who were diagnosed older than 50 years of age.[4,5] In addition, the risk of breast cancer is much greater in women with two or more affected first-degree relatives than in women with one affected relative. Relatives with bilateral breast cancer suggest greater risk than do relatives with unilateral breast cancer.[6]

Another important feature of inherited breast cancer is its association with ovarian cancer. Risk of ovarian cancer is moderately increased in first-degree relatives of breast cancer cases, and vice versa.[5,7,8] Because inherited breast cancer makes up only 5% to 10% of all breast cancer cases, the majority of women with breast cancer or a family history of breast cancer do not need specialized counseling. A family history is usually sufficient to arrive at a preliminary determination of whether risk is substantially increased and if so, to either begin counseling or refer the patient to a specialized center for counseling.

## SUSCEPTIBILITY GENES

BRCA1, the locus of a gene that predisposes women to breast and ovarian cancer, was initially identified in 1990.[9] Colon cancer in men and women and prostate cancer are also increased in BRCA1 carriers.[10] A second gene for hereditary breast and ovarian cancer, BRCA2, was found in 1994.[11] The latter has also been associated with male breast cancer, as well as with pancreatic, fallopian tube, laryngeal, and uterine cancer.[12,13]

BRCA1 and 2 are large genes on chromosomes 17 and 13, respectively. Hundreds of different mutations in the nucleotide sequences of these genes have been detected; many of them present in only a single family. These mutations may be *missense* (change in a single nucleotide not affecting the translation of the remainder of the protein), *nonsense* (change resulting in termination of protein translation at that point), or *frameshift* (deletion or insertion of one or a few nucleotides in the coding region resulting in a change in the reading frame for the remainder of the sequence). Mutations in the noncoding region of the gene and splice site mutations at intron/exon boundaries may also cause reduction in protein synthesis or production of a nonfunctioning protein. However, not all mutations result in a qualitative or quantitative change in protein production. Therefore some families carry "mutations" of no clinical significance; these are known as variants. Other families have a nucleotide change, but it is not clear whether the change is associated with the cancers in the family. These changes are known as "variants of uncertain significance." The significance of the latter depends on finding the change in affected family members and whether other families have been reported with the same change in affected individuals.

A further dilemma in interpretation of genetic testing results is determining the "penetrance" of a mutation. Certain mutations are more likely to result in breast cancer in carriers (80% by age 75), whereas other mutations show a weaker association (56%) with the development of cancer.[14]

Certain ethnic groups are more likely to have mutations than others. For example, two mutations in BRCA1 (185delAG, 5382insC) and one in BRCA2 (617delT) are found in 2.5% of the Eastern European (Ashkenazi) Jewish population.[15-17] These mutations account for 70% to 80% of mutations found in Ashkenazis. Initial genetic testing for those three mutations alone may be appropriate in this population. Other specific mutations have been described in French-Canadians, Icelanders, Dutch, and African-Americans.[18-21] For patients who test negative for a BRCA mutation, a variety of interpretations are possible (Table 4-2). To clarify the interpretation, it is best if an affected family member is tested before testing unaffected members.

## MANAGEMENT

After the initial pedigree analysis and determination that the family history is appropriate for genetic testing, attention must be given to the psychological and social issues that make testing desirable or not. Several aspects of testing need to be considered before the test is performed. These include (1) implications and limitations of the test, (2) test accuracy, (3) risk of passing a mutation to offspring, (4) options for risk management, (5) possibility of psychological distress to the patient and other family members, (6) possibility of insurance or employment-related discrimination, and (7) cost of testing and counseling.

If the patient proceeds with testing and is positive for a mutation, options include intensive surveillance, chemoprevention, and prophylactic surgery. Intensive surveillance for breast cancer would include monthly breast self-examinations (BSE), annual diagnostic mammograms, and semiannual physician breast examinations (Table 4-3). Despite the lack of evidence of the effectiveness of this approach in reducing breast cancer mortality in high-risk women, 60% to 90% of breast cancers in young women are evident by mammography, suggesting that surveillance will likely result in earlier detection and decreased mortality.[22-25]

Carriers of BRCA mutations have a 10% to 40% risk for ovarian cancer. Unfortunately, surveillance for ovarian cancer is much less successful than surveillance for breast cancer. Semiannual pelvic examinations, transvaginal ultrasounds, and CA-125 levels are recommended for high-risk women, but no data support their effectiveness in reducing mortality.

| TABLE 4-2 | | |
|---|---|---|

## Interpretation and Possible Consequences of Genetic Test Results

| If an Alteration is Found | If an Alteration is *Not* Found in a Woman With Breast/ Ovarian Cancer | If an Alteration is *Not* Found When One is Known to Be in the Family |
|---|---|---|
| There is an increased risk for developing cancer. Appropriate surveillance/ management should be established. | A genetic form of cancer cannot be ruled out; other genes that were not tested for or have yet to be identified may have caused the cancer in the family. | The individual is not at increased risk of developing cancer due to an alteration in the BRCA1 or BRCA2 gene. |
| Psychological consequences may result from knowing one is at increased risk for developing cancer or passing it on to children. | Specific management options should be discussed with the physician. | This does not mean that the individual will not develop cancer in his or her lifetime; the general population risk and screening guidelines still apply. |
| Insurability could be compromised. | The individual may have psychological difficulties knowing that there is no genetic explanation for the cancer in the family. | The individual may experience mixed feelings of relief or guilt that he or she is spared in the family. |
| Relatives are at risk for carrying the mutation and should be informed and offered genetic counseling, surveillance, or testing. | The woman tested could be a sporadic case of breast cancer within a BRCA1 or BRCA2 family; another affected woman in the family may need to be tested. | |
| | Relatives may still be at risk of developing cancer and should discuss the family history with the physician. | |

## CHEMOPREVENTION

The National Surgical Adjuvant Bowel and Breast Project (NSABP) showed a 50% reduction in invasive and in situ breast cancer in high-risk women (5-year risk, 1.67% or higher) who took tamoxifen for 5 years.[26] Effectiveness in BRCA1 and BRCA2 mutation carriers specifically is unknown.

Oral contraceptives are known to decrease the risk of ovarian cancer in the general population.[27] The same reduction (50%) is seen in women with BRCA mutations.[28]

TABLE 4-3

## Management Options for Cancer Prevention in Women with BRCA Mutations

| Treatment Option | Frequency |
|---|---|
| Breast self-examination | Monthly beginning at age 18 years |
| Clinical breast examination | Annually or semiannually beginning at age 25 years |
| Mammography | Annually beginning at age 25 years |
| Pelvic examination | Semiannually beginning at age 25 to 35 years |
| Transvaginal ultrasound with color Doppler and CA-125 | Semiannually |
| Prophylactic bilateral simple mastectomy | Personal decision |
| Prophylactic bilateral oophorectomy | Personal decision |

## PROPHYLACTIC SURGERY

Prophylactic mastectomy is a reasonable option for women at very high risk (BRCA carriers) who wish to be aggressive in reducing this risk. Data from the Mayo Clinic suggest that breast cancer incidence and mortality are reduced by 90% in high-risk women after mastectomy.[29] The same was true for the subset of high-risk women who were BRCA mutation carriers.[30] Total mastectomy and reconstruction are preferable to subcutaneous mastectomy, which leaves behind some breast tissue. Psychological counseling should be offered to women considering prophylactic mastectomy.

In contrast to mastectomy, prophylactic oophorectomy performed laparoscopically is more acceptable to many women because of the minimal cosmetic effects and the less arduous nature of the surgery. Prophylactic oophorectomy decreases the risk of both ovarian cancer (by at least 50%) and breast cancer (by 50%) in high-risk women.[31-33]

Women who test negative for a BRCA mutation, particularly if a mutation has been identified in an affected family member, will not be at increased risk for breast or ovarian cancer. They need reminding, however, that the general population cancer screening guidelines should be followed to reduce their risk for a sporadic cancer. Many of these patients with risk factors for other, nonneoplastic diseases may also want to consider postmenopausal hormone replacement therapy to reduce their risk of cardiac disease and osteoporosis (Figure 4-1).

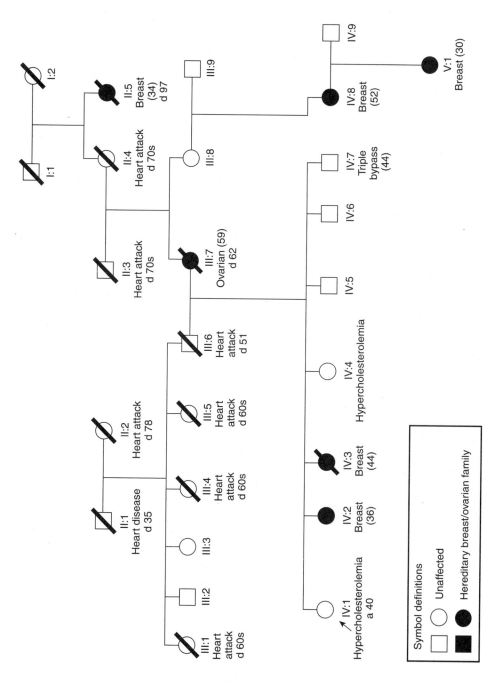

FIGURE 4-1  Pedigree of hereditary breast/ovarian cancer family.

### Colorectal Cancer Syndromes

Familial segregation of colon cancer may involve either a rare inherited syndrome or more commonly, familial clustering of cases. The genes associated with familial adenomatous polyposis (FAP) syndrome and hereditary nonpolyposis colorectal cancer (HNPCC) syndrome have been identified, and genetic testing to find gene carriers in affected families is commercially available. Research addressing the cellular mechanisms by which these genes operate and the proper application of genetic testing in these families is underway. However, the common familial clustering of cases appears to arise from the interaction of multiple, inherited susceptibility factors with environmental factors, giving rise to colorectal cancer when the cumulative "cancer factors" reach a particular level. The research in this area involves identification of these susceptibility genes and determination of how each interacts with environmental factors to give rise to cancer.

Colorectal cancer is the second most common cause of cancer death in the United States. The general population risk for colon cancer is 6%. Race, social class, residence, and diet are correlated with risk: white, upper-class, urban individuals with a high-fat diet are at greatest risk. Ninety percent of all colon cancer appears to be sporadic, arising from adenomatous polyps. Genetic predisposition has a significant role in approximately 10% of cases.[34,35] NPCC syndrome (Lynch syndrome) accounts for 5% to 8% of colon cancer, whereas the more aggressive form of colon cancer, FAP syndrome, is responsible for only 1% of colon cancer cases.[36] Like the breast/ovarian cancer syndrome, hereditary colon cancer is transmitted in an autosomal dominant fashion with each offspring having a 50% chance of inheriting the mutant gene from a parent who has the gene. Approximately 30% of cases are due to new genetic mutations (Figure 4-2).

## FAMILIAL ADENOMATOUS POLYPOSIS SYNDROME

FAP syndrome is an autosomal dominant condition characterized by the presence of hundreds or thousands of adenomatous polyps throughout the colon and rectum.[37,38] These polyps start appearing during adolescence and almost invariably undergo malignant transformation, usually by age 40. Most FAP cases are diagnosed by age 50 because of gastrointestinal bleeding, abdominal pain, or colon cancer.[37] Polyps may also be present in the distal stomach or antrum, duodenum, and terminal ileum. Some individuals with FAP syndrome also have multiple mandibular osteomas or congenital hypertrophy of the retinal pigment epithelium (CHRPE). The latter abnormality (single- or multiple-pigmented ovoid lesions) can be diagnosed with routine funduscopic examination. Individuals with Gardner syndrome have the features of FAP syndrome with more prominent extracolonic manifestations (osteomas of the skull, mandible, and long bones; desmoid tumors; dental abnormalities; epidermoid and sebaceous cysts; lipomas; fibromas; neoplasms of the thyroid, adrenals, biliary tree, and liver; upper gastrointestinal polyps, and CHRPE).[37,39]

The APC (adenomatous polyposis coli) gene has been located on chromosome 5, and multiple mutations are known.[40,41] Presymptomatic testing is available to close relatives of an individual with FAP syndrome. A protein truncation assay detects 90% of mutations; others can be detected with allele-specific assays.[42] Once a mutation has been detected in the affected individual or a family member, other members of the family can be tested for that specific mutation. Individuals carrying the mutation have a lifetime risk of colon cancer greater than 90%.[37] In such individuals, colonoscopy should begin at age 12 and repeated every 2 years.[37,43] Once colonic polyps are seen, colectomy is the treatment. If the

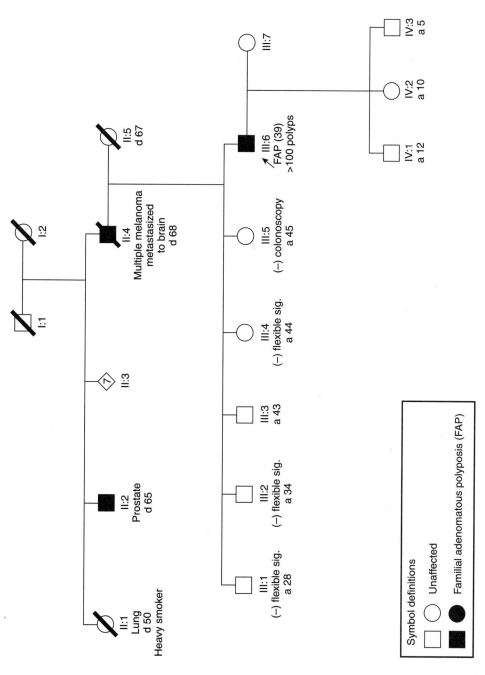

FIGURE 4-2   Pedigree of familial adenomatous polyposis family. (−), Negative; *sig.*, sigmoidoscopy.

at-risk individual elects not to undergo genetic testing, colonoscopy should be repeated every 2 years. If no polyps are found by age 40, it is unlikely that the individual carries the FAP gene and colonoscopic screening can be decreased to every 5 years. If genetic testing has shown the individual not to be a gene carrier, routine guidelines of the American Cancer Society for screening after age 50 should be followed. Therefore genetic testing can significantly benefit at-risk individuals by reducing their need for frequent colonoscopy.

## HEREDITARY NONPOLYPOSIS COLORECTAL CANCER SYNDROME

HNPCC syndrome, an autosomal dominantly transmitted condition, is also characterized by the presence of adenomatous polyps, although fewer (less than 100) than seen in patients with FAP syndrome. The polyps are generally found in the proximal colon. Mean age at diagnosis of colon cancer is 44 years, and mucinous or poorly differentiated cancers are common.[36] A family is generally considered to have HNPCC syndrome if (1) three or more relatives have verified colorectal cancer, one of whom is a first-degree relative of the other two; (2) colorectal cancer is seen in at least two generations; and (3) at least one case of colorectal cancer was diagnosed before are 50.[44] However, some families may have HNPCC syndrome but not meet these criteria because of small family size or a new mutation (Figure 4-3). Gene penetrance is very high, with virtually 100% of males and 54% of females developing colorectal cancer by age 70.[45] Extracolonic tumors, such as endometrial (60% of females), gastric (13%), ovarian (12%), ureteral, kidney, biliary tract, and brain, also occur frequently in individuals with HNPCC syndrome. The Muir-Torre variant of HNPCC syndrome includes sebaceous gland neoplasms and keratoacanthomas.

Several different genes on chromosomes 2, 3, and 7 have shown mutations in families with HNPCC syndrome.[46,47] These genes (MLH1, MSH2, MSH6, PMS1, and PMS2) have the common function of repairing DNA mismatches that occur during replication. Tumors from patients with HNPCC syndrome often demonstrate the replication error defect by showing microsatellite instability (MSI). Therefore initial testing for HNPCC syndrome is usually by analysis of a tumor for MSI, followed by mutational analysis of repair genes if MSI is present. Such testing, however, does not identify all mutations; the false-negative rate is 30%.[36]

Individuals who have a family history of HNPCC syndrome or who have positive genetic testing should have colonoscopy starting at age 21, with a repeat every 1 to 2 years until age 40 and every year thereafter. Potentially affected women should also have annual gynecological examinations with measurement of endometrial thickness with ultrasound or endometrial biopsies. For maximal risk reduction, subtotal colectomy is an option; for women, total abdominal hysterectomy and bilateral salpingoophorectomy should also be seriously considered.

### Prostate Cancer

Prostate cancer is the most common cancer in men and occurs most often in men over age 65, in African-American men, and in those with a family history of the disease. Average lifetime risk for prostate cancer is 10%; of these, 5% to 10% may be attributable to inherited susceptibility genes.[48] Most family aggregates of prostate cancer show an autosomal dominant pattern, with penetrance as high as 88% by age 85 in some families. Familial prostate cancer accounts for 43% of prostate cancers diagnosed before age 56 and 9% by age 85.[49]

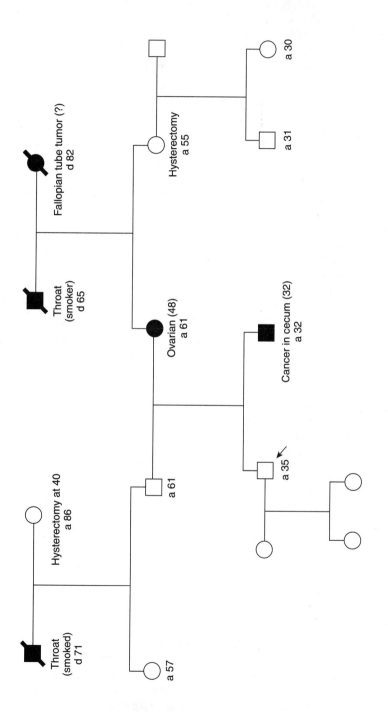

FIGURE 4-3    Pedigree of hereditary nonpolyposis colorectal cancer (HNPCC) family.

Whereas only 2% of prostate cancers in the general population are diagnosed before age 56, this number will likely increase with the introduction of new screening tools.[50] Whether the additional cases diagnosed before the age of 56 are due to genetic syndromes or are just sporadic cases diagnosed early is still unknown.

Recent evidence suggests that hereditary prostate cancer is a complex disease involving multiple susceptibility genes and variable phenotypic expression. A number of candidate genes for familial prostate cancer have been isolated on chromosomes 1 (HPC1, PCAP, CAPB) and X (HPCX). Overall, these four loci appear to account for only a minority of familial prostate cancer cases, and none of the putative genes has been identified so far. Studies have shown that families demonstrating male-to-male transmission, early average age at diagnosis (under 65 years), and five or more affected family members are more likely to be linked to HPC1 than are families without these findings.[51,52] Another genome-wide search on 162 families affected with prostate cancer identified a genetic susceptibility locus on chromosome 20 (HPC20).[53] It is well recognized that prostate cancer is heterogenous and that multiple genetic and environmental factors likely play a role in its etiology. Because of this complexity, clinical testing is not yet available for prostate cancer genes.

There has been much debate over the benefits of screening and treatment for early-stage prostate cancer, primarily because the aggressiveness of prostate cancer varies widely. Some tumors progress to invasive, potentially life-threatening disease, whereas others remain latent for the individual's lifetime. In the setting of a strong family history, there is less controversy about screening and treatment. Individuals at increased risk stand to benefit the most from screening. Men with a strong family history of prostate cancer (two or more first- or second-degree relatives) should have prostate-specific antigen (PSA) testing and a digital rectal examination annually between ages 50 to 70. Screening should start earlier (in their 40s) for men from families with a history of early-onset prostate cancer.[54] Future options for those at risk for hereditary prostate cancer include hormonal chemoprevention with antiandrogens and possibly, prophylactic prostatectomy.

In some families, prostate cancer may be associated with other known cancer predisposition syndromes. For example, excess cases of prostate cancer are found in families with mutant BRCA1 and BRCA2 genes; the relative risk among carriers is approximately 3. Prostate cancer can also be a component of the Li-Fraumeni syndrome, associated with a germline mutation in the p53 gene. Prostate cancer is not associated with hereditary melanoma or the HNPCC syndromes.

## SUMMARY

One of the most famous cancer family histories in the early nineteenth century was that of Madame Z, described by the French physician, Broca.[55] In this family, 16 of 26 members died at or before the age of 30 from breast or "liver" (probably metastatic breast) cancer. The prevailing belief at the time was that cancer resulted from acquired, not inherited, factors. Now it is known that genes and environmental factors interact in determining whether individual patients develop cancer. Cancer genetics is still in its infancy, but the rapid pace of development suggests that effective therapeutic and preventive measures can be anticipated. Eventually, such interventions may be routinely provided, extending the reach of clinical genetics far beyond the domain of pediatrics and obstetrics.

## REFERENCES

1. Gail MH, Brinton LA, Byar DP, et al: Projecting individualized probabilities of developing breast cancer for white females who are being examined annually, *J Natl Cancer Inst* 81:1879, 1989.

2. Gail MH, Benichou J: Assessing the risk of breast cancer in individuals. In DeVita VT Jr, Hellman S, Rosenberg SA, editors: *Cancer prevention,* Philadelphia, 1992, JB Lippincott.

3. Benichou J: A computer program for estimating individualized probabilities of breast cancer, *Comput Biomed Res* 26:373, 1993.

4. Claus EB, Risch NJ, Thompson WD: Genetic analysis of breast cancer in the cancer and steroid hormone study, *Am J Hum Genet* 48:232, 1991.

5. Claus EB, Risch NJ, Thomson WD: Age at onset as an indicator of familial risk of breast cancer, *Am J Epidemiol* 131:961, 1990.

6. Bernstein JL, Thompson WD, Risch N, et al: The genetic epidemiology of second primary breast cancer, *Am J Epidemiol* 136:937, 1992.

7. Cramer DW, Hutchinson GB, Welch WR, et al: Determinants of ovarian cancer risk. I. Reproductive experiences and family history, *J Natl Cancer Inst* 71:711, 1983.

8. Miki Y, Swensen J, Shattuck-Edens D, et al: A strong candidate for the breast and ovarian cancer susceptibility gene BRCA1, *Science* 266:66, 1994.

9. Hall JM, Lee MK, Newman B, et al: Linkage of early onset familial breast cancer to chromosome 17q21, *Science* 250:1684, 1990.

10. Ford D, Easton DS, Bishop DT, et al: Risks of cancer in BRCA1 mutation carriers, *Lancet* 343:692, 1994.

11. Wooster R, Neuhausen S, Mangion J, et al: Localization of a breast cancer susceptibility gene, BRCA2, to chromosome 13q1243, *Science* 265:2088, 1994.

12. Berman DB, Costalas J, Schultz DC, et al: A common mutation in BRCA2 that predisposes to a variety of cancers is found in both Jewish Ashkenazi and non-Jewish individuals, *Cancer Res* 56:3409-3414, 1996.

13. Tonin P, Narod S, Ghardirian P, et al: A large multisite cancer family is linked to BRCA2, *J Med Genet* 32:982-984, 1995.

14. Moslehi R, Chu W, Karlan B, et al: BRCA1 and BRCA2 mutation analysis of 208 Ashkenazi Jewish women with ovarian cancer, *Am J Hum Genet* 66:1259-1272, 2000.

15. Struewing JP, Abeliovich D, Peretz T, et al: The carrier frequency of the BRCA1 185delAG mutation is approximately 1% in Ashkenazi Jewish individuals, *Nat Genet* 11:198-200, 1995.

16. Roa BB, Boyd AA, Volcik K, et al: Ashkenazi Jewish population frequencies for common mutations in BRCA1 and BRCA2, *Nat Genet* 14:185-187, 1996.

17. Hartge P, Stuewing JP, Wacholder S, et al: The prevalence of common BRCA1 and BRCA2 mutations among Ashkenazi Jews, *Am J Hum Genet* 64:963-970, 1999.

18. Simard J, Tonin P, Durocher F, et al: Common origins of BRCA1 mutations in Canadian breast and ovarian cancer families, *Nat Genet* 8:392-398, 1994.

19. Thorlacius S, Olafsdottir S, Tryggvadottir L, et al: Study of a single BRCA2 mutation in male and female cancer families from Iceland with varied cancer phenotypes, *Nat Genet* 13:117-121, 1996.

20. Gao Q, Neuhausen S, Cummings S, et al: Recurrent germ-line BRCA1 mutations in extended African-American families with early onset breast cancer, *Am J Hum Genet* 60:1233-1236, 1997.

21. Peelan T, van Viet M, Petrij-Bosch A, et al: A high proportion of novel mutations in BRCA1 with strong founder effects among Dutch and Belgian hereditary breast and ovarian families, *Am J Hum Genet* 60:1041-1049, 1997.

22. Meyer JE, Kopans DB, Oot R: Breast cancer visualized by mammography in patients under 35, *Radiology* 147:93, 1983.

23. Morrow M: Identification and management of the woman at increased risk for breast cancer development, *Breast Cancer Res Treat* 31:53, 1994.

24. Cohen MI, Mintzer R, Matthies HJ, et al: Mammography in women less than 40 years of age, *Surg Gynecol Obstet* 160:220, 1985.

25. McSweeney MB, Egan RL: Breast cancer, not just a disease of middle age, *Diagn Imag* 1:48, 1984.

26. Fisher B, Costantino JP, Wickerham DL, et al: Tamoxifen for prevention of breast cancer: Report of the National Surgical Adjuvant Breast and Bowel Project P-1 Study, *J Natl Cancer Inst* 90:1371-1388, 1998.

27. Whittemore AS, Harris R, Itnyre J: Characteristics relating to ovarian cancer risk: collaborative analysis of 12 US case-control studies. II. Invasive epithelial ovarian cancers in white women, *Am J Epidemiol* 136:1184-1203, 1992.

28. Narod SA, Risch H, Moslehi R, et al: Oral contraceptives and the risk of hereditary ovarian cancer, *N Engl J Med* 339:424-428, 1998.

29. Hartmann LC, Schaid DJ, Woods JE, et al: Efficacy of bilateral prophylactic mastectomy in women with a family history of breast cancer, *N Engl J Med* 340:77-84, 1999.

30. Hartmann LC et al: Prophylactic mastectomy cuts cancer risk in women with BRCA mutations. Presented at the annual meeting of the American Association of Cancer Research, San Francisco, April 2, 2000.

31. Piver MS, Goldberg JM, Tsukada Y, et al: Characteristics of familial ovarian cancer: a report of the first 1,000 families from the Gilda Radner Familial Ovarian Cancer Registry, *Eur J Gyn Oncol* 17:169-176, 1996.

32. Rebbeck TR, Levin AM, Eisen A, et al: Breast cancer risk after bilateral prophylactic oophorectomy in BRCA1 mutation carriers, *J Natl Cancer Inst* 91:1475-1479, 1999.

33. Eisen A, Rebbeck TR, Wood WC, et al: Prophylactic surgery in women with a hereditary predisposition to breast and ovarian cancer, *J Clin Oncol* 18:1980-1995, 2000.

34. Bodner W, Bishop T, Karran P: Genetic steps in colorectal cancers, *Nat Genet* 6:217, 1994.

35. Slattery ML, Kerber RA: Family history of cancer and colon cancer risk: the Utah population database, *J Natl Cancer Inst* 86:1618, 1994.

36. Lynch HT, de la Chapelle A: Genetic susceptibility to non-polyposis colorectal cancer, *J Med Genet* 36:801-818, 1999.

37. Rustgi AK: Hereditary gastrointestinal polyposis and nonpolyposis syndromes, *N Engl J Med* 331:1694-1702, 1994.

38. Herrera L, editor: Familial adenomatous polyposis, New York, 1990, Alan R Liss.

39. Olschwang S, Tiret A, Laurent-Puig P, et al: Restriction of ocular fundus lesions to a specific subgroup of APC mutations in adenomatous polyposis coli patients, *Cell* 74:959, 1993.

40. Kinzler KW, Nilbert MC, Su LK, et al: Identification of FAP locus genes from chromosome 5q21, *Science* 253:661, 1991.

41. Nishisho I, Nakamura Y, Miyoshi Y, et al: Mutations of chromosome 5q21 genes in FAP and colorectal cancer patients, *Science* 253:665, 1991.

42. Powell SW, Petersen GM, Krush A, et al: Molecular diagnosis of familial adenomatous polyposis, *N Engl J Med* 329:1982, 1993.

43. Neal K, Ritchie S, Thompson JPS: Screening of offspring of patients with familial adenomatous polyposis: the St. Mark's Hospital Polyposis Register experience. In Herrera L, editor: Familial adenomatosis polyposis, New York, 1990, Alan R Liss.

44. Vasen HFA, Mecklin J-P, Khan PM, et al: The International Collaborative Group on hereditary non-polyposis colorectal cancer (CICG-HNPCC), *Dis Colon Rectum* 34:424, 1991.

45. Aarnio M, Sankila R, Pukkala E, et al: Cancer risk in mutation carriers of DNA-mismatch–repair genes, *Int J Cancer* 81:214-218, 1999.

46. Rhyu MS: Molecular mechanisms underlying hereditary nonpolyposis colorectal cancer, *J Natl Cancer Inst* 88:240-251, 1996.

47. Miyaki M, Konishi M, Tanaka K, et al: Germline mutation of MSH6 as the cause of hereditary nonpolyposis colorectal cancer, *Nat Genet* 17:271-272, 1997.

48. Narod S: Genetic epidemiology of prostate cancer, *Biochim Biophys Acta* 1423:F1-F13, 1998.

49. Carter BS, Beaty TH, Steinberg GD, et al: Mendelian inheritance of familial prostate cancer, *Proc Natl Acad Sci* 89:3367-3371, 1992.

50. Potosky AL, Miller BA, Albertsen PC, et al: The role of increasing detection in the rising incidence of prostate cancer, *JAMA* 273:548-552, 1995.

51. Gronberg H, Zu J, Smith JR, et al: Early age at diagnosis in families providing evidence of linkage to the hereditary prostate cancer locus (HPC1) on chromosome 1, *Cancer Res* 57:4707-4709, 1997.

52. Xu J: Combined analysis of hereditary prostate cancer linkage to 1q24-25: results from 772 hereditary prostate cancer families from the International Consortium for Prostate Cancer Genetics, *Am J Hum Genet* 66:945-957, 2000.

53. Berry R, Schroeder J, French A, et al: Evidence for a prostate cancer-susceptibility locus on chromosome 20, *Am J Hum Genet* 67:82-91, 2000.

54. Gronberg H, Wiklund F, Damber J-E: Age specific risks of familial prostate carcinoma, Cancer 86:477-483, 1999.

55. Broca P: *Traite des tumeurs,* Paris, 1866, Asselin.

# CHAPTER 5

# Prenatal Testing and Interventions

*Cathleen M. Harris*
*Marion S. Verp*

The fundamental ethical dilemmas engendered by genetic advances have not changed appreciably over the past two decades. What has changed instead is the level of knowledge of the general public regarding health matters and the technology available to assist in screening for genetic diseases and diagnosing them. Physicians and patients have seen improvements in the technology available to answer clinical genetics questions, although the principles guiding clinicians who offer genetic testing remain much the same.

This chapter outlines approaches to prenatal diagnosis currently in wide use and describes ways in which genetics is incorporated into prenatal screening and diagnostic strategies, including molecular testing methods and novel forms of in utero treatment. Chapter 12 discusses how new genetic testing methods might impact ethical considerations in the management of genetic problems during pregnancy and suggests ways in which clinicians who provide obstetric care may incorporate the knowledge acquired in the Human Genome Project (HGP) into general practice.

## TRADITIONAL APPROACHES TO PRENATAL DIAGNOSIS

The American College of Obstetricians and Gynecologists (ACOG) recommends that all pregnant women be offered maternal serum alpha fetoprotein (MSAFP) and multiple-marker screening and that women who will be 35 years or older at delivery be offered fetal karyotype analysis using amniocentesis or chorionic villus sampling.[1] Ultrasound markers of chromosome disorders are also an important component of many prenatal genetic screening programs.[2]

The MSAFP test is the most commonly employed prenatal genetic screening, aside from maternal age. The fetus synthesizes alpha fetoprotein (AFP) early in development and reaches high concentrations in the fetal blood. AFP also appears in amniotic fluid and maternal serum but in concentrations much lower than that of fetal blood. Maternal serum screening for AFP was initially used to detect fetal open neural tube defects such as anencephaly and meningomyelocele. Subsequently, Merkatz and colleagues[3] recognized that MSAFP values tend to be decreased among women whose fetuses are affected with Down syndrome, or trisomy 21. However, it became clear that a threshold approach, such as that used for the detection of open neural tube defects, was not appropriate for use in the detection of trisomy 21. Although the median of MSAFP values is lower in pregnant women whose fetuses have Down syndrome, the separation between the median for normal pregnancies and that for Down syndrome pregnancies is small. Subsequently, investigators have found that the sensitivity of serum screening can be improved by incorporating values of additional serum analytes, in particular human chorionic gonadotropin and unconjugated estriol, as part of the Down syndrome screening test.[1]

The approach of multiple-analyte analysis has been tested in large populations and has good clinical results.[4,5] When using maternal age alone as a screening method, only 20% of cases of fetal Down syndrome are identified. In contrast, if one screens for fetal Down syndrome using maternal age and MSAFP, the sensitivity is 35%. Using three or four analytes increases the sensitivity for fetal trisomy 21 to 60% to 80%. Some cases of fetal trisomy 18 (Edwards syndrome) can be detected using the multiple-marker screening approach, with relatively low levels of all three analytes being the typical pattern in an affected pregnancy.

In addition to multiple-marker screening, sonographic markers of fetal chromosome abnormalities have been used as an adjunct for improving detection rates of Down syndrome and other conditions. Nicolaides and others[6] reported that first-trimester measurements of fetal nuchal lucency are reported to have good sensitivity for detecting fetal aneuploidy, including Down syndrome and Turner syndrome. During the second trimester, sonographic indicators for Down syndrome include short femur and humerus, cerebral ventriculomegaly, fetal cardiac abnormalities, renal pelvis dilation (pyelectasis), echogenic bowel, and increased nuchal skinfold thickness. Using a combined approach that includes maternal age, multiple-marker screening, and ultrasound parameters, risk assessments for fetal Down syndrome can be refined.[7]

Although serum screening for fetal chromosome disorders came into widespread use in the 1990s, prenatal genetic diagnosis was available 15 years earlier. Tissue suitable for prenatal diagnosis has been obtained in several ways. Initially, prenatal genetic diagnosis was confined to midtrimester amniocentesis, which was performed at 16 weeks' gestation. Amniotic fluid was analyzed for AFP level or karyotype. Pregnancy loss rates after midtrimester amniocentesis have been evaluated in several large studies in the United States, Canada, and Europe. The risk of pregnancy loss due to amniocentesis is estimated to be approximately 0.5%.[8-10] With high-resolution ultrasound equipment available, as well as a growing number of experienced sonographers, some physicians have begun to offer amniocentesis before 14 weeks' gestation. However, the safety of early amniocentesis is less than that of midtrimester amniocentesis.[11,12]

Although midtrimester amniocentesis is thought to be reliable and safe, there has long been interest in developing methods for genetic testing during the first trimester to allow clinicians and patients earlier access to genetic information. In the 1980s, chorionic villus sampling (CVS) became available at numerous sites. CVS, performed at 10 to 13 weeks' gestation, involves removal of a small amount of placental tissue through a catheter that is introduced transcervically or a needle placed transabdominally or rarely, transvaginally.

The chorionic villi obtained may be used for karyotype analysis, biochemical testing, or DNA testing, as with amniotic fluid cells. In contrast to amniocentesis, however, AFP cannot be measured in villous samples. Several large randomized controlled trials of CVS versus midtrimester amniocentesis showed that there was a loss rate after CVS of approximately 1% over that of controls.[13-15] Previously, there had been speculation that a small increase in the risk of limb defects occurred as a result of CVS.[16,17] However, when CVS is performed at 10 weeks' gestation or later by an experienced operator, there appears to be no increase in these abnormalities.[18]

In some cases, rapid results of genetic testing are desirable. Fetal lymphocytes in fetal blood provide an excellent source of cells for such analysis. Fetal lymphocytes can be collected via cordocentesis, which involves aspiration of a specimen of fetal blood from the umbilical vein under direct ultrasound visualization.[19] In addition to its quick turnaround time for karyotype analysis, cordocentesis allows the clinician to clarify results found by amniocentesis or CVS. However, cordocentesis is the most invasive of the common testing methods, and the rate of fetal loss is approximately 1% to 2%.[20] In rare circumstances, sampling fetal tissues, such as skin, liver, or muscle, can be used to aid in determining whether a fetus is affected with a genetic condition, such as Duchenne muscular dystrophy.[21] In most cases, however, it is possible to diagnose genetic disorders by DNA analysis of amniotic fluid or villous cells.

Overall, amniocentesis offers the advantage of highly reliable results and a low rate of pregnancy loss. CVS is attractive because results are obtained early in pregnancy, so that decisions regarding pregnancy continuation or termination can be made in a timely fashion. In contrast, cordocentesis allows for rapid determination of fetal karyotype at advanced gestational ages but at the cost of requiring specialized skills and a potentially higher rate of fetal loss. Table 5-1 displays the various modalities for prenatal diagnosis currently available.

### TABLE 5-1

## Current Technologies Available for Prenatal Diagnosis

| Procedure | When Test is Performed | Method and Accuracy | Risks to Mother | Risks to Fetus or Embryo |
|---|---|---|---|---|
| Ultrasonography | During first or second trimester | Ultrasound waves emit from a transducer in pulses; sound waves bounce off structures and return to transducer. Accuracy depends on examiner and on nature of defect. | No physical risks | No known physical risks |

Modified from Mahowald MB, Levinson D, Cassel C, et al: *Milbank Q* 74(2):239-283, 1996.

*Continued*

TABLE 5-1

## Current Technologies Available for Prenatal Diagnosis—cont'd

| Procedure | When Test is Performed | Method and Accuracy | Risks to Mother | Risks to Fetus or Embryo |
|---|---|---|---|---|
| Multiple-marker screen | 15-21 weeks' gestation | Maternal serum sample is screened for AFP, estriol, and HCG. Sensitivity for Down syndrome is 60%; false-positive rate is 6%. | Usual risks of venipuncture | None |
| Midtrimester amniocentesis | 15-20 weeks' gestation | Needle inserted into uterus to aspirate 20 ml of amniotic fluid. False-positive and false-negative rates <0.5%. | Vaginal bleeding, amniotic fluid leak, infection | Fetal loss rate 0.5%; other risks: needle puncture, Rh sensitization |
| Chorionic villus sampling | 10-13 weeks' gestation | Transcervical catheter or transabdominal needle inserted into placenta, followed by tissue aspiration. Diagnostic success rate 99.6%. | Vaginal bleeding, infection | Fetal loss rate 0.5%-1.0% |
| Early amniocentesis | Before 14 weeks' gestation | Same method and accuracy as midtrimester amniocentesis, with less fluid aspirated. | Same as midtrimester amniocentesis, with increased risk of amniotic fluid leak | Fetal loss rate 1.7%, talipes equinovarus 1.2%, culture failure 1.3% |
| Percutaneous umbilical blood sampling | 18 weeks' gestation to term | Ultrasound guides needle into umbilical cord; fetal blood is aspirated. Accuracy approaches 100%. | Fetal-maternal hemorrhage, infection, premature rupture of membranes, labor | Fetal loss rate 1%-2%, fetal bleeding, umbilical cord hematoma, fetal bradycardia, fetal trauma, placental abruption |

*AFP,* Alpha fetoprotein; *HCG,* human chorionic gonadotropin.

**TABLE 5-1**

## Current Technologies Available for Prenatal Diagnosis—cont'd

| Procedure | When Test is Performed | Method and Accuracy | Risks to Mother | Risks to Fetus or Embryo |
|---|---|---|---|---|
| Fetal skin or liver biopsy | 17-20 weeks' gestation | Ultrasound used to guide biopsy of fetal tissues. Accuracy not established. | Bleeding in uterus, infection, premature rupture of membranes, labor | Fetal loss rate probably <5%, scarring |
| Preimplantation genetic testing | Before implantation | IVF performed; cells biopsied from zygote are analyzed before transfer into uterus. Polar bodies can be analyzed before oocyte insemination. Accuracy high, but errors reported. | Risks related to IVF procedure | No increase in anomalies, but loss rate in vitro and after transfer uncertain |
| Fetal cells in maternal serum | First trimester: currently investigational | Maternal blood sample drawn; fetal cells separated and analyzed using FISH with chromosome-specific DNA probes. | Usual risks of venipuncture | None |

*IVF,* In vitro fertilization; *FISH,* fluorescence in situ hybridization.

With the development of molecular methods of fetal DNA analysis, the number of possible diagnoses and treatments available for the embryo and fetus increase dramatically. The remainder of this chapter outlines certain technical advancements that have improved prenatal diagnosis.

## DNA-BASED PRENATAL DIAGNOSIS

Although it is the mainstay of prenatal diagnosis using amniocentesis and CVS, conventional cytogenetic analysis does not allow detection of specific mutations and does not indicate from whom genetic material has been inherited. On the other hand, DNA obtained from fetal tissues can also be used for other types of genetic analyses. Restriction enzymes, allele-specific oligonucleotide probes, and polymerase chain reactions (PCRs) allow direct mutational analysis and linkage analysis. All these modalities have permitted prenatal genetic diagnosis for a variety of conditions.[22]

When the molecular basis of a disease is known, precise tests can be designed to detect particular mutations. Cystic fibrosis (CF) testing is available for a large number of mutations. An example of direct mutational analysis is testing for mutations in the CF transmembrane conductance regulator (CFTR) gene. Fetal DNA can be obtained via amniocentesis or CVS. When a couple are at risk for a fetus with CF because they both carry CF mutations, prenatal diagnosis can assist them with decisions about pregnancy.

Another example of molecular diagnostics used for prenatal diagnosis is the detection of a point mutation present among individuals with sickle hemoglobin. Testing for this condition is greatly facilitated because all persons with sickle hemoglobin have the same mutation. To determine if a fetus will have normal hemoglobin A, will be a sickle carrier, or will be affected, a small amount of fetal DNA is obtained from CVS or amniocentesis. A portion of the beta-globulin gene around the site of the mutation responsible for sickle hemoglobin is then amplified using PCR. This product is then cut into fragments using endonucleases, and the fragments are separated by electrophoresis. If the fetus is a homozygote for hemoglobin A (normal), there are two bands of 100 and 150 base pairs (bp). If the fetus is affected and a homozygote for hemoglobin S, only the uncut 250-bp band is seen. If the fetus is a carrier, however, all three bands are visualized. Another form of hemoglobin DNA testing uses PCR to amplify normal and mutant DNA selectively. The amplified pieces are then marked directly with a radioactive probe. The presence of a mutant gene is visualized as a "dot" corresponding to the appropriate PCR sample. Molecular genetic testing allows couples at risk for having a child with sickle cell disease to obtain an unambiguous result regarding their fetus.[23]

At the University of Chicago, patients are offered customized diagnostics for prenatal evaluation for rare diseases. A family with a child affected by a rare disease undergoes mutational analysis using DNA sequencing methods. Clinical assays for specific mutations are developed. In a subsequent pregnancy, either CVS or amniocentesis is used to obtain fetal cells for DNA analysis with the customized clinical assay.

## FLUORESCENCE IN SITU HYBRIDIZATION

Fluorescence in situ hybridization (FISH) is a powerful technology that is becoming more popular in prenatal diagnosis. FISH involves hybridizing DNA probes representing specific chromosomes or chromosomal regions to target DNA, where the probes bind to homologous sequences. DNA probes can be used to paint an entire chromosome, to bind to chromosome-specific repetitive sequences, or to bind to unique sequences.[24] One of the most common applications of FISH has been in prenatal detection of common fetal aneuploidies. Commercially available FISH assays utilize probes for chromosomes 13, 18, 21, X, and Y. The number of signals for each of these chromosomes is analyzed in interphase nuclei, obviating the need for cell culture and allowing results within 24 hours. Such assays can reliably detect trisomies 13, 18, and 21, as well as certain sex chromosome abnormalities. FISH is not a substitute for conventional cytogenetics, however, since FISH fails to detect other cytogenetic abnormalities, such as deletions, translocations, and marker chromosomes. Evans and colleagues[25] estimated that the FISH assay would detect only 65% of all chromosome abnormalities in their high-risk pregnant population. Thus FISH is currently being used as a rapid and inexpensive preliminary assessment of aneuploidy status, with results confirmed by standard cytogenetics.

In addition to using FISH for detection of aneuploidy, FISH can aid in the detection of structural chromosome abnormalities. Prader-Willi syndrome (PWS) is the result of absence of the paternal copy of the PWS gene, which is located on chromosome 15. Most cases are caused by inheritance of two copies of chromosome 15 from the mother and none from the father. Sometimes a deletion may be too small to be visualized with routine cytogenetics. FISH analysis with the small nuclear ribonucleoprotein N (SNRPN) gene probe can show whether the patient has inherited a normal copy of the gene from the father.

## PREIMPLANTATION GENETIC DIAGNOSIS

Another approach to prenatal diagnosis is preimplantation genetic diagnosis (PGD). In 1990, Handyside and colleagues[26] reported the first successful PGD of embryonic sex. Couples at risk for X-linked disease in their offspring underwent in vitro fertilization (IVF), embryo biopsy, Y chromosome–specific DNA testing of the biopsied cells, and subsequent transfer of female embryos. These couples established viable pregnancies, which ultimately resulted in healthy female infants.

Since then, PGD has been used by a relatively small number of patients. Techniques vary in different centers. In most cases, zygotes fertilized in vitro are biopsied at the six- to ten-cell stage. One or two cells are removed through an opening created in the zona pellucida. The cells are analyzed using PCR or FISH; unaffected embryos are identified and transferred to the uterus. A report from 29 centers summarized the results obtained from 1200 patients who had undergone PGD: 231 pregnancies developed from 965 embryo transfers. From these pregnancies, 166 babies were born, yielding a success rate of 14% per patient. In this report, two thirds of the analyses were performed for chromosomal disorders, and one third were performed for single-gene disorders such as Duchenne muscular dystrophy, CF, Tay-Sachs disease, hemophilia A, and severe combined immunodeficiency (SCID).[27]

It is possible to biopsy other cells from the preembryo. The trophoectoderm can be biopsied on day 5 to 6. Alternatively, the polar body may be studied before oocyte fertilization. Depending on the indication for testing, the first polar body is analyzed for chromosome number or for the presence of a particular mutation. Under certain circumstances in which crossing over of chromosomes may have occurred, the second polar body may need to be analyzed as well.

To date, studies have not shown an increased risk of pregnancy loss or malformations after PGD. However, a post-PGD pregnancy rate equal to that from IVF does not prove that PGD does not interfere with embryonic development. In general, PGD patients are fertile and would therefore be expected to have a higher pregnancy rate than patients undergoing IVF because of infertility. In addition, the reliability of diagnosis is important in determining whether PGD will become more widely used in clinical practice. The few reports of false-negative diagnoses were likely caused by contamination of the oocyte with DNA from a nonfertilizing sperm or from another source (laboratory worker or pipette). Most fertilizations are now performed with intracytoplasmic sperm injection before PGD, thus reducing the possibility of contamination from other sperm.

## FETAL CELLS IN MATERNAL CIRCULATION

Many clinicians have wished for a *noninvasive* method of prenatal diagnosis that would allow prenatal diagnosis to be offered to all pregnant women rather than just to those at increased risk for fetal genetic problems. In 1969, Walkonowska and colleagues[28] demonstrated that fetal lymphocytes appear in the maternal circulation during pregnancy. To be used for analysis, however, the small number of fetal cells must be separated from the vast number of maternal cells in a blood sample.

Recent developments in cell-sorting techniques and in amplification and analysis of genetic material have given new impetus to the effort to achieve fetal genetic diagnosis via a maternal blood sample. For example, researchers have learned which fetal cells are most suitable for study. Although fetal lymphocytes were the first type of cell to be extracted from maternal circulation, they have a long half-life and can persist in the maternal circulation for many years. Thus a fetal lymphocyte in the maternal circulation may reflect a prior pregnancy rather than an ongoing pregnancy. Trophoblast cells have also been detected in maternal serum, but these are difficult to isolate. Instead, recent attention has focused on isolating fetal erythroblasts from maternal blood. Because fetal erythrocytes are nucleated, fetal DNA can be extracted and amplified by PCR reactions or can be studied using FISH probes.

In 1994, Simpson and Elias[29] reported the successful detection of trisomies 18 and 21, as well as Klinefelter syndrome, in seven of eight pregnancies at 10 to 19 weeks' gestation using maternal blood samples taken at amniocentesis or CVS. Other investigators reported that the number of fetal cells in the maternal circulation is increased in aneuploid pregnancies, which may prove useful as an initial screen. The sensitivity and specificity of this method in screening for fetal chromosome abnormalities remain uncertain. The National Institute of Child Health and Human Development (NICHHD) is conducting a multicenter clinical trial of this method of prenatal diagnosis for fetal aneuploidy.

In addition to chromosome diagnosis, detection of single-gene disorders may also be possible by analyzing fetal cells in the maternal serum for paternal alleles. Cheung and associates[30] reported the successful diagnosis of normal hemoglobin genes in two pregnancies at risk for fetal sickle cell disease and β-thalassemia. In each case, fetal cells were separated from maternal blood cells using differential cell characteristics and antibodies to embryonic or fetal hemoglobin. Fetal cells could then be selected visually from prepared slides. DNA was extracted from the fetal cells, amplified, and tested for the hemoglobin mutations of interest.

In a similar fashion, Lo and colleagues[31] determined the fetal Rh D type by analyzing fetal cells in the maternal circulation. They extracted DNA from the plasma of 57 pregnant women who were Rh D negative and used a PCR-based test that was sensitive enough to detect the Rh D gene in a single cell. Twelve of the women were tested in the first trimester and 45 in the second or third trimesters. Ultimately, 39 fetuses were determined to be Rh D positive by standard serological testing of cord blood, and 18 were Rh D negative. In the samples obtained from women in the second or third trimester, the results of Rh D PCR analysis of maternal plasma DNA were completely concordant with the infant serological status. Among the maternal plasma samples collected in the first trimester, two contained no Rh D DNA, despite the fetuses being Rh D positive. The results in the other ten samples were all concordant and correct.[31]

## TABLE 5-2

## Conventional Cytogenetics and DNA-Based Analyses

| Procedure | Type of Tissue Used for Analysis | Method of Analysis | Examples |
|---|---|---|---|
| Conventional cytogenetics | Amniotic fluid Chorionic villi Fetal lymphocytes | Metaphase nuclei are lysed and chromosomes stained with Giemsa solution. Chromosome number and banding patterns are inspected. | Amniocentesis for advanced maternal age to exclude fetal trisomy |
| DNA analysis | Amniotic fluid Chorionic villi Fetal lymphocytes Other fetal tissues | Fetal DNA is extracted. Molecular techniques are used to investigate specific areas of the genome. | Rh D typing Mutational analysis for sickle cell disease Analysis for common mutations found in CF |
| FISH | Amniotic fluid Chorionic villi Fetal lymphocytes | Specific DNA probes are used to bind to unique sequences or to entire chromosomes. | Aneuvysion screening test for aneuploidies involving chromosomes 13, 18, 21, X, and Y |

*FISH*, Fluorescence in situ hybridization.

As researchers gain more knowledge and experience, the problems of fetal cell type, gestational age, separation of the small number of fetal cells from the maternal circulation, and specificity of testing methods may be overcome. Table 5-2 compares the types of genetic analysis that are currently available. In the future, blood samples may be drawn from all consenting pregnant women early in gestation, with analyses performed according to each woman's risk for an offspring with a chromosome abnormality, single-gene disorder, or blood antigen to which she is sensitized.

## TREATMENT OF EMBYRO/FETUS FOR GENETIC DISORDERS

An underlying assumption in the development of prenatal genetic diagnosis is that physicians would be able to prevent the negative consequences of genetic disease by diagnosing and treating human embryos before irreversible changes that lead to disability. In past years, prenatal diagnosis was criticized as merely a "search and destroy mission," since the only options available to parents were selective abortion and delivery of an affected fetus. Recent successes in the treatment of fetuses using pharmacological, surgical, and other interventions demonstrate that the goal of prenatal diagnosis for the amelioration of fetal disease can be realized.

One approach to treating genetic diseases prenatally has been to administer medications to the pregnant women or to the embryo/fetus to bypass a deficient enzymatic pathway. Several disease processes have been addressed in this fashion, but success is mixed. One example is the treatment of pregnant women at risk for bearing a child with congenital adrenal hyperplasia. This disorder is most often caused by a deficiency in the 21-hydroxylase enzyme, which results in virilization of female fetuses (ambiguous genitalia). To diminish the virilizing effects of the disease, a pregnant woman is given dexamethasone before 9 weeks' gestation. Prenatal diagnosis (with mutational analysis) is then performed by collecting fetal cells via CVS or amniocentesis, and dexamethasone is continued until term only if an affected female is diagnosed. This regimen has been successful at diminishing the expected masculinization of some affected female fetuses, but success has not been universal.[32] The optimal dose and duration of therapy are not certain. Also, dexamethasone treatment addresses only the virilization; glucocorticoid and mineralocorticoid deficiencies persist in the child and require lifelong treatment. Other diseases amenable to in utero medical therapy include multiple carboxylase deficiency, methylmalonic acidemia, galactosemia, and phenylketonuria.

More recently, ingestion of folic acid before conception was shown to decrease the risk of open neural tube defects. Open neural tube defects, such as spina bifida and anencephaly, occur in approximately 1 in 1000 births in North America. In at least some fetuses, a defect is present in the enzymes needed for homocysteine metabolism.[33] These enzymes are necessary for DNA synthesis and the production of myelin, which is the fatty sheath that insulates nerve axons. Defects lead to abnormal accumulation of homocysteine. Because folic acid metabolites act as cofactors in normal homocysteine metabolism, folic acid administration during neural tube formation should decrease the likelihood of fetal spinal defects. However, a direct link between folic acid and reduction of neural tube defects has not been established for most families. Clinical studies show that folic acid supplementation does reduce spina bifida and anencephaly for women with no prior history of affected children (0.4 mg/day) and for women who have had previous children or family members with such defects (4.0 mg/day).[34,35] Many food products are now fortified with additional folic acid in an effort to provide women of childbearing age with additional amounts in their diet.

Other approaches to fetal therapy include invasive procedures aimed at correcting anatomical defects or reducing the morbid effects of defects. One area of success is in the treatment of fetal urinary tract obstruction. Fetal urethral obstruction can result in severe impairment in kidney function and a lack of amniotic fluid. In this setting, inadequate fetal lung development is common and usually fatal. These renal and pulmonary effects can be prevented or ameliorated through urinary tract decompression with shunts placed in the fetal bladder under ultrasound guidance. A normal volume of amniotic fluid can be restored if fetal renal function still exists. The utility of this approach is limited by the risk of infection, catheter obstruction or dislodgement, and possible fetal injury. Several hundred fetuses have been treated in this way, and experience indicates in many cases that fatal pulmonary hypoplasia can be prevented.[36] Other lesions that can be treated in an analogous way include fetal hydrothorax, fetal cystic adenomatoid malformation of the lung, and large fetal ovarian cysts.

Open fetal surgery has been used to treat several types of malformation of the fetus. The most extensive experience with fetal surgery is in the management of fetal congenital diaphragmatic hernia (CDH). Most infants with CHD die because of lack of proper lung development due to the presence of fetal abdominal contents in the chest. Harrison and others[37] performed antenatal surgery for fetal CHD. The woman's uterus is incised to expose the fetal chest, which is then opened. The herniated viscera is returned to the fetal abdomen, and the diaphragm is repaired. This approach can treat affected fetuses because it allows the fetal lungs and gut to develop normally and prevents the evolution of pulmonary hypoplasia, which is the most likely cause of death. With surgery, however, there are significant complications, including amniotic fluid leak, premature labor, maternal blood transfusion, and pulmonary edema due to tocolytics. Additionally, all the women must be delivered by cesarean section. Nonetheless, there have been a number of survivors with CDH treated with fetal surgery.

## GENE THERAPY

Much optimism surrounds the possibility of ameliorating disease by manipulating genes to treat medical disorders. Somatic gene therapy, which is the insertion of single genes into somatic cells, can be seen as a natural extension of common medical procedures such as administering medications or transplanting organs. In this type of therapy, desired genes are inserted into somatic cells by way of a delivery system of retroviruses, adenoviruses, liposomes, naked DNA, or hematopoietic stem cells. Both in vivo and ex vivo approaches to gene therapy have been successful in experimental animal models of prenatal gene therapy. Using the in vivo approach, researchers injected foreign gene/liposome complexes into pregnant mice and detected gene transfer across the placenta. Gene expression was found in the fetuses and in pups postpartum, with no evidence of germline transmission.[38] DNA incorporated into retrovirus vectors can also be injected directly into the umbilical vein of the fetus or into the fetal liver. Ex vivo methods may also be applicable for prenatal gene therapy. For example, after partial fetal hepatic resection, hepatocytes would be grown in cell culture and transduced with retroviral vectors. Fetuses with inherited metabolic diseases could thus be treated by injection with their own modified hepatocytes. Other work in animals using fetal gut, skin fibroblasts, bone marrow cells, and muscle tissue indicates several possible approaches to somatic gene therapy in the prenatal period. The safety and efficacy of prenatal somatic gene therapy, however, are not yet established.

In humans, in utero hematopoietic stem cell transplantation has been performed successfully. The goal of this therapy is to introduce a substitute DNA in the form of blood progenitor cells into the cells of an affected individual, with the hope of symptomatic improvement or cure. Tissue can be obtained from an allogeneic stem cell donor or by removing the fetuses' own stem cells, inserting a desired gene in vitro, and returning the treated cells to the fetus. Studies of the fetal immune system suggest that fetuses younger than 18 weeks' gestation are able to tolerate foreign antigens, and engraftment of allogeneic cells occurs without rejection. Since the late 1980s, in utero hematopoietic stem cell transplantation has been achieved in several cases, including cases of bare lymphocyte syndrome, SCID, and thalassemia.[39]

Finally, germline gene therapy involves inducing a genetic change in somatic and germ cells, which can be passed on to subsequent generations. To some, germline gene therapy represents a preventive health strategy for future generations. It is important to realize that any gene alterations made to preembryos will result in genetic changes that will be passed through the germline to future generations. The potential for unanticipated adverse effects with this type of therapy has caused researchers to call for restraint in developing germline gene therapy. At present, research on germline gene therapy is prohibited, pending the study of the ethical, social, and legal implications of such interventions.

## SUMMARY

Because of their history of involvement in prenatal testing and interventions, clinicians who practice obstetrics are probably more familiar than others with the complex issues that these options represent. This chapter identifies many of the options, but the list will multiply as advances in genetics proliferate. For busy clinicians, the most daunting challenge of genetics is to keep current on the alternatives available and to acquire the skills necessary to make them safely available to patients, either in the clinician's practice or through referral.

## REFERENCES

1. American College of Obstetricians and Gynecologists: *Maternal multiple marker screening,* ACOG Educational Bulletin Number 228, Washington, DC, 1996, ACOG.
2. Lockwood CJ, Lynch L, Berkowitz RL: Ultrasonographic screening for the Down syndrome fetus, *Am J Obstet Gynecol* 165:349, 1991.
3. Merkatz IR, Nitowsky HM, Macri JN, et al: An association between low maternal serum α-fetoprotein and fetal chromosomal abnormalities, *Am J Obstet Gynecol* 148:886, 1984.
4. Haddow JE, Palomaki GE, Knigh GJ, et al: Prospective prenatal screening for Down's syndrome using maternal markers, *N Engl J Med* 327:588, 1992.
5. Wald NJ, Densem JW, Smith D, et al: Four marker serum screening for Down's syndrome, *Prenat Diagn* 14:707-716, 1994.
6. Nicolaides KH, Brizot ML, Snijders RJM: Fetal nuchal translucency: ultrasound screening for fetal trisomy in the first trimester of pregnancy, *Br J Obstet Gynaecol* 101:782-786, 1994.
7. Vintzileos AM, Egan JF: Adjusting the risk for trisomy 21 on the basis of second trimester ultrasonography, *Am J Obstet Gynecol* 172(3):837-844, 1995.
8. NICHHD National Registry for Amniocentesis Study Group: Midtrimester amniocentesis for prenatal diagnosis: safety and accuracy, *JAMA* 236:1471, 1976.
9. Simpson NE, Dallaire L, Miller JR, et al: Prenatal diagnosis of genetic disease in Canada: report of a collaborative study, *Can Med Assoc J* 15:739, 1976.
10. United Kingdom Medical Research Council: Working party on amniocentesis: an assessment of the hazards of amniocentesis, *Br J Obstet Gynaecol* 85(suppl 2):1, 1978.
11. Sundberg K, Bang J, Smidt-Jensen S, et al: Randomised study of risk of fetal loss related to early amniocentesis versus chorionic villus sampling, *Lancet* 350(9079):697-703, 1997.
12. Nicolaides K, Brizot M, Patel F, et al: Comparison of chorionic villus sampling and amniocentesis for fetal karyotyping at 10-13 weeks' gestation, *Lancet* 344(8920):435-439, 1994.
13. Rhoads GG, Jackson LG, Schlesselman SE, et al: The safety and efficacy of chorionic villus sampling for early prenatal diagnosis of cytogenetic abnormalities, *N Engl J Med* 320:609, 1989.
14. Canadian Collaborative CVS-Amniocentesis Clinical Trial Group: Multicentre randomised clinical trial of chorion villus sampling and amniocentesis, *Lancet* 1:1, 1989.
15. MRC UK: MRC European trial of chorion villus sampling, *Lancet* 337:1491, 1991.
16. Firth HV, Boyd PA, Chamberlain P, et al: Severe limb abnormalities after chorion villus sampling at 56-66 days gestation, *Lancet* 337:762, 1991.

17. Burton BK, Schulz CJ, Burd LI: Limb anomalies associated with chorionic villus sampling, *Obstet Gynecol* 79:726-30, 1992.

18. Kuliev AM, Modell B, Jackson L (World Health Organization): Limb abnormalities and chorionic villus sampling, *Lancet* 340: 668, 1992.

19. Daffos F, Capella-Povolsky M, Frestier F: Fetal blood sampling during pregnancy with use of a needle guided by ultrasound: a study of 606 consecutive cases, *Am J Obstet Gynecol* 153:665, 1985.

20. Ludomirsky A: North American PUBS Registry 1986-1991. Abstract presented at the Society for Perinatal Obstetricians Annual Meeting, San Francisco, 1993.

21. Evans MI, Greb A, Kunkel LM, et al: In utero fetal muscle biopsy for the diagnosis of Duchenne muscular dystrophy, *Am J Obstet Gynecol* 165:728, 1991.

22. American College of Obstetricians and Gynecologists: Genetic technologies, ACOG Technical Bulletin Number 208, Washington, DC, 1995, ACOG.

23. Bishop CE: DNA-based prenatal diagnosis. In Simpson JL, Elias S, editors: *Essentials of prenatal diagnosis,* New York, 1993, Churchill Livingstone.

24. Trask B: Fluorescence in situ hybridization, *Trends Genet* 7:149, 1991.

25. Evans MI, Ebrahim SA, Berry SM, et al: Fluorescent in situ hybridization utilization for high-risk prenatal diagnosis: a trade-off among speed, expense, and inherent limitations of chromosome-specific probes, *Am J Obstet Gynecol* 171:1055-1057, 1994.

26. Handyside AH, Kontogianni EH, Hardy K, et al: Pregnancies from biopsied human preimplantation embryos sexed by Y-specific DNA amplification, *Nature* 344:768-770, 1990.

27. Kuliev A, Rechitsky S, Verlinsky O, et al: Birth of healthy children after preimplantation diagnosis of thalassemias, *J Assist Reprod Genet* 16(4):207-211, 1999.

28. Walkonowska J, Conte FA, Grumbach MM: Practical and theoretical implications of fetal/maternal lymphocyte transfer, *Lancet* I:1119-1122, 1969.

29. Simpson JL, Elias S: Isolating fetal cells in maternal circulation for prenatal diagnosis, *Prenat Diagn* 14:1229-1242, 1994.

30. Cheung MC, Goldberg JD, Kan YW: Prenatal diagnosis of sickle cell anemia and thalassemia by analysis of fetal cells in maternal blood, *Nat Genet* 14:264-268, 1996.

31. Lo YMD, Hjelm NM, Fidler C, et al: Prenatal diagnosis of fetal RhD status by molecular analysis of maternal plasma, *N Engl J Med* 339(24):1734-1738, 1998.

32. David M, Forest MG: Prenatal treatment of congenital adrenal hyperplasia resulting from 21-hydroxylase deficiency, *J Pediatr* 105:799, 1984.

33. Mills JL, Scott JM, Kirke PN, et al: Homocysteine and neural tube defects, *J Nutr* 126(3):756S-760S, 1996.

34. MRC Vitamin Study Research Group: Prevention of neural tube defects: results of the Medical Research Council Vitamin Study, *Lancet* 2:131, 1991.

35. Milunsky A, Jick J, Jick SS, et al: Multivitamin/folic acid supplementation in early pregnancy reduces the prevalence of neural tube defects, *JAMA* 262:2847, 1989.

36. Manning FA, Harrison MR, Rodeck C: Catheter shunts for fetal hydronephrosis and hydrocephalus—report of the International Fetal Surgery Registry, *N Engl J Med* 315: 336, 1986.

37. Harrison MR, Adzick NS, Longaker MT, et al: Successful repair in utero of a fetal diaphragmatic hernia after removal of herniated viscera from the left thorax, *N Engl J Med* 322:1582, 1990.

38. Tsukamoto M, Ochiya T, Yoshida S, et al: Gene transfer and expression in progeny after intravenous DNA injection into pregnant mice, *Nat Genet* 9(3):243-248, 1995.

39. Touraine JL: In utero transplantation of stem cells in humans, *Nouv Rev Fr Hematol* 32: 441, 1990.

40. Mahowald MB, Levinson D, Cassel C, et al: The new genetics and women, *Milbank Q* 74(2):239-283, 1996.

# PART II

# GENERAL TOPICS FOR PRIMARY CAREGIVERS

# CHAPTER 6

# Implications of Genetics for Concepts of Disease

*Dan W. Brock*

Until recently, new knowledge of human genetics has mainly impacted reproductive medicine, prenatal care, and developmental pediatrics. In the future, genetic testing will increasingly be done by primary care practitioners, bringing with it difficult clinical issues such as appropriate genetic counseling and confidentiality of genetic information to primary care practice. The new genetic medicine also will create two greater challenges for primary care practitioners involving (1) the concept of disease and (2) how that concept defines and delineates the scope of their practice.

The first part of this chapter largely draws on work in philosophy of science and philosophy of medicine on the concept of disease. The prevention and treatment of disease are the guiding aims of medical practice. Will increased knowledge of human genetics necessitate important changes in this concept of disease? How can genetic disease be distinguished from other diseases?

The second part addresses the concept of disease in primary care and other medical practice, as well as in social and policy contexts. How will this concept change with increased genetic knowledge and increased capacity to make genetic and other interventions? How is the concept of disease used to demarcate the proper scope and aims of medicine, or what physicians ought to be and ought not to be doing? The concept of disease distinguishes between treatment and enhancement, which in turn helps to determine, for example, what should be covered by health insurance. New genetic knowledge and expanded capacities for genetic interventions put pressure on medical, social, and policy uses of the concept of disease. The impact of advances in genetics on primary care and other medical practice may be profound.

## CONCEPTS OF HEALTH AND DISEASE

A conception of disease should be broader than the common notion of disease and should encompass all the physical and mental conditions of living organisms that are incompatible with health. This would include injuries, for example, even though an injury is not usually considered a disease. To understand the concepts of both health and disease, the conception of disease must be broad enough that health could be seen as the absence of disease. It must also encompass what primary care medicine treats or prevents. The philosophy of medicine has many proposals on how to understand the notions of health and disease.[1-3]

Health is sometimes taken to be equivalent to a condition of well-being, a beneficial or valuable condition of a person; healthy conditions are "valuable" conditions, and diseases are "disvaluable" conditions. For example, the World Health Organization[4] has characterized health as "a state of complete physical, mental, and social well-being." Although health is valuable and valued and disease is disvaluable and disvalued, health and disease are not simply equivalent to valuable and disvaluable conditions.[5] Other conditions besides health are valuable and contribute to well-being. Having an IQ of 150 and many friends does not make one healthier than a person with an IQ of 120 and fewer friends. Conceptions of health and disease become too broad by defining them simply as valued and disvalued conditions of a person.

In examining the social connection between disease and the medical profession, some sociologists suggest that disease is simply whatever physicians treat. Some diseases have no treatment, however, such as Alzheimer or Huntington disease. Also, physicians treat conditions that are generally not considered diseases, as with cosmetic surgery and contraception. A concept of disease independent of what physicians *happen* to treat is needed in order to argue that disease is what physicians *ought* to treat.

Sometimes health is identified with statistical normality; disease would then be abnormal conditions of an organism. Normality has a role, whether statistical or biological, in a concept of health, but health cannot simply be identified with normality and disease with abnormality. Some abnormal conditions are not diseases or unhealthy, such as blood type O, red hair, and a 7-foot height. Also, some essentially univeral diseases are statistically normal but not healthy, such as dental caries.

Sometimes disease is identified with conditions that cause pain or suffering. Disease typically causes pain and suffering, but it is not equivalent to conditions that do so. Some diseases are asymptomatic and cause no pain or suffering; others never cause pain or suffering, such as minor skin warts. Also, life contains other sources of pain and suffering besides disease.

Sometimes disease is equated with disability. The concept of disability is a part of disease, but it is not possible simply to identify disease with disability. Minor diseases such as skin warts are not disabling, and disabilities in some contexts are too dependent on social roles.

Sometimes the health of an organism is equated with its adaptation to its environment. However, this makes health and disease too relative to a particular environment in which an organism happens to be, whereas health and disease concern normal environments and organisms' normal function in them.

Finally, sometimes disease is understood as the mechanism that disrupts homeostasis in an organism. Some diseases do cause changes in body temperature, such as pneumonia. However, many functions of organisms affected by disease are not naturally understood in homeostatic terms, such as growth, reproduction, and locomotion.

## Objective Conception

Properly understood and qualified, most of these unsatisfactory conceptions of disease do play a role in a more satisfactory account. In an objective conception of disease, health is the normal or the natural, and disease impairs health. Ascriptions of health and disease are relative to a particular reference class of organisms or parts of organisms, differentiated in terms of uniform functional design. Organisms are differentiated at least by species, as well as by sex and age in the case of humans. According to Boorse,[3] "The normal function of either a part or process of members of a relevant reference class is the statistically typical contribution that that part or process makes to the survival, and the expectation of survival and reproduction, of the organism." *Health* in a member of that reference class is normal functional ability, or the readiness of each part or process to perform its normal function. Health of an organism or organ is the readiness to perform its typical functional role, on typical occasions, with at least typical efficiency. *Disease* is an internal state of an organism that impairs health, or reduces the functional ability of an organism below its typical functional level.

This conception of disease and determination of what constitutes a disease rest on no value judgments. One of the principal controversies in the philosophy of medicine is whether diseases can be understood and identified without at least implicit appeal to value judgments. In this account, what constitutes a disease is an empirical question to be settled by the science of biology. The causal roles of the lungs or liver in the design of organisms, as well as their effect on increasing the probability that organisms survive and reproduce, are empirical determinations, not value judgments. Health and disease in this account presuppose no more value judgments than does biological science itself.

Latent or asymptomatic disease does not limit the functional capacities, typically the behavioral capacities, of the organism as a whole, but it does cause dysfunction in the organism at a lower level in the functional structure. Where a condition varies in a reference class, such as height, eye color, or blood type, no one version of that trait will be necessary for health.

Boorse's account of disease has the following strengths:

1.  It helps distinguish what is a disease from what is "bad" for an organism. Hemophilia is typically bad for humans, and it is a disease. Other conditions, however, are bad but are not diseases. The inability to regenerate damaged brain tissue is bad, at least for some individuals on some occasions, but it is not a disease. Boorse's account, with its reliance on normal species function, shows why that is the case.
2.  This account fits cases with a disease at both abnormal ends of a particular range of function. For example, both hyperthyroidism and hypothyroidism, or hypertension and hypotension, are diseases because normal functional ability is to secrete hormones, or to maintain blood pressure, within a given range.
3.  This account fits cases that seem the same at a gross physical level; it helps explain why some are viewed as disease and others are not. For example, a small and weak person cannot lift heavy weights. A strong man with Addison disease also cannot lift heavy weights. Behaviorally, these cases appear similar, but the second is a dysfunction caused by Addison disease, whereas the first is not disease, but only one end of the range of normal function.

Possible problems with understanding disease in this way include the following:

1. Boorse's conception does not consider abnormal structural conditions without a functional role as diseases. For example, congenital absence of an appendix is not a disease.
2. This account needs further refinement for cases of essentially universal disease, such as dental caries. An environmental disaster also might affect everyone's germ cells such that all that is understood as disease would be passed on to all successors.
3. Some philosophers of medicine believe that this account wrongly omits the evaluative component of the concept of disease. Engelhardt,[6] Sedgwick,[7] and others have argued that infectious bacilli, lesions, and fractured bones do not become diseases or illnesses unless people take an interest in them, or more specifically, take an interest in being *without* them.

Boorse's account of disease is essentially the conventional view. Can we fit genetic diseases into the conventional view of disease, or do they force us to revise or abandon the conventional view? All disease results from the interaction between a physical organism, with its particular genetic endowment, and its environment. How can we distinguish between genetic and nongenetic diseases? Causal and environmental approaches can be used to address this question.

### Causal Approach

The first approach distinguishes genetic disease in causal terms; it is implicit in most primary care practitioners' understanding of what is a genetic disease. In genetic disease, genetic factors are more important in causing the disease than environmental factors. However, all disease occurs in organisms with a particular genome existing in a particular environment, typically from an interaction of genetic and environmental conditons. Phenylketonuria (PKU) occurs when a person without a gene that produces an enzyme needed to metabolize phenylalanine eats a normal diet that is high in phenylalanine. Arsenic poisoning occurs when a person lacking a gene to neutralize arsenic ingests arsenic from the environment. Why are genes the more important cause of PKU, whereas environment is the more important cause of arsenic poisoning?

The main problem for the causal approach is how to specify causal importance without being arbitrary. This is difficult, at least with only a causal analysis, since the relativity of what is identified as the most important cause, "the cause" of a particular event, in moral and legal contexts is familiar; causal inquiries are in part normatively guided.[8] Consider a patient who is respirator dependent and cannot be weaned, is fully competent, and has asked to be taken off the respirator, realizing that she will then die; her primary care physician is prepared to respect her wishes and remove her from the respirator.[9] In the first version of this case the physician extubates the patient, stops the respirator, and the patient dies. What is the cause of death, for example, for completing the death certificate? The physician and family typically would identify the patient's underlying disease, such as chronic obstructive pulmonary disease (COPD), as the cause.

In the second version of this case the situation is the same, except the patient has a greedy nephew who stands to inherit her resources and is afraid that his inheritance will be consumed by the hospitalization, not knowing that his aunt has decided to stop treatment. He goes into her room while she is sedated and does exactly what the physician does in the first version: he extubates the patient, stops her respirator, and she dies. What is the cause of death in this version of the case? A moral or legal inquiry into the cause of death now would focus not on the COPD, although its presence was necessary for the patient's death, but on what the nephew did. In the common-sense understanding of the cause of death, the nephew deliberately killed his aunt by removing her from the respirator. The moral or legal inquiry asks, among the causal conditions contributing to the patient's death, did anybody do something that was morally or legally prohibited? In the first version, no one did so. The physician acted appropriately and within his professional role, and thus the law accepts the disease and not the physician as the cause of death. In the second version, what the nephew did is morally wrong and legally prohibited, and thus for practical reasons, morality and the law pick out the nephew, not COPD, as the cause of death. In moral and legal contexts, what is singled out from all the causally relevant conditions as the cause is determined by what could be called "pragmatic concerns," and thus it is relative to those pragmatic concerns.

Now consider causal inquiries in medical science.[10] Suppose we find that four conditions, C1, C2, C3, and C4, are each necessary and jointly sufficient for some disease E in normal humans. We want to know what is the cause of E not occurring on a particular occasion. We find that C2, C3, and C4 are present, but not C1. Then the fact that C1 was not present is the cause of E not occurring; in that instance, C1 is the most important causal factor for E. However, this does not enable us to pick out one cause, such as C1, as generally more important for a disease. Since each of C1, C2, C3, and C4 is necessary for E, we could pick out each of the other three causal conditions in the same way when only they are not present. Which causal factor is most important depends on which other causal factors are present or absent on a particular occasion.

Fruit flies illustrate the more specific relativity of determining the most important cause of a particular condition as genetic or environmental (Figure 6-1).[10] Suppose the causal question is why M1 has smaller wings than N1. If N1 is a normal fruit fly, M1 is a mutation, and they are raised in the same environment, the cause of M1's shorter wings is apparently genetic. Suppose instead that you have only seen M1, M2, and M3, and not N1, N2, or N3. You know that M2 and M3 were raised in increasingly higher temperatures than M1. What is the cause of the shorter wings of M1? Now the answer is that the cause is environmental, not genetic. Both the genetic and the environmental answers are correct in their different contexts. The important point is that you obtain a different answer to whether the cause of a particular condition is genetic or environmental depending on the reference class to which the particular individual is being compared.

Figure 6-2 illustrates this point in a human context. Lactose accumulation in the intestines causes the symptoms of diarrhea and cramping (S). S occurs in infants who consume milk and do not produce enough lactase to avoid lactose accumulation. Consider two examples, *A* and *B*. In the top line, each L represents an individual who does produce sufficient lactase to avoid S, and each dash represents an individual who does not. In the second line, each M or dash indicates whether or not that individual drinks milk. Example *A* consists of Scandinavians, nearly all of whom produce sufficient lactase and also drink milk. Why does the one middle individual develop S? The causal factor differentiating that individual from the others without S is lactase deficiency, which has a genetic cause, and so

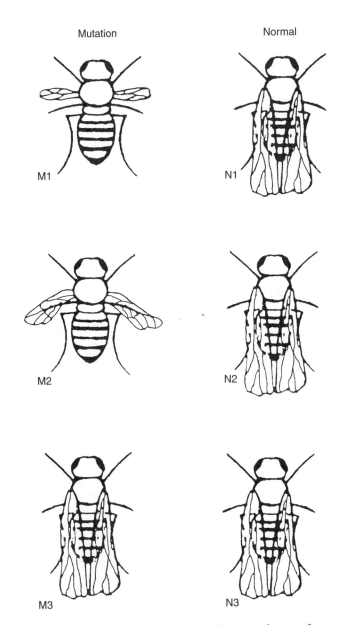

**FIGURE 6-1** Fruit flies in determination of genetic or environmental causes for certain conditions. See text.

(Redrawn from Itesslow G: What is a genetic disease? On the relative importance of causes. In Nordenfelt L, Lindahl B, editors: *Health, disease and causal explanation in medicine,* Dordrecht, The Netherlands, 1984, Reidel.)

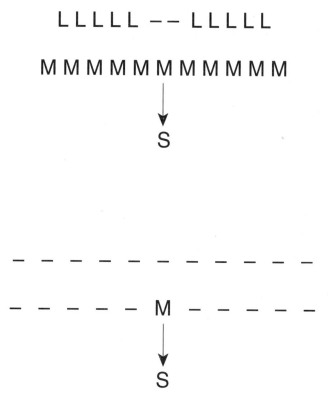

FIGURE 6-2   Determination of environmental and genetic causes for diarrhea and cramping *(S)*. *L*, Lactase; *M*, milk. See text.

(Redrawn from Itesslow G: What is a genetic disease? On the relative importance of causes. In Nordenfelt L, Lindahl B, editors: *Health, disease and causal explanation in medicine,* Dordrecht, The Netherlands, 1984, Reidel.)

the cause of S is genetic. Now consider example *B,* in which the individuals are from certain parts of Africa where lactase deficiency is common but drinking milk is rare. S occurs in the middle individual because S has an environmental, not a genetic, cause; S is a result of drinking milk.

Again, the relative importance of conditions causing a particular disease depends on the frequency of the conditions and the objects of comparison. It is uncertain whether genetic and environmental disease can be distinguished in terms of the most important cause being genetic or environmental without using this built-in relativity. A genetic or environmental classification of disease is not based only on the disease itself, the causal mechanisms at work, and the strength of the causal connections.

**Environmental Approach**

A more promising way of distinguishing genetic from nongenetic diseases depends on a normal environment (NE) and a normal genome (NG) for an organism,[11] versus an abnormal environment (AE) and abnormal genome (AG). Figure 6-3 represents the four possibilities and allows us to classify diseases as environmental or genetic. In the first box (NE, NG) there is no disease. In the second box (NE, AG) the disease is genetic, for example, PKU. In the third box (AE, NG) the disease is environmental, for example, malaria. In the fourth box (AE, AG) the disease is overdetermined, for example, hypoxia in a patient with sickle cell disease who is also in a low-oxygen environment. In this case, more must be known to sort out the relative importance of the genetic and environmental contributions to the particular patient's condition. This is the most natural way of distinguishing genetic from environmental diseases, although it requires knowledge of an organism's NG and NE and is complex.[12] The Human Genome Project provides that knowledge of the normal human genome.

**Contribution of Genetics to Disease Concept**

New genetic knowledge about many conditions will change the understanding of what is and is not disease; for example, some conditions thought to be part of normal aging are diseases. New genetic knowledge will also change the classification of particular diseases as environmental or genetic; for example, Laing's theory[13] that schizophrenia is primarily an environmental disease is now widely rejected in favor of the view that schizophrenia's cause is primarily genetic. New genetic tests will change the way primary care physicians attempt to treat or prevent many diseases, but it will not require a new conceptual understanding of disease itself. Instead, new genetic knowledge and new understanding of genetic compo-

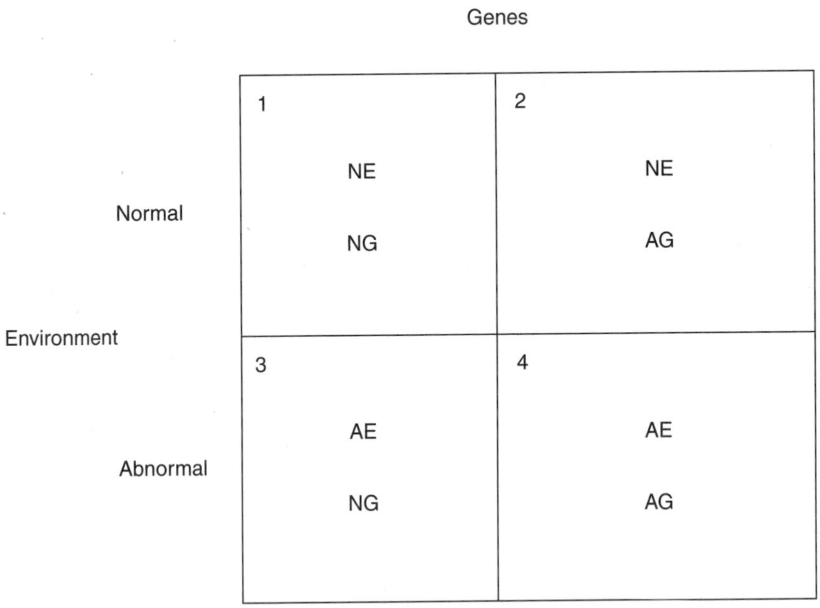

FIGURE 6-3 Classification of disease as environmental or genetic. *N,* Normal; *A,* abnormal; *E,* environment; *G,* genome. See text.
(Redrawn from Wachbroit R: *Am J Med Genet* 53:236-240, 1994.)

nents in the causation of disease can be incorporated into the conventional conception of disease in the philosophy of medicine. Different causal components of disease can be sorted out to distinguish genetic from nongenetic diseases, although not always without a context-dependent relativity.

## MEDICAL, MORAL, AND POLICY CONTEXTS

Primary care, more than most areas of medicine, is pressured to expand beyond medicine's traditional domain and define and limit its proper domain. Health is typically taken to be the proper aim of medicine.[14] If diseases are conditions that result in adverse departures from normal species function, that is, conditions that impair health, prevention or treatment of disease is where physicians should apply their skills. By contrast, improving human function above normal levels is *enhancement,* not treatment of disease, and thus does not serve the goal of health and does not fall within the proper goals of medicine. Future advances in genetic knowledge and intervention will put pressure on this use of the concept of disease to define and delimit the aims of medicine.

### Self-Determination and Well-Being

Suppose that health, and in turn the treatment and prevention of disease, is the only proper aim of medicine, meaning (1) health is the only goal for which physicians should strive, and (2) no other goal or value should constrain their striving for the health of their patients. If this is the aim of medicine, physicians should be experts about when individuals need treatment and about which modality would best treat their disease and promote their health. Moreover, if no other goals or values should limit physicians' pursuit of health, an extremely paternalistic account of the goals of medicine and of physicians' proper role would follow. In this view, physicians would not offer treatment to patients, but instead *provide* it to patients, even imposing it against patient's wishes, whenever it is necessary to treat patients' disease and promote their health.

Physicians should not impose unwanted treatment on competent patients, however, because another important value is at risk in decisions about a patient's treatment: respecting the patient's self-determination or autonomy.[15] *Self-determination* means simply the interest of ordinary persons in making important decisions about their lives for themselves, according to their own values or conception of a good life and not according to someone else's idea of what would be best for them. Self-determination is the principal moral basis for the requirement that treatment not be rendered without the patient's informed consent; it serves as a side constraint on physicians' pursuit of their patients' health. If respecting a patient's self-determination is added to, or put as a constraint on, the pursuit of the goal of health and the treatment or prevention of disease, physicians should not impose unwanted treatment on patients. Even qualified by the constraint of respecting patients' self-determination, however, health and the treatment of disease are not the proper goal of medicine.

Health and disease, as briefly characterized earlier, can be objectively determined by biological science, at least in principle, even if medical science is often uncertain how best to achieve health and treat disease. In its reports on health care treatment decision making, however, the President's Commission for the Study of Ethical Problems in Medicine and

Biomedical and Behavioral Research[15] characterized the proper goal of medicine not as health and the absence of disease, but as *promoting the patient's well-being*. The notion of well-being is complex, and a patient's well-being is not served by always giving them whatever they want, since patients can be mistaken for a variety of reasons about what will best promote their well-being. The goal of promoting patients' well-being is broader than health and properly places medical care within the context of other valued components of patients' lives besides health. It makes perfect sense to say of someone, "Well, his health is fine, but his marriage is falling apart, his career is in shambles, his investments have plummeted in value, and to make matters worse, he is pretty miserable these days." This description is sensible because health is only one component of the broader notion of well-being.

Physicians should use their medical knowledge, training, and experience to help promote their patients' well-being. The optimal intervention often cannot be determined simply by the biologically based concepts of health and disease. In many decisions about treatment, judgments must be made about the relative importance of complex effects on patients and their lives. For example, is it worthwhile to undergo the side effects of another round of chemotherapy for a 25% chance of remission of the patient's cancer for 6 months? Such trade-offs cannot be made by biological and medical science alone and thus do not fall entirely within the province of physicians' expertise; patients must weigh, according to their own values, the relative importance of those different effects.

These are the principal reasons why objective, biologically based notions of health and disease should not be used to demarcate the proper goals and scope of medicine, particularly in primary care. The patient's self-determination and the subjectively determined place of health and specific health interventions must also be considered in a patient's well-being. The fast-approaching age of genetic medicine will place further but different pressure on defining the goals of medicine solely by the notions of health and disease.

### Genetic and Pharmacological Enhancements

Two especially serious and feared diseases often encountered in primary care practice are acquired immunodeficiency syndrome (AIDS) and Alzheimer disease. AIDS attacks and destroys a patient's immune system. Alzheimer disease attacks and destroys a patient's cognitive function, in particular memory. Treatments that would protect and preserve the immune systems of AIDS patients or the memory of Alzheimer patients would be appropriate goals of medicine. Each would help preserve or restore an important normal function, but even normally functioning immune systems and memories function much lower than their capability. A healthy person's immune system is far from optimal in its capacity to fend off many diseases and their harmful effects. A healthy person's memory is also far from optimal. The genetic bases of the immune system and of memory are complex and poorly understood, but at some point in the future with improved understanding, genetic or pharmacological interventions to enhance them above their normal level may become possible.

At that point it will be difficult to restrict genetic or pharmacological interventions to the treatment of disease. Enhancements of normal function will seem just as important a benefit as treatment or prevention of disease that restores or preserves normal function. If medical means are expanded to include enhancements of normal function, medicine will have much less well-defined and limited aims, because there is no natural or clear endpoint in how effective our immune system or memories might become.

Genetic manipulations to enhance human functions are many years in the future, but similar pressure on the use of the concept of disease to define the proper aims and limits of medicine already exists in primary care practice. Allen and Fost[16] use growth hormone (GH) to illustrate this point. Consider two children. Johnny is a short 11-year-old boy with documented GH deficiency resulting from a brain tumor. His parents are of average height. His predicted adult height without GH treatment is approximately 160 cm (5 feet, 3 inches). Billy is a short 11-year-old with normal GH secretion, but his parents are quite short, and so he is said to have "genetic short stature." His predicted adult height is the same as Johnny's. Billy is at the low end of the normal curves for growth and height. He has no disease, but his adult height, like Johnny's, might be increased with GH treatment. Short height is associated, at least in American society, with a variety of disadvantages. Billy has the same disadvantages as Johnny, and he might also benefit from GH treatment.

What should physicians do when Billy's parents ask for GH treatment for him? Early consensus in pediatrics was that Johnny should receive treatment because he has a disease—GH deficiency—but Billy should not. Billy's parents might not be persuaded by this position and its rationale, however, since their child has the same disadvantage and could receive the same benefit from GH treatment as Johnny. Now consider Tommy, who has an expected height of 175 cm (5 feet, 9 inches), the norm for adult males in American society, and whose parents want GH for him. It is a well-documented advantage in American society, they argue, to be of above-average height, and they want to secure this advantage for their child. This would clearly be enhancement, not treatment, but are there persuasive grounds for refusing GH to Tommy?

As physicians gain new capacities for enhancements, either by direct genetic interventions or by using new genetic knowledge to make pharmacological interventions, they are likely to find it increasingly difficult to justify refusing these interventions to patients who want them on the grounds that medicine's job is only to treat disease. The early professional consensus that Johnny but not Billy should receive treatment has already eroded substantially. Some pediatricians would now treat Billy as well, although GH treatment appears to produce only limited height gains for children with idiopathic short stature.

## Access and Equality of Opportunity

Even if the concept of disease cannot be used to delineate and limit the proper domain of medicine, it might at least be used to limit what society must pay for through health insurance. Health insurance policies and managed care plans typically limit coverage to all "medically necessary care," which is defined as care expected to be effective in the prevention, treatment, or palliation of disease.[17] Whether particular care is medically necessary is often controversial, as illustrated by the recent "drive-by delivery" controversy over whether only 1 day of hospitalization after normal delivery is medically necessary for women giving birth, as some managed care and insurance plans claimed. Despite these controversies, most agree that (1) health insurance should cover all care that is medically necessary to treat disease, and (2) justice requires securing access to medically necessary care for individuals who cannot secure it for themselves.

Why is lack of access to medically necessary health care an injustice? Daniels[18] cites health care's moral importance; justice requires access to health care because this protects or restores fair equality of opportunity. Diseases are conditions resulting in impairments of normal species function. Health care needs comprise the care necessary to protect, restore, or compensate for loss of normal function. The moral role of normal species function is to secure for individuals a fair share of the range of opportunites normal for their particular society. Equality of opportunity is fundamental to American moral and political culture and most theories of justice. Because of disease's link to normal function and equality of opportunity, treatment of disease has been widely accepted as delimiting the social obligation to secure health care for all.

How might the genetic revolution affect this social obligation to secure health care for all in the service of equality of opportunity?[19] Equality of opportunity requires the following:

1. Elimination of formal barriers, whether overt or covert, to some groups competing for scarce roles and benefits; practices that barred African-Americans or Jews from competing for positions violated this component.
2. Provision of all available means for people to develop the qualifying conditions needed in competing for scarce roles and benefits; education for all and its public funding are fundamental to this component.
3. Elimination of qualifying conditions for roles that are not related to successful performance; tests for promotion that are not reasonably related to successful performance in those roles violate this component.

These different components of equality of opportunity operate in the context of background differences in people's natural talents and abilities. Even with full equality of opportunity, some people still do better than others in the genetic lottery, with much better expectations and opportunities.

Genetic interventions or pharmacological interventions made possible by new genetic knowledge may reduce or even eliminate many of these fixed natural differences between people that result in substantial inequalities in their expectations and opportunities in life.[20,21] The medical profession will develop and control these genetic and pharmacological interventions, and patients will seek them from their primary care physicians. Why not use medicine for enhancements that reduce or remove these natural inequalities? Egalitarians will state that our commitment to equality of opportunity requires doing so, instead of simply accepting the unequal and now unfair results of the genetic lottery; results will be seen as unfair, not merely unfortunate, because they will have come under social control. Further advances in genetics may challenge the meaning and strength of society's moral and social commitment to equality of opportunity and medicine's role in helping to achieve it.

**Treatment Versus Enhancement**

Whether or not health insurance and other social welfare programs continue to fund only the treatment of disease, society will still face the policy issue of whether and when genetic enhancements should be permitted. Can physicians justifiably say to Tommy's or Billy's parents, "You cannot use your own resources to try to increase your child's height"? The issue will be more pressing when potential enhancements are more important and beneficial than just increasing height. Would it be good public policy to permit widespread enhancements of human function?[22]

Many potential enhancements will produce positional or competitive benefits; enhancing some people's condition will benefit them only if a condition in others is not similarly enhanced. If these enhancements are expensive and not available to all, for example, through universal health insurance, only wealthy people will be able to afford them. Permitting such enhancements but not subsidizing them for less wealthy persons will increase inequality and unfairness. On the other hand, some competitive enhancements might be inexpensive or funded for everyone; the unfairness of unequal access is elimimated, but now the enhancements would be self-defeating. If everyone becomes 4 inches taller, for example, no one has gained a competitive or positional benefit or advantage; all would still have their same relative place in the distribution of height. The costs and risks of universal competitive enhancements could not be justified. Public policy could reasonably prohibit or limit competitive enhancements that would typically be either unfair or self-defeating.

The problem for public policy, however, is that many enhancements may not produce solely competitive benefits. Consider enhancing people's capacity to focus their attention; some normal adults already use methylphenidate (Ritalin) for this purpose.[23] This would benefit people in many competitive contexts, such as education and employment, but would also have noncompetitive or intrinsic benefits unrelated to the relative position of others, such as increasing people's ability to enjoy and appreciate music. To the extent that genetic enhancements produce intrinsic benefits, no fairness or self-defeating reasons exist to prohibit them. Many genetic enhancements may have complex benefits, however, both competitive and intrinsic, and thus public policy will be pulled in two incompatible directions on whether to permit them.

## SUMMARY

New genetic knowledge will not require fundamental changes in the concept of disease, and genetic disease can be distinguished from nongenetic disease. Genetic advances may change medical, moral, and policy uses, however, with implications for the concept of disease. For primary care physicians, these issues do not have the direct clinical impact of ethical dilemmas, such as when to breach confidentiality regarding genetic information or when to use the results of genetic tests, but they engage some of the most fundamental assumptions of medicine that determine the aims and limits of clinical practice.

## REFERENCES

1. Boorse C: Health as a theoretical concept, *Philosophy Sci* 44:542-573, 1977.
2. Boorse C: On the distinction between disease and illness, *Philosophy Public Affairs* 5(2):49-68, 1975.
3. Boorse C: Concepts of health. In Regan T, Van DeVeer D, editors: *Health care ethics,* Philadelphia, 1987, Temple University Press.
4. World Health Organization: Preamble to WHO constitution.
5. Callahan D: The WHO conception of health, *Hastings Center Studies* 3, 1973.
6. Engelhardt HT Jr: Human well-being and medicine: some basic value judgments in the biomedical sciences. In Engelhardt HT Jr, Callahan D, editors: *Science, ethics and medicine,* Hastings-on-Hudson, NY, 1976, Hastings Center.
7. Sedgwick P: Illness—mental and otherwise, *Hastings Center Report* 1:30-31, 1973.
8. Hart HLA, Honore AM: *Causation in the law,* Oxford, 1959, Oxford University Press.
9. Brock DW: Death and dying. In Veatch R, editor: *Medical ethics,* ed 2, Boston, 1996, Jones & Bartlett.

10. Hesslow G: What is a genetic disease? On the relative importance of causes. In Nordenfelt L, Lindahl B, editors: *Health, disease and causal explanation in medicine,* Dordrecht, The Netherlands, 1984, Reidel.

11. Wachbroit R: Distinguishing genetic disease and susceptibility, *Am J Med Genet* 53:236-240, 1994.

12. Lloyd EA: Normality and variation: the Human Genome Project and the ideal human type. In Cranor CF, editor: *Are genes us? The social consequences of the new genetics,* New Brunswick, NJ, 1994, Rutgers University Press.

13. Laing RD: *The divided self,* London, 1959, Tavistock.

14. Kass L: Regarding the end of medicine and the pursuit of health, *The Public Interest* 40:11-42, 1975.

15. President's Commission for the Study of Ethical Problems in Medicine and Biomedical and Behavioral Research: *Making health care decisions,* Washington, DC, 1982, US Government Printing Office.

16. Allen DB, Fost NC: Growth hormone therapy for short stature: panacea or Pandora's box, *J Pediatr* 117:16-21, 1990.

17. Sabin JE, Daniels N: Determining "medical necessity" in mental health practice, *Hastings Center Report* 24(6):5-13, 1994.

18. Daniels N: *Just health care,* Cambridge, 1985, Cambridge University Press.

19. Brock DW: The Human Genome Project and human identity, *Houston Law Review* 29:7-22, 1992.

20. Buchanan AE, Brock DW, Daniels N, Wikler D: *From chance to choice: genes and social justice,* Cambridge, 2000, Cambridge University Press.

21. Kitcher P: *The lives to come: the genetic revolution and human possibilities,* New York, 1996, Simon & Schuster.

22. Brock DW: Enhancement of human function: some distinctions for policy makers. In Parens B, editor: *Technologies for the enhancement of human capacities,* Georgetown, 1998, Georgetown University Press.

23. Diller LH: The run on Ritalin: attention deficit disorder and stimulant treatment in the 1990's, *Hastings Center Report* 26(2):12-18, 1996.

# CHAPTER 7

# Normality and Functionality: A Disability Perspective

*Anita Silvers*

At age 33, Jenny Morris was a mother, a winning politician, and an activist in a flourishing feminist movement. Then she fell off a wall in her garden and injured her lower spine. She lost the ability to walk but retained all her political knowledge and skills, her relationship with her child, and her disposition to fight for social justice. Her social value changed little after the fall.

Transitioning from the class of able-bodied people to the class of disabled persons, Morris was shaken to find people without disabilities shunning her new standpoint. She discovered that her peers—the Marxist and feminist reformers with whom she previously identified ardently—had no interest in extending their theories to reflect the life of the kind of person she had become, that is, a nonwalking person.[1]

Identifying with her new social class, Morris became threatened by how little value was placed on their lives. She cites the following three public policies as evidence of the low regard in which disabled people's lives are held:

1.  American court rulings that it is entirely rational for a person with a serious physical impairment to choose to die
2.  British legislation excepting fetuses who are liable to be impaired from a prohibition against terminating pregnancies past 24 weeks
3.  The 1939 German decree authorizing physicians to accord a mercy death to impaired persons who could not be cured

"The explicit motivation for these occurrences," according to Morris, "is the notion that physical and intellectual impairment inevitably means a life which is not worth living."[2]

This chapter discusses a familiar conception that encourages the deprecation of people because they have disabilities. Neither a medical notion nor a scientifically substantiated one, this political idea influences the practice of health care pervasively and perversely. It shapes policies on the medical uses of human genetics knowledge. Clinicians who permit their practice to be guided by this idea may be induced by nonmedical considerations to depreciate the lives of people with genetic disabilities.

## PERSPECTIVES ON DISABILITY

In prescientific times, disability was thought to originate from offensive or unnatural individual behavior, although the offspring of the offender, rather than the offender, often incurred the disability.[3] In this so-called moral model of disability, a person's impairment constitutes evidence of some moral failing. A vestige of the moral model remains in the blame directed at individuals whose noncompliance or lack of self-control is thought to have contributed to their illness or injury.

### Medical Model

The second half of the nineteenth century saw a wholesale transition from moral to scientific explanations for the limited achievement that typified certain groups of people. The dire economic and social status of persons of African heritage was attributed to defects in their biology rather than to their spiritual deprivation; the new concept of race was the biological correlative of moral character. In about the same era, disability was medicalized. Its meaning was explained in "scientific" and "objective" terms as biological dysfunction. Despite the hope that the medicalized perspective would be morally neutral, it has often invited intolerance of physical and mental difference. The medical model of disability simply opens another avenue of failure for those who are impaired; their failing lies in the inability to recover fully normal function.

By focusing on whether their disabilities are reparable or incurable, the medical model further exacerbates the repudiation of disabled people. When disability is seen in this light, the very existence of people with disabilities is construed to signify not only their own inadequacies, but also the current limitations of the medical community in realizing repairs. In a culture that detests and fears limits, medicine has traditionally aimed to reduce such dysfunction in individuals, with the eventual goal of eliminating disability from the population.

Genetic technology is expected to help achieve this goal. By applying knowledge of genetics, physicians can identify at-risk individuals, who may be dissuaded from reproducing when apprised of their liability of having a disabled child, thereby preventing the conception of people who are biologically anomalous. Genetic technology also can mitigate a biological anomaly's impact by creating compensatory organic products, such as insulin for people with diabetes. In the future, some disabling conditions may be treated by altering genetic irregularities in single-gene disorders such as Duchenne muscular dystrophy.[4]

Although at present the success of therapies to refashion anomalies in a person's genes is problematic, high hopes and equally sizable resources have been invested in developing these therapies. From a medicalized point of view, the optimal medical intervention enables the patient to become genetically typical. "One kind of intervention against disability is uncontroversially right. This is any treatment that does not prevent the existence of the person with the disability but aims to alleviate or cure the disability."[5]

## Social Model

Although many accept the medicalized view of disability, people with disabilities often interpret their situation differently. They understand their limitations in terms of social rather than personal deficits. This social model of disability transforms the notion of "handicapping condition" from a biological state that disadvantages unfortunate individuals to a state of society that disadvantages an oppressed minority. The social model attributes the dysfunction experienced by people with disabilities primarily to obstructive social arrangements. People who do not function in "species-typical" ways often are impeded in the expression of their capabilities by socially constructed barriers. The barriers range from discriminatory practices, such as denial of employment to qualified persons with disabilities, to thoughtlessly inaccessible design of the workplace. Some theorists on disability rights construe the absence of adequate support services and health care benefits as another barrier to the effective functioning of people with impairments.[3]

In contrast to the medicalized perspective, the experience of people with disabilities suggests that reforming social arrangements to achieve equitable opportunity and accessibility is often the most effective way of reducing their dysfunction. The preeminent strategies of the medical model—preventing the existence of biologically anomalous people or altering them to make them species typical, or normal—unfairly disparages personal traits central to the identity of people with disabilities. Controversy thus arises about whether it is right to use medical means to restore people to species-typical functioning.

## Medicine's Shortcomings

By placing a premium on the goal of conformity with species-typical functioning, the medicalized approach to disability may not only be coercive but may expose biologically anomalous individuals to risky, costly, and ineffective treatment. To illustrate, deaf cultural community members believe that implanting cochlear devices in prelingually deaf children hazards their future by supplanting the proven effectiveness of communication in sign language with a device whose success is unpredictable. They charge that such risky intervention is impelled by an unproven assumption, namely, that living as a hearing person is necessarily better than living as deaf.[6,7]

This problem is not new. Medicine has a mixed record in treating disabled persons. Its progress in reducing mortality rates from disabling disease and accidents has swelled the number of people with disabilities, but the historic record also reveals the institutionalization of many biologically anomalous people merely because they did not seem normal. For example, when a new superintendent had inmates at the Iowa Home for Feeble-Minded Children tested in the early 1950s, he found more than 50 testing higher than some of the employees, with normal IQs ranging to at least 120. Apparently, these individuals were institutionalized solely because their anomalies were disturbing to those empowered to make decisions regarding their placement. One man was institutionalized as a child nearly 60 years earlier because of his peculiar eye rolling.[8]

At times, medicine has imposed unnecessary risk and suffering on competent but biologically anomalous individuals through interventions aimed at making them look more normal. For instance, when surgical accidents occurred during male circumcision, some physicians advised parents to raise the young victims as girls, since cosmetic surgery could alter the child's genitals to give the appearance of a normal girl but could not restore them to look like a normal boy.[9] Appearing as a normal girl was thus regarded as better than looking like a defective boy, even though the former course would require decades-long hormone treatments. Similarly, children with Down syndrome are sometimes subjected to procedures to make them look less anomalous, that is, to look like what they are not.

In another example, walking, rather than "wheeling," is the most typical way humans gain mobility. Individuals with walking limitations may be discouraged from atypical but effective compensatory modes of functioning, such as the use of a wheelchair, and to be subjected to dangerous, ineffective surgery so that they mobilize in the species-typical mode. Similarly, individuals in whom thalidomide caused congenital anomalies of the upper limbs report that, throughout their childhood, medical professionals forced them to wear dysfunctional prosthetic arms and disparaged the superior function they could achieve using their feet to pick up and manipulate objects; the prosthetic arms were thought to make them look more normal.[10] Such practices assume there is a biological mandate for functioning in "normal" ways. This mandate often is invoked to argue that restoring anomalous individuals to species-typical functioning is a preeminent social good.[11] In the experience of many people with disabilities, however, policies that magnify the status of biological norms too often damage disabled persons by disallowing acceptance of their alternative modes of functioning. In their experience, medical practice traditionally has been dominated by policies that discount alternative approaches to functioning and that damage disabled persons by devaluing their differences.

## DOES GENETIC TECHNOLOGY INHERENTLY DEVALUE DISABLED PERSONS?

From a disability perspective, especially from the viewpoint prompted by the social model of disability, genetic medicine raises questions about medical practices that can reduce the natural variety of functional capacities in humans. By enabling medicine to prevent the birth of children who are biologically anomalous, genetic testing can greatly diminish human diversity. Altering genes associated with biological anomaly can do the same. Genetic technology deployed according to a standard of normality could reduce variation from species-typical function significantly, thereby exacerbating the isolation of individuals who depart from the species' biological norms. Indentifying individuals as disabled implies that they are exceptions among normal people. Although being normal is not unquestionably valuable, people with disabilities often accept medicine's traditional goal of normalizing them. However, because modern genetic medicine can effect a more thorough program of normalizing than traditional drug and surgical interventions, continuing to acquiesce is problematic.

Some people with disabilities conclude that the burgeoning uses of genetic technology in medicine must eventually prevent the existence of people such as themselves. Disability activists insist that genetically testing people to eliminate or disadvantage anomalous individuals and genetically altering people to surmount inherited biological flaws are tantamount to denying the worth of the lives of people with disabilities.[12] Some also contend that altering their inherited traits changes who they are.[13] At least one application of human genetics knowledge, genetic testing, inherently devalues people with disabilities. According to Kass,[14] genetic testing programs equate deviation from "species typicality" with failure to be fully human. As evidence, he cites the widely accepted practice of terminating pregnancies if genetic testing indicates a propensity for certain genetic diseases.

> *As a result of our knowledge of genetic diseases, we know that persons afflicted with certain diseases will never be capable of living the full life of a human being. . . so a child or fetus with Down's syndrome will never be truly human. There is no reason to keep them alive. This standard, I would suggest, is the one which most physicians and genetic counselors appeal to in their hearts, no matter what they say or do. Why else would they have developed genetic counseling?*[14]

Because the medical framework for genetic testing treats genetic anomalies as deviations from the definitive human genome, society concludes that individuals with such anomalies fall short of being truly human.[14] Is this premise unavoidable in programs of genetic testing? If so, people who use genetic testing would routinely equate genetic anomaly with truncated humanity.

Consider, however, what people with achondroplasia, the most common form of dwarfism, think about genetic testing. Some people with this condition oppose genetic testing on the grounds that the practice risks the collective future of the dwarf community. Because three quarters of achondroplastic children are born to average-size parents who are unprepared for them, fetal testing could result in dramatically fewer dwarf children. Nevertheless, such testing benefits dwarf couples, who can avoid bringing to term high-risk pregnancies. In 1995, after the achondroplasia gene was identified, the Little People of America (LPA), the main support group for individuals with dwarfism and their families, held a series of forums. Few of its members urged a position opposing the test.[15]

A fatal form of achondroplasia (homozygous achondroplasia) occurs when both parents are achondroplastic dwarfs. Of the 10% to 15% of achondroplastic babies born to achondroplastic parents, one fourth have this condition. Because of skeletal design, most dwarf women have high-risk pregnancies necessitating cesarean deliveries, adding to the seriousness of family-planning decisions. In one view, people with achondroplasia who terminate pregnancies because the fetus has homozygous achondroplasia must be persuaded that their child is not truly human in view of its genetic anomaly.[14] This is an implausible analysis of their motive. The genetically anomalous parents not only know they are fully human, but also know their children have an even chance of being similarly anomalous. This illustrates that genetic technology is not inherently devaluing to biologically anomalous people. After all, achondroplastic parents employ it to promote rather than prevent the existence of individuals who are atypical members of the species.

## MEDICALIZATION AND NORMALIZATION

Many LPA members who want genetic information remain apprehensive about the general public having similar access to their personal information. Fueling this fear is the recognition that genetic knowledge could be an instrument for imposing homogenization and reducing the diversity in capabilities of humankind. This concern is especially prevalent among those who see similarities between dwarfism and other genetic conditions historically regarded as disabilities. Former LPA president Ruth Ricker states, "We have historically been viewed through the medical model of disability. In that light we are concerned about health policies which emphasize victimization and suffering and devalue human variation."[15]

Why does the conventional medical approach to disability promote such policies? Medicine's mission is conventionally described as the maintenance of health. A person is healthy if she or he functions as is typical for the species. The claim that no value judgments enters into this account of medicine is based on empirical determination of what modes and levels of functioning are species typical, a subject for research in the biological sciences. If this claim withstands scrutiny, we may have confidence in the objectivity of clinical decisions that aim to restore patients to normal functioning.

But is it perspicacious, unbiased, and harmless to appeal to species-typical functioning as the standard that justifies medical intervention? First, that standard is vague. Discussions of species-typical function in the medical ethics literature often conflate biological states with modes of performing functions and functional outcomes of such performance. That is, it is not clear whether the goal of medical intervention is to approximate biological typicality (such as a hand transplant might achieve), or to bring about normal ways of performing functions (as might be achieved equally well by a cosmetically correct and mechanically dexterous electronic hand), or to effect common levels of functional outcomes (as might be achieved by a skilled hook wearer).

Second, because normal performance is defined with reference to familiar modes and levels of performance, what is regarded as normal often is artificially skewed by patterns of social domination that favor some performances over others and consequently ensure that those will continue to be the most common and seemingly normal ones. For instance, the domination of individuals for whom text is the most efficient conveyer of information has led to social arrangements that presume the ability to read text as normal. This bias disadvantages people who perform the activities of reading and writing texts badly, even when these individuals excel at aural or pictorial communication. When this bias is medicalized, energy and expenditures are applied to developing therapies meant to transform these individuals into normal readers and writers, even if it is more efficient for them to communicate in alternative ways.

Similarly, in treating children exposed prenatally to thalidomide, medical professionals biased toward manipulating objects with upper rather than lower extremities insisted, to the disadvantage of their patients, that mechanical hands necessarily are better than fleshy feet for manipulating objects. To suppose that anomalous performance must be functionally inferior to species-typical levels and modes of performance is to make two mistaken assumptions about human biological functioning: (1) human biological organization is functionally rigid, when instead it is immensely adaptive, and (2) human social organization is functionally rigid, when instead it can be flexible in expanding the opportunities of different types of people.

The drive to normalize can lead to misperceptions about dysfunction. Acknowledging or ignoring differences in social context affects whether a genetic anomaly is considered a genetic disease. For example, mild mental retardation does not disable women in low-technology environments or simple societies who clean, cook, and bear children. Murray[16] insists it would be inequitable to allocate resources to rich societies to prevent mental retardation but not to poor ones. Consequently, the burden of mental retardation must be assessed uniformly from nation to nation, regardless of significant national differences in how mental retardation affects people's lives. The same impairment may be differentially disabling or not disabling, depending on the environment; "in many cases, allocating resources to avert disability could exacerbate inequalities."[16] Regardless of the realities of functioning in different social environments, equality demands uniformity in assessing the burden of an impairment so that differences in context do not suggest that exalted functioning is reserved for the most privileged persons. A normal level of cognitive functioning must be designated and medical interventions deployed to reduce the incidence of individuals whose cognitive performances are anomalous.

However, there is nothing inequitable in acknowledging that an anomaly is no burden at all if it is not experienced as one. There is no inequity in refraining from intervening where intervention has little or no benefit. It is inequitable, however, to treat people as dysfunctional when they actually are not, and on that basis to impose medical treatment that alters them.

Arguably, the functionality of the "fit" between any person and the environment is crucial to the person's well-being and derivatively to health. It is therefore misleading to define the aim of medical intervention in abstract terms that refer to "normal" environments and "normal" functions. Successfully functional fit is determined not by abstract averages but by actual particularities. So it is unclear whether a dominating standard of normalization should be built into the policies that guide medical interventions.

Inescapable dangers exist, however, from policies that fail to disentangle *natural* functional disadvantage from *artificial* social disadvantage. Public policy should not further privilege, fix, and fortify common or dominant modes of functioning by favoring medical practice that privileges the modes of functioning typical of our species over anomalous but comparably efficient modes. The prevalence of this mistake in discussions about the deployment of medical technology is an understandable cause of wariness among people with genetic disabilities. The allure of bringing about a population free of genetic anomaly could induce clinicians to be aggressive in advising patients to seek genetic repair.

## BIOLOGICAL DIFFERENCE AND DYSFUNCTION

People with disabilities have reason to fear being subjected to genetic homogenization in attempts to relieve society from the responsibility of adjusting to their differences, even when their differences do not make them especially ill or dependent. Historically, the dominant class's fashion of functioning often has been adopted as a standard for assessing other kinds of people. To illustrate, Herbert Spencer, the Darwinian sociologist whose writing promoted eugenics, argued against efforts to restore function similar to those of the dominant group in those who are biologically "defective." Such attempts, he said, would result in "a puny, enfeebled and sickly race."[17]

This example suggests that distinguishing benign from baleful genetic alterations requires avoiding interventions made primarily for the purpose of homogenization. Drawing this distinction is especially important for primary care physicians because they are the usual gatekeepers for interventions that aim at reducing a patient's difference from species typicality. For example, parents most likely will turn to the primary care physician, at least initially, to discuss the feasibility and the advisability of treating a child for shortness of stature.

In considering what to advise, primary care physicians should reflect on whether their viewpoint is shaped by a conviction about the inferiority of disabled people's lives. Among the most powerfully limiting environmental elements endured by people who are not species typical is devaluation of others. This and other constrictions engendered by social environments hostile to biological anomaly can reduce a disabled person's function.

Medical practice conventionally has equated such functional limitation with reduced quality of life. It is conventional to assign priority to curing anomalies that reduce the ability to achieve physical, cognitive, or emotional performance, because such lowered function cannot help but diminish the quality of life (see Chapter 6). The influence of atypical functioning on people s quality of life is not self-evident.

> *Even serious physical limitations do not always lower quality of life if the disabled persons have been able or helped sufficiently to compensate for their disabilities so that their level of primary functional capacity remains essentially unimpaired; in such cases it becomes problematic even to characterize those affected as disabled.*[18]

Because the individuals Brock describes just before writing the passage above are persons born without arms and legs, this last remark is quite revealing. To believe that persons with no arms and no legs are not disabled just because they can do what others do (in this case, can eat, drive, paint pictures, raise a family) reveals how Brock views failure in life as an inescapable feature of disability.

One's self-respect, a critical component of a good quality of life, depends on one's measuring one's own capacities and capabilities favorably against the standard of normal human functioning.[19] The regard of others influences how we regard ourselves, and we are especially sensitive to our physicians' regard. Medical applications of our knowledge of human genetics thus may compromise a person's self-assuredness by revealing potential, as well as already actualized, departures from this standard.

> *[P]eople who feel healthy and who as yet suffer no functional impairment will increasingly be labeled as unhealthy or diseased. . . . For many people, this labeling will undermine their sense of themselves as healthy, well-functioning individuals and will have serious adverse effects both on their conceptions of themselves and the quality of their lives.*[19]

Being medically regarded or labeled as dysfunctional, not the malfunctioning itself, impairs an individual's sense of self and reduces quality of life. Biological anomaly damages people's self-regard mostly because it depreciates how other people regard them. The Americans With Disabilities Act recognizes this fact with disability discrimination protections not only for individuals who are substantially limited in executing major life activities, but also for individuals who are regarded as being so.[20]

## DOES MEDICINE INHERENTLY DISVALUE DISABLED PERSONS?

As stated earlier, genetic technology can be used to promote or to prevent the existence of people with disabilities. If promoting species typicality is the aim of medicine, however, then medical applications of knowledge about genetics inherently devalue the disabled, who are by definition atypical. The conventional view follows:

> *The dominant conception of the appropriate aims of medicine focuses on medicine as an intervention aimed at preventing, ameliorating, or curing and thereby restoring, or preventing the loss of, normal function or of life. . . . Problematic though the dis-*

*tinction may be, quality of life measures in medicine and health care consequently tend to focus on individuals' or patients' dysfunction and its relation to some such norm.*[18]

The allure of being normal is so strong as to warrant no interventions that improve people's functioning beyond the commonplace.

*Whether the norm be that of the particular individual, or that typical in the particular society or species, the aim of raising people's function to above the norm is not commonly accepted as an aim of medicine of equal importance to restoring function up to the norm.*[18]

Conventional medicine's reverence for normality is expressed as well in the President's Commission report used to guide federally supported medical research into altering genes. The report urged a ban on "interventions aimed at enhancing 'normal' people." These were construed as problematic because "the difficulty of drawing a line suggests the danger of drifting toward attempts to 'perfect' human beings once the door of 'enhancement' is opened."[21]

In this future, individuals who come by advantageous biological traits adventitiously, as the result of natural processes, will be rare. It will be common practice to acquire advantageous biological traits through applications of genetic engineering, so biological advantage will become the product of social forces that determine the development and allocation of the technology.

Until now in our democratically organized competitive society, where vigor, industry, and talent constitute the primary determinants of success, individuals' natural biological and moral endowments have been regarded as relatively impervious to the influence of social position, offering an antidote to artificially induced social privilege. Gene transfer technology purportedly makes humans' most fundamental biological characteristics so malleable that biological superiority could be realigned to be a product of, rather than a constraint on, the privilege that social rank or power bestows. From a perspective influenced by our growing power to uncouple individuals' destiny from their biological endowment, laboring under a biological disadvantage could become identified with inferior social rank. In other words, as the President's Commission warned, genetic engineering could transform the "natural lottery" into a new kind of "social lottery," one in which being left with a genetically unrepaired disability is the sign of a social loser.[21] This consideration, however, is political, not medical. That is, the tie between being normal and enjoying a high quality of life furthers a political standard, as does the instruction to eschew enhancement. The goal here is to secure an egalitarian social system against manipulation through the use of medical techniques.

On this scheme, functioning typically appears to be more important in escaping social limitations than in escaping personal ones. Many atypical individuals can achieve this benefit independent of medicine's power to normalize them. Environments are revisable, and people may successfully negotiate them by functioning in both unusual and commonplace ways. One strategy is to enhance an atypical individual's strengths to compensate for limitations, that is, to enhance some performances above the normal level. To pursue such a strategy usually is thought to exceed the aims of conventional medicine (see Chapter 6), but this may not be the case from a disability perspective.

# BEYOND THE TYRANNY OF NORMALIZING

The source of medicine's goal of normal functioning is a political conviction that attempts to promote equality but imposes homogeneity instead. Whether all of an individual's modes of functioning are species typical is not decisive for the individual's capabilities. Although restoring patients to genetic normality may be the medically conventional goal, other strategies exist for improving function.

Medical interventions derived from knowledge of human genetics should not be governed by the aim of imposing species typicality on patients but instead by the goal of enhancing functionality by whatever strategy is most effective. From a disability perspective, enhancing the functionality of alternative modes of performance to compensate for a limitation of the species-typical mode may be a better approach. The overall outlines of this comprehensively versatile approach to biological anomaly are presented by the World Health Organization in the *International Categorization of Impairments, Disabilities and Handicaps.*[22] For policy purposes, this document attempts to integrate medical and social interpretations of disability. Dysfunction is understood to emerge from a mismatch between the individual's mode and level of biological performance and the demands of the environment. No single strategy is made central to the medical interventions recommended for disability. The strategy of repair, which restores dysfunctional individuals to species-typical mode and level of functioning, is acknowledged as one medical approach to disability. Compensatory strategies are equally recommended. A compensatory strategy differs from a reparative strategy in that effective functioning may be achieved without seeking or accomplishing restoration of species typicality. In compensatory efforts, anomalies remain but need not compromise functional success.

Thus, for example, individuals who experienced successful postpolio rehabilitation often developed an exquisite sense of balance to compensate for one of the disease's typical sequelae, the marked disparity of strength between right and left sides and upper and lower parts of the body. Similarly, nonoral deaf communicators often surpass other people in their ability to express themselves in body language.[23] Applications of biotechnology can be similarly compensatory. The gene transfer that boosts the low-density lipoprotein receptor above normal range compensates for the effects of familial hypercholesterolemia, and the gene transfer that induces capillary formation compensates for the effects of arterial blockage.

Already of importance at the level of rehabilitative medicine, compensatory interventions appear to be similarly important at the level of genetic medicine. There appears to be no medical basis for thinking that interventions designed to eliminate biologically atypical individuals, or to restore them to species-typical biological condition, have a natural priority over compensatory interventions, that is, over applications that improve the level of one biological performance mode to compensate for dysfunctional deficit in another. Although disability advocates may be concerned that engineering their genes would threaten disabled people's identities,[13] compensatory biotechnology no more does so than wheelchairs, sign language, or talking computers. All these enhance the functionality of one kind of performance (arm movement, gesturing, listening) to compensate for limitations in another kind of performance (leg movement, speaking and hearing, seeing). It thus appears that compensatory genetic alterations are compatible with both medical and disability perspectives.

It sometimes is argued that enhancing any biological function above its species-typical level, regardless of whether such an intervention is compensatory, at best falls outside the proper goals of medicine and at worst is a source of social danger.[21] Conventional medicine, however, improves on nature through enhancement. Immunization programs enhance physical performance beyond the level that is native to our species. Because certain organisms or events can initiate damaging biological processes in the body, immunization compensates by enhancing other biological processes so that persons can defend against such damage. Although now used routinely to provide the protection deserved by fragile populations such as the elderly and the very young, immunization protocols originally were denounced as dangerous because they boosted individuals' resistance to disease above the level that then was typical of the species.

Not only are enhancements such as immunization now conventional, but analogous strategies have been pursued in genetic medicine. For instance, research into genetic analogs of vaccination abounds. Ironically, refraining from interventions that enhance performance may further disadvantage those who have not been favored by the natural lottery. Promoting the primacy of natural limitations over biotechnically engineered enhancements may not be fair to disabled persons. At one time, for example, lower leg amputees were deemed noncompetitive because their prostheses made them run too slowly. Currently, however, new materials and designs have created special sports prostheses that permit skilled and talented wearers to run faster than can be done with fleshy feet. Using these corrective devices is now banned in competitive running to prevent unfairly disadvantaging nondisabled runners in the competition. Some shapes and strengths of fleshy feet are better for running than others, but athletes who have the best kinds of feet are not banned for disadvantaging the common-footed runner. Arguably, it is unfair to exclude runners when prostheses render them uncompetitive and to exclude them when better prostheses make them very competitive.[24] In general, it is unfair to exclude people from being benefited by medical knowledge because they can be more functional by becoming less typical.

## SUMMARY

Although conventional medicine and the ethics reflecting its values assume interventions that achieve species typicality are uncontroversially good, the prospect of genetically eliminating or altering individuals simply to achieve this standard is threatening when considered from a disability perspective. The concern is not that applications of genetic knowledge inherently endanger the disabled, but that political considerations will continue to hold medical interventions to the arbitrary standard of normality. No clinical reasons have emerged, however, for making the pursuit of normality the preeminent strategy for using genetic information in medicine. Important ethical considerations warn that privileging such a strategy may be coercive.

When medical ethicists and medical policymakers assume the aim of genetic medicine is to transform anomalous people so that they will function according to species-typical norms, they beg a most important question from a disability perspective: can genetic technology improve disabled people's functioning without coercively attempting to normalize them? Current research into techniques for therapeutic gene alteration suggests an affirmative response to this question. Ultimately, however, clinicians' decisions about facilitating exceptional functioning, rather than focusing on species-typical functioning, will determine whether people with disabilities are embraced rather than marginalized by the practice of genetic medicine.

# REFERENCES

1. Morris J: *Pride against prejudice,* Philadelphia, 1991, New Society Publishers.
2. Morris J: Tyrannies of perfection, *New Internationalist,* July 1992.
3. Silvers A, Wasserman D, Mahowald M: *Disability, difference, discrimination: perspectives on justice in bioethics and public policy,* Lanham, Md, 1998, Rowman & Littlefield.
4. Satz A, Silvers A: Disability and biotechnology. In Mehlman M, Murray T, editors: *Encyclopedia of biotechnology: ethical, legal and policy issues,* New York, 2000, Wiley & Sons.
5. Glover J: Future people, disability, and screening. In Fishkin J, Laslett P, editors: *Justice between age groups and generations,* New Haven, Conn, 1992, Yale University Press.
6. Davis D: Genetic dilemmas and the child's right to a open future, *Hastings Center Report* 27(2), 1997.
7. Silvers A: An open future: exchange with Dena S. Davis, *Hastings Center Report* 27 (5), 1997.
8. Trent J: *Inventing the feeble mind,* Berkeley, Calif, 1994, University of California Press.
9. Colapinto J: *As nature made him: the boy who was raised as a girl,* New York, 2000, HarperCollins.
10. Baughn B, Degener T, Wolbring G: Personal communications, 2000.
11. Daniels N: Justice and health care. In Van deVeer D, Regan T, editors: *Health care ethics: an introduction,* Philadelphia, 1987, Temple University Press.
12. Kaplan D: Prenatal screening and diagnosis: the impact on persons with disabilities. In Rothenberg K, Thomson E, editors: *Women and prenatal testing: facing the challenges of genetic technology,* Columbus, 1994, Ohio State University.
13. The Campaign Against Human Genetic Engineering (CAHGE): E-mail, 1998.
14. Kass L: Implications of the human right to life. In Munson R: *Intervention and reflection: basic issues in medical ethics,* Belmont, Calif, 1983, Wadsworth.
15. Ricker R: Do we really want this? Little People of America Inc. Comes To Terms With Genetic Testing: a project to study the ethical and social implications of genetic screening for the dwarf and short stature community, Website of Little People of America, 1995.
16. Murray C. Lopez A: *The global burden of disease,* Cambridge, 1996, Harvard School of Health.
17. Miles R: *A women's history of the world,* London, 1988, Michael Joseph.
18. Brock D: *Life and death,* Cambridge, 1993, Cambridge University Press.
19. Brock D: The Human Genome Project and human identity. In Weir R, Lawrence S, Fales E, editors: *Genes and human self-knowledge: historical and philosophical perspectives on modern genetics,* Ames, 1994, University of Iowa Press.
20. Public Law 101-336, Section 3, Definitions 2c.
21. President's Commission for the Study of Ethical Problems in Medicine and Biomedical and Behavioral Research: *Splicing life: the social and ethical issues of genetic engineering with human beings,* Washington, DC, 1982, US Government Printing Office.
22. World Health Organization: *International categorization of impairments, disabilities and handicaps,* Geneva, 1999, WHO, //www.who.int/msa/mnh/ems/icidh/icidhtrg/sld033.htm.
23. Corker M: *Deaf or disabled or deafness disabled?* Buckingham, UK, 1998, Open University Press.
24. Recombinant DNA Advisory Committee (RAC): Discussion regarding the use of normal subjects in human gene transfer clinical trials, Bethesda, Md, 1997, National Institutes of Health.

# CHAPTER 8

# Cultural and Ethnic Differences in Genetic Testing

*James E. Bowman*

The primary care physician is in an awkward position with respect to genetic testing. Formerly, patients and their families sought health care only after trauma, the onset of symptoms or signs of disease, or because of communicable disorders within the family or community. Later, routine checkups became part of ordinary care. An increased focus on public health meant that the physician was responsible not only for diagnosing illness, but also for predicting disease. Immunizations, contraception, and presymptomatic screening tests gradually became part of the medical armamentarium.

Although the genetic revolution suggests the next step in preventive health care, medical genetics has not yet evolved to be part of routine practice. Instead, a multitude of professionals and nonprofessionals invade the domain of the primary care physician. The genetically "ill" but clinically well patients are tested and diagnosed in various settings, including community programs, synagogues, churches, mosques, public health departments, and medical centers. Primary care physicians, if they are involved, are frequently the last to know about the genetic status of their patients.

To complicate the problem further, the media, single-interest genetics pressure groups, bioethicists and their commissions, and legal experts all explore the latest advances in science and inundate what was once the sacrosanct domain of the practitioner. National and international human genome programs now descend on practitioners with their cadres of medical geneticists, genetic counselors, ethicists, philosophers, lawyers, and politicians, as if practitioners are not trained to deal with the complex problems of medical genetics. It is rarely mentioned, however, that most of the nonphysician *experts* in genetic public policy had no training in genetics. If nonphysicians can become knowledgeable about genetics and join the cacophony of self-proclaimed experts, why not primary care physicians? The best relationships between primary care providers and genetics specialists occur when each recognizes the other's limitations.

Medical genetics is not the only field of medicine to come under the aegis of a variety of groups. Practitioners formerly decided individually what to do for patients, but increasingly their decisions are directed by others who are self-appointed or appointed by authoritative and recognized bodies.[1] Interestingly, however, the field of medical genetics has become so complex that genetic counselors and medical geneticists themselves are often general practitioners in an expanding field. No medical geneticist is expert in all of the thousands of genetic disorders. Many also need continuing genetics education even in their own narrow field.

Directly or indirectly, genetic screening and policy are influenced by diverse groups and organizations. For physicians, the American College of Medical Genetics serves to define and support a "standard of care" for genetic medicine. The American Society of Human Genetics and related genetics organizations provide parallel guidance to basic science researchers, clinical researchers, and genetic counselors. There are also numerous community groups such as disease-of-the-month organizations, National Institutes of Health, Food and Drug Administration, other Health and Human Services departments, Department of Energy, the academic university medical establishment, National Academy of Sciences Institute of Medicine, Office of Technology Assessment of the U.S. Congress, and a plethora of other public and private organizations, many of which ignore the primary care physician—the focus of this book. Another important organization is the National Association of Genetic Counselors, whose members form the backbone for genetic interpretation and support for patients and families with genetic disorders. The family is not the endpoint, however, because race, a discredited word or concept, and ethnic and religious groups are also major factors in genetic diversity.

## VAGARIES OF ETHNIC AND CULTURAL DISTINCTIONS

In the United States, common ethnic classifications include Native American (now American Indian once again), White, African-American, Hispanic, Asian, and Other. African-Americans were once categorized as Colored, then Negro, then black and various pejorative terms.[2] Hispanic is too broad a categorization because Mexican-Americans, early (immediately post-Castro) Cuban-Americans, and recently arrived Cuban-Americans, Central and South Americans, and Puerto Ricans (Mainland and Islander) are quite different from one another, and there are diverse groups within these categories as well. Most immigrants from Southeast Asia arrived after the Vietnam War, but most Chinese and Japanese have long-standing ancestry in the United States.

The historical categorization of African-Americans emanates from slavery, by the rule of hypodescent.[3] To perpetuate slavery in succeeding generations, the offspring of Black-White matings and their descendants have been classified variously as Colored, Negro, Black, or African-American. Paradoxically, according to this scheme, an African-American mother cannot have a White child, but a White mother can have an African-American child.

In other countries, African ancestry is not as stringently defined. For example, I could fly to Brazil today and be classified into one of about 40 divisions, from Black to White, and other African-Americans might be classified into as many as 40 different other categories. In Brazil a Black person who is educated or wealthy is "White." (There is an old Brazilian aphorism, "Money whitens.") Next I could fly to South Africa and be classified as Coloured, but other African-Americans might be classified as Black, Coloured, or White.[2] I could subsequently fly to the Middle East and be categorized as Iranian, Lebanese, Saudi Arabian, Iraqi, or Turk, then fly home and be African-American once more.

In defining race, physical appearance is not precise enough to be used as a categorical variable. Hammerschmidt[4] and other editors of scientific publications have therefore agreed to reject papers in which human categories are not precisely defined. Characterizing a group of study subjects as "a Black Chicago population," for example, is imprecise by this criterion. The editors argue that if a population is only described as Black or White, it is unclear that the study can be replicated. As one editor stated:

> *The laudable objective to find means to improve the health conditions for all or for specific populations must not be compromised by the use of race or ethnicity as pseudobiological variables. From now on,* Nature Genetics *will therefore require that the authors explain why they make use of particular ethnic groups or populations, and how classification was achieved. We will ask reviewers to consider these parameters when judging the merits of a manuscript—we hope that this will raise awareness and require more rigorous design of genetic and epidemiological studies.*[5]

To complicate matters further, even though genetic variation is used to delineate populations and ethnic groups, there is often more intragroup variance than intergroup variance. Clearly, we all belong to the same species *(Homo sapiens)* because diverse peoples have met and mated, producing fertile offspring.

Cavalli-Sforza,[6] the principal organizer of the Human Diversity Project, states unequivocally that races do not exist. With such continuity in variation from place to place, defining race, except in very general terms, is practically impossible; precision would require thousands of racial categories. Also, there are as many racial classifications as investigators.[2] Despite the vagaries of classification, primary care physicians must realize that yesterday's category may not apply today. Offspring of mixed ethnic or religious origins frequently pick and choose how they want to be classified. Mixed categories are common; some African-Americans adopt white categories, and about one half of Jews marry outside their religious group. From the standpoint of genetics, fine distinctions should be made among Oriental, Sephardic, Ashkenazi, and Ethiopian Jews because genetic disorders common to one group are rare in the others.

## SICKLE HEMOGLOBIN TESTING

Sickle hemoglobin testing was initiated in the United States in the early 1970s after the commercialization of a solubility test for sickle hemoglobin by a major pharmaceutical company.[7] Although widely advertised as such, this test did not delineate sickle cell trait from sickle cell disease. Most educational brochures implied that sickle cell anemia is confined to Blacks, even though sickle hemoglobin is also prevalent in populations other than Africans and their descendants, such as Greeks, southern Italians, Arabs, southern Iranians, and Asian Indians. Educational brochures, including some from the National Institutes of Health (NIH), were replete with misinformation, even equating sickle cell trait with sickle cell disease.[7] A 1971 Heart and Lung Institute news release claimed that sickle cell disease was the most common inherited disorder in the United States and affected more than 2 million Black citizens.[8]

At least 12 states passed mandatory sickle hemoglobin screening laws, usually under pressure from Black community organizations. Many laws were restricted to the testing of Black children and couples planning to marry; one law included inmates of mental and correctional institutions. Major corporations began selectively screening Blacks. Black flight attendants—who had just been admitted to these jobs—were screened for sickle hemoglobin, and those who tested positive were discharged. A majority of the major life insurance companies raised rates as high as 25% for persons with sickle cell trait, even though the life expectancy of such individuals is the same as for those who do not have sickle hemoglobin. Sickle cell organizations proliferated and vied for funds, and many disseminated misinformation in the Black community.[7,9]

Community pressure and politics resulted in the passage of the National Sickle Cell Anemia Control Act in 1972, Omnibus Genetics Bill in 1976, and Health Services Amendments in 1978.[10-12] Use of "control" in the title of the National Sickle Cell Anemia Control Act was unfortunate because control of sickle cell anemia is only possible with eugenics practices reminiscent of Nazi Germany. Sickle hemoglobin misinformation even infiltrated the language of the act, which stated erroneously that more than 2 million Blacks in the United States have sickle cell anemia; it should have said that 2 million U.S. Blacks have sickle cell trait.

Ostensibly, the major objective of these programs was to enable the community to make informed decisions about reproduction. Counseling was allegedly nondirective—a standard caveat in genetic screening programs. Before the availability of prenatal diagnosis, all the alternatives that might follow a positive test were distasteful: abstinence, artificial insemination, genetic roulette, or abortion. Since these programs occurred before the 1973 *Roe v. Wade* decision of the U.S. Supreme Court, however, abortion was illegal in most states.[13]

The development of techniques for newborn screening and prenatal diagnosis of sickle cell disease ushered in a new phase of hemoglobin screening. This was important because morbidity and mortality in infants with sickle cell disease were reduced by penicillin prophylaxis to prevent infections, particularly those of pneumococcal origin[14]—a major accomplishment of the National Sickle Cell Disease Program.

In 1990, under the leadership of Dr. Charles F. Whitten, the National Association for Sickle Cell Disease developed a position on prenatal diagnosis of sickle cell anemia.[15] Whitten's program emphasizes sickle hemoglobin rather than hemoglobinopathies, and only Black pregnant women are screened. The program involves testing all pregnant Black women to determine whether they are carriers of the sickle gene. Each woman found to be a carrier is counseled that her partner should be tested to determine whether he is also a carrier. If both are carriers, prenatal tests can determine if the fetus has sickle cell anemia. If the partners elect to continue the pregnancy, their decision must be supported. Postabortion counseling should also be offered. No mention is made of options for the woman if her partner refuses testing or is unavailable.

Screening pregnant women for hemoglobinopathy results in the detection of a significant number of individuals who do not know they have sickle cell disease. Because of the relevance of this information to reproductive and medical decisions, obstetricians who do not screen for hemoglobinopathies may be at risk for medical malpractice if a pregnant woman with sickle cell disease is overlooked and has complications from the disease. Further, obstetricians and other health workers who fail to inform, counsel, or use improper techniques to detect genetic disorders in high-risk groups expose themselves to wrongful birth suits.[16,17]

As illustrated by the history of sickle cell disease testing in the United States, the development of a rational public policy for human genetics depends on a host of factors, including economic status; the presence or absence of minority religious, ethnic, or racial groups that have been subject to discrimination; the availability and complexity of techniques for prenatal diagnosis; the accessibility and cost of prophylactic, medical, or surgical therapy; the psychosocial and economic effect on the family; and the overall impact on society.

Predictably, the development of genetics programs is most advanced in Western countries, but once technology has been introduced, its use frequently becomes widespread. To understand better how ethnic and cultural differences influence the development of programs for genetic services in other countries and cultures, the next section describes programs or practices in Italy, Greece, Saudi Arabia, parts of Africa, India, and China.

## INTERNATIONAL PERSPECTIVES

Because of the high incidence of thalassemia, extensive surveys for abnormal hemoglobins and thalassemias have been conducted in Italy.[18] Prenatal diagnosis for thalassemia is well organized and has apparently led to significant reductions in the birth of children with thalassemia. This was accomplished despite the opposition of the Catholic Church to abortion. For example, in one screening program for the prevention of thalassemia in the province of Latium, the average frequency of heterozygous $\alpha$- or $\beta$-thalassemia was 2.4%.[2] This figure was ascertained from a study of 289,763 students. At a single center, 50,000 students a year were examined. Beginning in 1980, at-risk couples were evaluated. Some of these couples (51 of 161) were already parents of an affected child and came to the center during or before a new pregnancy. The majority of couples (110 of 161) had no affected children and came for counseling before conception because of the school screening program. In the latter group, 37 women became pregnant, and 6 of 31 monitored pregnancies had a homozygous fetus that was aborted. In general, this population approved of the screening program, and at-risk couples accepted prenatal diagnosis and abortion.

The experience of prenatal testing for thalassemia in Greece is comparable to that of Italy. In a study at the University of Athens, 50% of couples requested prenatal testing in 1977-1978, which increased to 78% in 1984.[19] The proportion of couples who sought repeat prenatal testing also steadily increased. The annual number of newborns with thalassemia major decreased by almost 50%, and the cost of carrier identification and prenatal diagnosis was much less than the estimated expense of treatment for newborns with thalassemia. During an extensive registry study by the World Health Organization of prenatal testing for thalassemia in countries with high-risk populations, the number of couples who requested prenatal diagnosis also increased steadily.

Although studies in Canada and the United Kingdom, as well as Italy and Greece, show general acceptance of prenatal diagnosis for thalassemia, the acceptance of prenatal diagnosis for sickle cell anemia in the Middle East and in Africa is yet to be demonstrated. Falciparum malaria, tuberculosis, schistosomiasis, yellow fever, hookworm, trypanosomiasis, typhoid fever, cholera, *Loa loa,* malnutrition, and other disorders may so overwhelm the health care delivery system that genetic disorders may not have a high priority.

The acceptability of prenatal diagnosis for sickle cell anemia in Moslem countries is unknown. At an international meeting in Riyadh, Saudi Arabia, in 1984, however, sickle cell disease in Saudi Arabia was said to be much milder than in other parts of the world. Accordingly, prenatal diagnosis with abortion may not have the priority seen in countries where more severe forms of the disease are common. Nonetheless, because some couples may not want to have a child with sickle cell disease, some participants suggested that widespread population screening programs for sickle cell disease should be instituted so that couples would know their sickle hemoglobin status before marriage. Importantly, abortion is rejected by many Moslem theologians, even though the Koran is ambiguous about induced abortion in early pregnancy. The approach of genetic screening and genetic planning without prenatal diagnosis thus appears to be the present course for Saudi Arabia. Even so, Islam, as with Christianity and Judaism, has many religious divisions. Other Moslem countries or different Moslem groups may choose divergent approaches.

In many countries in Africa, complex problems of the prevention and treatment of communicable and nutritional diseases are further complicated by the birth of thousands of children with sickle cell disease each year. The frequency of this disorder at birth may be as high as 1 in 25 to 1 in 50 in some regions.[2] Investigators in various countries of Africa, the Middle East, and the Far East have contributed to the development of technology for ascertaining abnormal hemoglobins and thalassemias. They have cooperated with Western scientists in anthropological studies using restriction enzyme analysis of DNA, techniques also used for prenatal diagnosis. Accordingly, scientists in these countries are now confronted with ethical, economic, and legal issues similar to those of some Western countries.

Western scientists have suggested that programs for selective abortion of fetuses with sickle cell disease may be indicated in African countries. African investigators retort that this policy would be a misuse of scarce health funds, and that such proposals are merely subtle efforts by Western governments to control the growth of non-Western populations. For example, with respect to sickle cell disease, for at-risk couples alone, 140,000 amniocenteses per 1 million conceptions would be required to detect all cases of hemoglobinopathy, and the population increases by 1 million every 4 months in this region.[20] In much of Africa, ethical prohibitions against abortion are similar to those found in other countries. Nevertheless, views are widely divergent.

In China, the most populous country in the world, the government has taken many measures to decrease population growth, including a restriction on birth of one child for urban couples and two children for rural couples. In 1994 the Chinese government also acted to decrease the incidence of children with severe genetic disorders through a law on maternal and infant health care. Unlike the United States, however, China mandates that mothers and infants receive medical and health care services. Marriage is allowed for couples with a serious genetic disease only if they agree to take long-term contraceptive measures or to be sterilized. When applying for marriage, the couple must produce their premarital checkup certificates. If a physician detects or suspects that a married couple of childbearing age have a serious genetic disorder, the physician gives medical advice that the couple are expected to heed. The physician also provides medical advice for termination of pregnancy, which is performed free of charge.

Although the most common reason for prenatal testing is the avoidance of disease in offspring, genetic testing can also be undertaken for nonmedical reasons, such as gender selection. Culture influences such decisions. In many countries, for example, males are preferred over females; Asian Indians may lead in this preference. In India a male child is preferred because the oldest male child must light a parent's funeral pyre to ensure access to the afterlife. Females are expensive. Although a marriage dowry is now illegal, it is still practiced, and often the family must incur debt to meet this marriage obligation. Gender selection is often requested by Asian Indians living in the United States, where this practice often is viewed with abhorrence, even though abortion in the first trimester is legal.[13]

## OTHER RECESSIVE CONDITIONS WITH ETHNIC PREDILECTION

Although the history of sickle cell testing in the United States illustrates the potential for discrimination in the use of genetic information, other autosomal recessive diseases associated with specific ethnic groups include Tay-Sachs disease, Gaucher disease, and cystic fibrosis.

### Tay-Sachs Disease

Tay-Sachs disease (TSD) is a progressive neurogenerative disorder resulting from a deficiency of hexosaminidase A; its onset is at about 6 months of age, when symptoms of paralysis, dementia, and blindness become increasingly severe, leading to death by about the third year of life.[21] TSD has its highest frequency in Ashkenazi Jews, but French-Canadians and Cajuns are also at risk; Sephardic Jews are not at high risk for TSD. Kaback and O'Brien[21] introduced TSD screening into the Ashkenazi Jewish community in Baltimore in the 1970s. The program involved community education through the media, presentations at synagogues, and importantly, participation by rabbis. Extensive counseling followed testing. Gradually the program became a model for others throughout the United States and abroad. Kaback and colleagues[22] reviewed the experience of TSD carrier screening and prenatal diagnosis in testing centers throughout the world and found a marked decrease in the incidence of TSD.

The approach of the Orthodox Jewish community in Israel is novel because members eschew abortion. The purpose of the program is the prevention of marriage between carriers. The individuals tested mostly are engaged couples or students in religious high schools. Code numbers identify the individuals, and the tests are completed within a few days as part of the engagement process. The carrier frequency is 1:26, which is higher than that of the Ashkenazi Jewish population. Since the beginning of the screening program, however, no child with TSD has been born to newlywed couples of this community.[23] The program has expanded to include testing for Gaucher disease and cystic fibrosis.

### Gaucher Disease

Zimran and colleagues[24] found a high frequency of the Gaucher disease mutation at nucleotide 1226 among Ashkenazi Jews in Israel. The carrier frequency was 8.9%, and birth incidence was 1:450. Clinical manifestations range from asymptomatic to severe. Beutler and colleagues[25,26] identified 30 mutations in patients with Gaucher disease, and Brady[27] estimated that about 200,000 individuals in the United States have the disease. More than two thirds of patients are of Ashkenazi Jewish origin, and the prevalence in carriers is about 4.6%, similar to that found in the Ashkenazim in Israel.

Human placental glucocerebrosidase has been used as enzyme replacement therapy for Gaucher disease, with biochemical, hematological, and some clinical improvement. Estimated costs of treatment for the disease range from $100,000 to $382,200.[26,28] A recombinant form of glucocerebrosidase has decreased the infection risk associated with human-derived protein administration but has not reduced the cost. Because of the high cost, some argue that replacement therapy should be offered only to those with severe symptoms. It seems doubtful, however, that affected children of parents who can afford the treatment will be denied access to it.

## Cystic Fibrosis

Cystic firosis (CF) is the most common autosomal recessive genetic disease in Caucasians. In the United States, controversy still surrounds the efficacy and the ethics of routine prenatal diagnosis for pregnant women, especially in community-wide screening programs. In contrast, Europeans have few problems with this issue.

CF has its highest frequency in Northern Europeans; the most common mutation is the Δ508. When the CF locus was discovered, only 75% of carriers could be identified. At present, 80% to 90% of carriers may be found in European-American populations. Because of the uncertainty of negative tests for CF, however, even with more than 800 mutants identified, population screening and prenatal diagnosis have not been broadly supported in the United States. In contrast, Canada, the United Kingdom, and Denmark have all initiated community screening programs.[29] Even in the early days of CF testing, 75% of the health professionals and 75% of community members believed that the introduction of screening would be worthwhile.[29] Such a program is being considered in Brittany, France, where more than 98% of mutations causing CF may now be detected in a Celtic population.[30]

In the United States, several NIH and American Society of Human Genetics committees issued a consensus that mass CF screening should not be implemented, and that couples should be informed about available tests only when a mate had a close relative affected. They also recommended follow-up counseling and interpretation of test results, appropriate quality control, and population initiatives after pilot studies.

In 1992, Wilfond and Fost[31] suggested that routine prenatal testing for CF should cease until the detection rate reaches 95%. This point has been reached, but testing is still not routinely offered. The authors stated that the public's interest in carrier testing, prenatal testing, and pregnancy termination is uncertain because patients with CF have an uncertain survival, variable disability, and normal intelligence. Also, considerable cost is associated with CF testing. Accordingly, primary care physicians should inform patients of the availability of CF tests and refer interested patients to genetic counselors rather than provide the test themselves.

## Complex Disorders

Along with single-gene disorders, complex disorders also occur more prevalently in certain ethnic groups than in others. Certain Asian, Pacific, and Amerindian populations, for example, are at increased risk of type II diabetes. The Pima Indians of the United States have one of the highest world frequencies, 35% of the adult population.[32] As expected, type II diabetes is higher in Mexican-Americans (because of their Amerindian component) than in Anglo-Americans. The incidence of diabetes-related end-stage renal disease in Mexican-Americans, however, is greater than that predicted from their excess of type II diabetes.

The disease also has an earlier age of onset, greater severity, and poorer control of diabetes than that of other groups.[32] The higher morbidity and mortality of diabetes in the Mexican-American group could also be a reflection of inadequate medical care.

## SUMMARY

At present, primary care physicians are concerned about not only patients with genetic disease who may be stigmatized as unfit, but also individuals who carry a single dose (carriers) of a genetic defect, which causes little if any effect. Since we all have at least five recessive genes, we are all at risk for having "unfit" children. With the human genome now mapped, many more potentially harmful genes—recessive and otherwise—will be unveiled in each of us. Consequently, in this day of rapid advances in genetics, we all have the potential to pass "unfit" disorders on to the next generation. Because we are all similar in this regard, scientific advances in the understanding of the human genome *may* be one of the best defenses against eugenic discrimination. We rarely discriminate against those who are "like ourselves."

All ethnic and cultural groups have their own high-frequency genetic disorders. Primary care practitioners should understand some of these risks in relation to different ethnic groups to facilitate care of those whose differences are sometimes associated with discrimination. Boxes 8-1, 8-2, and 8-3 list common genetic disorders and variations that are prevalent in Africans, Europeans, and Jews, respectively.[33,34] Physicians must remember, however, that genetic disorders with an increased frequency in certain groups may be found in all populations.

---

### BOX 8-1 HIGH-FREQUENCY GENETIC VARIANTS AND DISORDERS COMMON TO AFRICANS AND THEIR DESCENDANTS

Sickle cell disease*
α- and β-Thalassemia
Glucose-6-phosphate dehydrogenase deficiency
Fy (Duffy) silent gene
Rh system RH positive (R0, cde)
Arcus cornea
Café au lait spots
Clubbing of digits
Polydactyly
Vitiligo
Abnormal separation of sutures
Earlobe absent
Keloid
Hereditary hypertropic osteoarthropy
Scapholocephaly

---

*Also present in high frequency in southern Italians, Greeks, Arabs, Egyptians, southern Iranians, Eti-Turks, and Asian Indians.[2]

## BOX 8-2 HIGH-FREQUENCY GENETIC VARIANTS AND DISORDERS COMMON TO EUROPEANS

Cystic fibrosis
Neural tube defects
Congenital spherocytic anemia
Phenylthiocarbamide (PTC) taster
Red-green color vision defect
$\alpha_1$-Antitrypsin deficiency
Baldness
Cleft lip and palate
Hemophilia A
Congenital dislocation of hip
Hereditary spherocytosis
Phenylketonuria
XYY syndrome

## BOX 8-3 HIGH-FREQUENCY GENETIC VARIANTS AND DISORDERS COMMON TO JEWS

**Ashkenazi**

Tay-Sachs disease
Niemann-Pick disease
Gaucher disease
Canavan disease
Torsion dystonia
Familial dysautonomia
Nonclassical 21-hydroxylase deficiency
Bloom syndrome

**Sephardi and Oriental**

Glucose-6-phosphate dehydrogenase deficiency
Familial Mediterranean fever
Gaucher disease
$\beta$-Thalassemia
Larson-type dwarfism

# REFERENCES

1. Sniderman AD: Clinical trials, consensus conferences, and clinical practice, *Lancet* 354:327-330, 1999.
2. Bowman JE, Murray RF Jr: *Genetic variation and disorders in peoples of African origin,* Baltimore, 1990, Johns Hopkins University Press.
3. Harris M: *Patterns of race in the Americas,* New York, 1974, Norton.
4. Hammerschmidt DE: It's as simple as black and white! Race and ethnicity as categorical variables, *J Lab Clin Med* 133:10-12, 1999.
5. Census, race and science, *Nat Genet* 24:97-98, 1999 (editorial).
6. Cavalli-Sforza LL: Race differences: genetic evidence. In *Plain talk about the Human Genome Project,* Tuskegee, Ala, 1997, Tuskegee University College of Agricultural, Environmental and Natural Sciences.
7. Bowman JE: Genetic screening programs and public policy, *Phylon* 38:117-142, 1977.
8. National Heart and Lung Institute, National Institutes of Health: *HEW News,* November 1971.
9. Reilly PR: *Genetics, law, and social policy,* Cambridge, Mass, 1977, Harvard University Press.
10. National Sickle Cell Anemia Control Act, Public Law 92-294, 1972.
11. Omnibus Genetics Bill, Title IV of Public Law 84-278, National Sickle Cell Anemia, Cooley's Anemia, Tay-Sachs, and Genetic Diseases Act, 1976.
12. Health Services Amendments, Section 205, Public Law 95-626, 1978.
13. *Roe v Wade,* 410 US 116, 1973.
14. Gaston MH, Verter JI, Woods G, et al: Prophylaxis with oral penicillin in children with sickle cell anemia, *N Engl J Med* 315:1593-1599, 1986.
15. National Association for Sickle Cell Disease: *Prenatal diagnosis of sickle cell anemia,* Los Angeles, 1990, The Association.
16. Capron AM: Tort liability in genetics, *Columbia Law Review* 79:619-684, 1979.
17. Shaw MW: Conditional prospective rights of the fetus, *J Leg Med* 5:63-115, 1984.
18. Tentori L, Marinucci M: Hemoglobinopathies and thalassemias in Italy and Northern Africa. In Bowman JE, editor: *Distribution and evolution of hemoglobin and hemoglobin loci,* New York, 1983, Elsevier.
19. Loukopoulos D: Prenatal diagnosis of thalassemia and of the hemoglobinopathies: a review, *Hemoglobin* 9:435-459, 1985.
20. Konety-Ahulu FID: Ethics of amniocentesis and selective abortion for sickle cell disease, *Lancet* 1:38-39, 1982.
21. Kaback MM, O'Brien JS: Tay-Sachs: prototype for prevention of genetic disease, *Hosp Pract* 8:107-116, 1973.
22. Kaback M, Lim-Steele J, Dabholkar D, et al: Tay-Sachs disease—carrier screening, prenatal diagnosis, and the molecular era: an international perspective, The International TSD Data Collection Network, *JAMA* 270:2307-2315, 1993.
23. Brodie E, Zeigler M, Eckstein J, et al: Screening for carriers of Tay-Sachs disease in the Ultraorthodox Ashkenazi Jewish community in Israel, *Am J Med Genet* 47:213-215, 1993.
24. Zimran A, Gelbart T, Westwood B, et al: High frequency of the Gaucher disease at nucleotide 1226 among Ashkenazi Jews, *Am J Hum Genet* 49:855-89, 1991.
25. Beutler E, Geilbert T, Kuhl W, et al: Identification of the second common Jewish mutation makes possible population-based screening for the heterozygous state, *Proc Natl Acad Sci* 88:10544-10547, 1991.
26. Beutler E, Kay AC, Saven A, et al: *N Engl J Med* 325:1809-1810, 1991 (letter).
27. Brady RO: Personal communication to McKusick VA, 1982.
28. Zimran A, Hafdas-Halpern I, Abrahamov A: Enzyme replacement therapy for Gaucher disease, *N Engl J Med* 325:1810-1811, 1991.
29. Watson EK, Williamson R, Chapple J: Attitudes to carrier screening for cystic fibrosis: a survey of health care professionals, relatives of sufferers and other members of the public, *Br J Gen Pract* 41:237-240, 1992.

30. Davies K: Genetic screening for cystic fibrosis, *Nature* 357:424, 1992.
31. Wilfond BS, Fost N: The introduction of cystic fibrosis carrier screening into clinical practice: policy consideration, *Milbank Q* 70:629-659, 1992.
32. Polednak AP: *Racial and ethnic differences in disease,* Oxford, 1989, Oxford University Press.
33. McKusick VA: *Mendelian inheritance in man,* ed 11, Baltimore, 1994, Johns Hopkins University Press.
34. Bonne-Tamir B, Adam A: *Genetic diversity among Jews: diseases and markers at the DNA level,* Oxford, 1992, Oxford University Press.

# CHAPTER 9

# Gender and Access Differences in Genetic Services

*Mary B. Mahowald*

Cultural and ethnic differences in genetics are often related to gender and class differences. For example, different cultures define different childrearing roles for men and women, and the childrearing role influences many women's economic situation. Physiological differences between the sexes are relevant to health care practice; ability to pay is relevant to people's access to genetic services. This chapter develops a conception of justice aimed at avoiding or reducing discrimination based on race, ethnicity, gender, ability, or class.

## GENDER DIFFERENCES IN GENETICS

Although gender is usually viewed as a social category and sex as a biological category, the two are related in both life and clinical practice. In general, social expressions of gender are rooted in sexual identity. The sex differences across the spectrum of genetic diseases can be categorized in five ways (Box 9-1):

1. Conditions that primarily or exclusively affect one sex
2. Conditions affecting the sexes in unequal ratios
3. Conditions influenced by the sex of the transmitting parent
4. Conditions affecting fertility differently in men and women
5. Conditions in which pregnancy poses particular risks to those affected

When the sex difference entails greater risk for affected men, as in fragile X syndrome, or for affected pregnant women, as in cystic fibrosis or sickle cell anemia, clinicians are obliged to inform patients of this sex-specific impact. In some cases, however, the burden of the disease is exacerbated by psychosocial factors, by gender rather than by sex, or by gender as influenced by sex.[1] For example, a positive test for breast cancer susceptibility will have different impact on women than on men. Clinicians need to attend to psychosocial as well as physiological sex-based differences in discussing test results and planning treatment with patients.

## BOX 9-1 SEX DIFFERENCES IN CLINICAL MANIFESTATIONS OF GENETIC DISEASE

1. Conditions affecting one sex only or primarily
   a. Most X-linked diseases (affected male, unaffected female carrier)
      Examples: Duchenne muscular dystrophy, Hunter syndrome, hemophilia A
   b. Sex-limited disease (from nature of the disease)
      Examples: breast cancer (mainly women), ovarian cancer (only women), prostate cancer and hypospadias (only men)
2. Conditions affecting the sexes in unequal ratios
   a. Male >female
      Example: posterior urethral valves
   b. Female > male
      Example: anencephaly
3. Conditions determined by sex or other characteristic of transmitting parent
   a. Triplet repeat expansion diseases
      Examples: fragile X syndrome and myotonic dystrophy (maternal inheritance increases severity), Huntington disease (paternal inheritance increases severity)
   b. Imprinting diseases
      Examples: Angelman syndrome (deficiency of maternal contribution), Prader-Willi syndrome (deficiency of paternal contribution)
   c. Parental age effect
      Examples: Down syndrome (older mothers), achondroplastic dwarfism and Marfan syndrome (older fathers)
   d. Mitochondrial inheritance (always transmitted by mothers)
      Examples: myoclonic epilepsy, ragged red muscle fiber disease
4. Conditions affecting fertility in males and females
   a. Infertility in males
      Example: cystic fibrosis
   b. Infertility in females
      Example: congenital adrenal hyperplasia
5. Conditions in which pregnancy exacerbates risks for affected women
   Examples: cystic fibrosis, sickle cell anemia, Marfan syndrome, neurofibromatosis

Significant sex-based and gender-based differences in genetics also result because men and women play disparate roles in the reproductive process. Although fetal conditions may be triggered by either parent or both, women alone undergo prenatal testing and interventions on behalf of their potential children. Legally and practically but not without moral controversy, women in the United States and elsewhere are also the only ones who may decide to terminate or continue a pregnancy after a positive genetic test.[2,3] Gender differences related to their different reproductive roles arise because women are held more responsible than men for the welfare of children and potential children. Some women are pressured to undergo tests or interventions they would otherwise avoid. Cultural, ethnic, religious, and familial influences may compromise the autonomy of some women in decisions about prenatal testing and interventions.[4] As genetic tests and possible interventions proliferate, pressures on women to avail themselves of these technologies are likely to increase.

TABLE 9-1

## Preference for Childlessness, Adoption, or Reproductive Assistance

Responses to the question:
If you cannot become a parent by the usual route of intercourse, conception, pregnancy, and childbirth, would you prefer to remain childless, or would you pursue medical assistance or adoption to become parents?

| Preference | Women (%) | Men (%) |
|---|---|---|
| Remain childless | 7 (13.5) | 4 (7.4) |
| Seek adoption | 8 (15.3) | 16 (29.6) |
| Seek medical assistance | 37 (71.1) | 34 (62.9) |

### Reproductive Roles

One seldom-considered gender difference that clinicians should bear in mind in dealing with couples, or even with individual men or women, is explicitly tied to their different roles in reproduction. Because men can only be biologically related to children through their genes, they may place greater emphasis on the genetic tie to children than women do. Women typically are biologically related to children through gestation as well. Advances in reproductive technology have provided means of separating the genetic tie from the gestational tie, allowing women in some cases to choose between the two. Two recent studies show that many women choose gestation over genetics. A survey of men and women in gynecology and postnatal wards in Leeds, England, about half of whom were health care personnel, found that a statistically insignificant majority of both viewed gestation as the more important biological tie for women.[5] In another study, this finding was only applicable to women; men favored the genetic rather than the gestational tie between women and their children.[6] This study population comprised patients and family members in a general medical clinic at an urban university hospital. The second study's results also show a preference for seeking reproductive assistance rather than adoption or childlessness if couples are unable to have a biologically related child by the usual route of sexual intercourse and gestation by the woman (Tables 9-1 and 9-2). Although differences in the study populations probably influenced the results, both studies show that gestation, which is gender specific, is more important than genetics to many people.

These data are important to clinicians who counsel patients about treatment modalities that may compromise their capacity to have a biologically related child. Clinicians should not assume (1) that biological or genetic parenthood is so significant that individuals would avoid the treatment, or (2) that a couple are united in their desire to be parents, whether biologically or by adoption. Although care of individuals affects family members, who often affect the care of patients, it is a mistake to view couples or families as if they have singu-

| TABLE 9-2 |

## Genetics or Gestation

If you could choose one of the following, which would you choose?

OPTION 1: GENETICS
*Women:* To be genetically related without carrying the pregnancy and giving birth to your child.
*Men:* You and your partner are genetically related to your child, but your partner does not carry the pregnancy and give birth.

OPTION 2: GESTATION
*Women:* To carry the pregnancy and give birth without being genetically related to your child.
*Men:* You are genetically related to your child, but your partner is not. Your partner carries the pregnancy and gives birth.

| Options ($p = 0.032$) | Women (n = 37) | Men (n = 34) |
|---|---|---|
| Genetics | 48.6% | 73.5% |
| Gestation | 51.4% | 26.5% |

lar views about available options. The autonomy, burdens, and benefits of each person should be addressed with recognition that these are often different and sometimes conflicting. Priorities may be set in cases of conflict according to two rules: (1) the autonomy of the one most affected has priority over that of others, and (2) when autonomy is lacking in that individual (e.g., a child), his or her best interests have priority.

### Caregiving Roles

Gender differences in genetics are also evident in a set of psychosocial issues related to but separate from sex differences. These issues generally involve women's caregiving role in formal and informal settings. Women tend to concentrate in positions of less prestige and income within the health care professions, although more women are in genetics than in other areas, perhaps because the newness of the field coincides with a greater influx of women into medicine.[7,8] This has led to a proportionately greater number of leadership positions for women in genetics. Nonetheless, most doctorally prepared geneticists and genetic counselors are men, and most master's-prepared genetic counselors are women.[9] Given the limited number of master's-prepared genetic counselors and the time required for adequate counseling in primary care settings, nurses may take on a greater role in providing relevant genetic information to patients.

The caregiving role of women is related to their reproductive role through social factors that link the two roles. Such factors include the limited number of providers of genetic services, required waiting periods for these services, transportation and child care needs, language barriers, and lack of awareness or education about the possibility, benefits, and risks of genetic testing.[1] Cultural assumptions about their caregiving role may lead to pressures on women to undergo or not undergo tests or interventions. To promote women's autonomy, clinicians must assist them in making decisions that reflect women's values.

As primary caregivers of children, disabled persons, and elderly people, women are more likely to experience depression than their male counterparts. Caregiving is also associated with a greater incidence of physical ills, anger, and guilt on the part of the caregiver.[10,11] Successful treatment of chronically ill patients has led to their extended life span, which has concomitantly increased caregivers' physical and psychological burden. Because outside activities are restricted for primary caregivers within the home, their economic and psychological welfare is often compromised. The economic burden of advances in genetics is probably greater for women than for men because the majority of the world's poor are women and their children.[12,13] Class-based differences, however, apply to men as well as women.

## CLASS-BASED DIFFERENCES IN GENETICS

Most primary caregivers are familiar with discrepancies in health care that result from the different economic capacities of patients and their families. Such discrepancies account for most differences in access to genetic services. Some patients already can afford genetic tests and treatments not available to others; this will increasingly be the case as new tests and interventions are introduced. However, being able to afford genetic services does not imply that those who buy them are thereby advantaged or that those who cannot afford the services are thereby disadvantaged. In some cases, utilization of genetic services clearly promotes the patient's autonomy and interests; in other cases, it may entail reduced autonomy and incremented risks for the patient. In other words, genetic inequality may occur through overdistribution as well as underdistribution of genetic services. It may also occur through distribution of the same resources to groups who have a different need for them.[14] Any of these ways of allocating genetic services may fail to account for the different and discrepant needs of patients (Table 9-3).

### Allocation of Resources

The inequality of underdistribution of health resources mainly affects poor persons and uninsured or underinsured groups. Access to genetic services for these groups is determined by the willingness of the government or private insurance to cover its cost. Technologies that have proved their cost-effectiveness to providers are typically covered; those that have not are available only to those who are able and willing to pay for them. For example, prenatal tests for women over 35 years of age and cancer risk testing of individuals with a family history of cancer may be covered solely because of their cost-effectiveness. If people can pay out of pocket, however, they may obtain prenatal testing or cancer risk testing even if the testing is not deemed cost-effective. Although testing some groups may not be cost-effective for the government or insurers, such testing is often relevant to individual patients and their care providers. Negative results are usually reassuring, and positive results en-

| TABLE 9-3 | | |
|---|---|---|

## Inequality in Distribution of Genetic Services

| Type of Distribution | Description | Example |
|---|---|---|
| Underallocation | Unavailability of genetic services to those who could benefit but cannot pay | Preimplantation genetic diagnosis |
| Overallocation for nonmedical reasons | Availability of genetic tests for any reason to anyone who can pay | Tests for sex selection |
| Same allocation | Distribution of same service to everyone | Mandatory testing of everyone, regardless of risk |

courage health practices that may prevent the onset of symptoms or lead to early discovery and successful intervention.

Besides new genetic tests, advances in gene therapy also are denied to those who cannot pay, including fetuses and children. The inequality of this denial is exacerbated by poverty, an environmental factor that may influence the expression of multifactorial genetic diseases.[15] Optimal care of individual patients thus supports the provision of genetic information and services to those who cannot pay as well as those who can pay for genetic tests.

The impact of poverty on access to genetic services is not simply a matter of who can pay for them. Access also requires social circumstances and supports that do not interfere with provision of services.[16] As with other health care services, poor people are less likely than others to be educated about the availability and usefulness of genetic tests or interventions. Immigrants are less likely to find practitioners who can speak their language. Many are unable to change work schedules to fit the only times available for medical appointments. Women who have positive prenatal test results may be denied access to abortion because they cannot obtain the procedure before viability.[17]

Primary caregivers are routinely asked to document the health status of patients for employers or insurance carriers. It is therefore crucial to inform patients about the risks to coverage from genetic tests and results. The history of sickle cell testing affirms that women and men have been denied access to jobs or insurance because of discriminatory practices associated with genetic disease or genetic susceptibility to disease.[18] In a free enterprise system, this will increasingly be the case as genetic tests proliferate.

Underallocation of services to poor people is one side of class-based differences in genetics. The other side involves two types of unjust allocation of genetic services: distribution of the same services to everyone and distribution of some services to recipients who do not need or desire them. Allocation of the same genetic services to everyone is unjust because individuals have different needs for them or have different burdens and benefits to be obtained through them. Treating patients justly does not mean treating them all the same; it requires recognition of and attention to their different needs.

Overallocation of genetic services may involve those who are affluent enough to pay, who may be disadvantaged rather than advantaged because the services entail disproportionate risks or complications. Social pressures to undergo experimental or novel genetic interventions may be greater for this group, as a potential but fallible means of optimizing their own or their children's health. At times the pressures may come from investigators who are insufficiently attentive to possible conflicts between research priorities and the best interests of patients who agree to experimental tests or treatment. Primary caregivers may play a significant role in recognizing when this occurs. They may also be in a better position than geneticists to critique the attempts of commercial testing companies to increase access to new tests, regardless of whether the tests are helpful to individual patients. People who can pay out of pocket may be increasingly subject to unjust overallocation of genetic services by overeager researchers and vendors of genetic tests or interventions.

### Provider-Patient Differences

Another class-based difference in genetics is evident in the contrast between the providers of genetic services, whether geneticists, genetic counselors, or primary caregivers, and many patients. The vast majority of providers are Caucasian, whereas patients belong to multiple ethnic groups.[9] When genetic services are covered by private or governmental insurance, typically the providers also belong to a more advantaged socioeconomic group than their patients. The class difference from this disparity is exacerbated by the vulnerability or dependence that patients typically experience in regard to their caregivers. For health professionals the ideal of the profession is to reduce such dependence.[19]

Although it is impossible to eliminate the economic gap that makes one group dependent on the other, it is possible to reduce the psychological gap by maximizing patients' knowledge and control of the decision-making process. Because their role usually entails an ongoing relationship and a wider range of interactions with patients, primary caregivers are better situated than geneticists and genetic counselors to reduce the psychological gap between themselves and patients. Such efforts may be facilitated by a conception of justice.

## GENETIC JUSTICE BETWEEN GENDERS AND CLASSES

Different conceptions of justice identify different goods to be distributed equally to individuals or groups.[20] Some conceptions give greater weight to individual liberty; others support equal distribution of material resources. A *libertarian* conception, for example, seeks to promote liberty for everyone through fair procedures of distribution, ignoring the often discrepant outcomes. A *liberal* conception of justice attempts to minimize discrepant outcomes and maximize individual liberty by focusing on equality of opportunity. However, some liberal conceptions stress the maximization of liberty more than the minimization of outcome discrepancies, and vice versa. The conception of justice best suited to address the differences previously identified attempts to reduce discrepant outcomes with minimal compromise of individual liberty. This is an *egalitarian* conception of justice,[18] well supported by the Nobel laureate philosopher and economist Amartya Sen.

For Sen, an egalitarian theory of justice emphasizes the capability of individuals and groups to achieve the goals they define for themselves. "Capability reflects a person's ability to choose between alternative lives, and its valuation need not presuppose unanimity regarding some one specific set of objectives."[21] In other words, capability is determined from the standpoint of the individual or group. Using Sen's concept, the ideal of genetic equality is a situation in which differences triggered or caused by genetics do not advantage an individual or group over others, despite the different capabilities with which they are associated. This may be expressed as follows:

$$\frac{\text{Capability of X}}{\text{Capability of Y}} = 1$$

When differences associated with genetics lead to one individual or group having advantage over the other, inequality results, which may be expressed as follows:

$$\frac{\text{Capability of X}}{\text{Capability of Y}} \neq 1$$

Differences associated with genetics may be unchangeable, such as those resulting from gender or genetic endowment. Other differences, such as those from gender socialization and socioeconomic status, are changeable. However, neither changeable nor unchangeable differences are necessarily associated with inequality. To the extent that differences related to genetics influence the capabilities and potential advantages of individuals and groups, genetic justice requires the following:

1. Identification of the differences
2. Determination of whether differences are associated with inequality
3. Efforts to eliminate or ameliorate resulting inequalities

All the differences added together for each individual or group would then be equal to the sum of differences in every other; in other words, a comparison of the advantages for individuals or groups would always produce a ratio equal to 1, or as close an approximation as possible to 1.

According to Sen, capabilities of individuals and groups are influenced by biological, social, and cultural factors that determine how and to what extent they can express their freedom. Unequal capabilities arise from overlapping characteristics, such as sex, socioeconomic status, and ability. These diverse characteristics "give us very divergent powers to build freedom in our lives even when we have the same bundle of primary goods."[21] The primary goods are self-respect, rights and liberties, powers and opportunities, income and wealth, health and vigor, and intelligence and imagination.[22] Overcoming the inequalities associated with the "divergent powers" of individuals or groups requires attention to different capabilities and their related advantages or disadvantages.

## SUMMARY

Primary caregivers are well aware of the different, often reduced capabilities of their patients, and physicians' typical goal is to help patients utilize their different capabilities to surmount the resulting disadvantages. Ironically, pursuit of this goal is at odds with the tendency in some segments of society to practice "political correctness" by ignoring differences on grounds that recognition of them involves prejudice or bias. Although clinicians usually focus on the capability of good health, health is often inseparable from capabilities determined by gender and class as well as other differences among individuals and groups. Advocacy for patient health thus demands advocacy for the conditions conducive to health. Taken together, these advocacies suggest a constructive complementarity between the dual roles of the primary caregiver as professional and as citizen.

# REFERENCES

1. Mahowald MB, Levinson D, Cassel C, et al: The new genetics and women, *Milbank Q* 74(2):248-270, 1996.
2. *Roe v. Wade,* 410 US 113, 1973.
3. Cook RJ: Abortion laws and policies: challenges and opportunities, *Int J Gynaecol Obstet* 3(suppl), 1989.
4. Rapp R: Women's responses to prenatal diagnosis: a sociocultural perspective on diversity. In Rothenberg KH, Thomson EJ, editors: *Women and prenatal testing: facing the challenges of genetic technology,* Columbus, 1994, Ohio State University Press.
5. Thornton JG, McNamara HM, Montague IA: Would you rather be a "birth" or a "genetic" mother? If so, how much? *J Med Ethics* 20:87, 1994.
6. Ravin AJ, Mahowald MB, Stocking CB: Genes or gestation? Attitudes of women and men about biological ties to children, *J Womens Health* 6(6):1-9, 1997.
7. Graduate medical education, *JAMA* 280(9): 836-837, 1998.
8. *Statistical abstract of the United States,* Washington, DC, 1995, US Government Printing Office.
9. National Society for Genetic Counselors: Professional status survey, *Perspect Genet Counsel* 18(suppl):1-8, 1996.
10. Eiser C: Psychological effects of chronic disease, *J Clin Psychol Psychiatry* 31(1):85-98, 1990.
11. Parks SH, Pilisuk M: Caregiver burden: gender and the psychological costs of caregiving, *Am J Orthopsychiatry* 61:501-509, 1991.
12. Phillips JM, Sexton M, Blackman JA: Demographic overview of women across the lifespan. In Allen KM, Phillips JM, editors: *Women's health across the lifespan,* Philadelphia, 1997, Lippincott-Raven.
13. *The world's women 1995 trends and statistics,* New York, 1995, United Nations.
14. Mahowald MB: Gender justice and genetics. In Hudson Y, Peden WC, editors: *The social power of ideas,* Lewiston, NY, 1995, Edwin Mellen Press.
15. Starfield B: Child health care and social factors: poverty, class, race, *Bull NY Acad Med* 5(3):300, 1989.
16. Nsiah-Jefferson L: Reproductive genetic services for low-income women and women of color: access and sociocultural issues. In Rothenberg KH, Thomson EJ, editors: *Women and prenatal testing: facing the challenges of genetic technology,* Columbus, 1994, Ohio State University Press.
17. Henshaw SK: Actors hindering access to abortion services, *Fam Plann Perspect* 27 (2):54, 1995.
18. Mahowald MB: *Genes, women, equality,* New York, 2000, Oxford University Press.
19. Mahowald MB: The physician. In Lawry R, Clarke R, editors: *The power of the professional person,* New York, 1988, University Press of America.
20. Beauchamp TL, Childress JF: *Principles of biomedical ethics,* New York, 1994, Oxford University Press.
21. Sen A: *Inequality reconsidered,* Cambridge, Mass, 1992, Harvard University Press.
22. Rawls J: *A theory of justice,* Cambridge, Mass, 1971, Harvard University Press.

# CHAPTER 10

# Genetic Counseling in the Primary Care Setting

*Shelly A. Cummings*

Clinical genetics is a young science. As recently as 100 years ago there was little scientific information for people concerned about their risk of an apparently hereditary disorder or birth defect occurring in themselves or their children. Such conditions were frequently ascribed to exogenous forces, such as punishment for past actions or a curse. On rare occasions the inheritance pattern was correctly interpreted, as in the Talmudic proscription against circumcising brothers of bleeders. It was known that men with hemophilia, a disease in which blood does not clot properly, tended to have male relatives with the same disease. Also, these male relatives were usually on the maternal side of the family. In Biblical times, women with a maternal uncle or brother affected with bleeding problems were advised not to have their sons circumcised. Although other diseases were also known to run in families, the process by which a disease could be transmitted from healthy parents to their children remained unclear.

Over the past century, understanding of genetic disorders, their variability, and mechanisms of the disease process has grown exponentially. In addition, but at a slower pace, important advances have occurred in the study of human behavior, health policy, ethics, counseling, and risk management. These advances have fostered a movement of activism for taking control of one's own health care. The field of genetic counseling emerged as a means by which this activism could be expressed in the relationship between primary care practitioners and their patients. Genetic counseling involves communicating complex medical information to families in a nondirective and appropriate manner that respects their individual and family goals and ethical and religious standards. Trained genetic counselors assist families in coping with the emotional, psychological, medical, social, and economic consequences of genetic disease.[1]

Until recently, genetic counseling has primarily taken place in the prenatal setting, often focusing on chromosome or single-gene etiology. Advances in the genetics of complex and adult-onset disorders have demonstrated the need for such services in other areas of medicine. This chapter discusses the diverse roles that trained genetic counselors can serve in the primary care setting.

## THE PROFESSION OF GENETIC COUNSELING

During the last 30 years the field of genetic counseling has expanded rapidly. The National Society of Genetic Counselors, formed in 1979, currently has over 1800 members. There are now more than 20 graduate-training programs for genetic counselors in the United States, with most programs accepting only four to seven students each year. The American Board of Genetic Counseling (ABGC) certifies training programs that grant master's degrees in genetic counseling. Graduates of these programs also can take a certifying examination administered by ABGC. Training programs for genetic counselors are 2-year master's level programs with course work and clinical field training in medical genetics and counseling. Most enter this field from a variety of disciplines including biology, chemistry, genetics, nursing, psychology, public health, and social work. The genetic counselor's training combines genetics, medicine, laboratory work, counseling, social work, and ethical analysis.

After completing their master's level training, genetic counselors continue their education by attending local, regional, and national educational meetings in the field of medical genetics and genetic counseling. They practice in a variety of settings, including hospitals, private offices, commercial laboratories, federal and state government offices, universities, and research laboratories. Genetic counselors also serve as educative resources for other health care professionals and the public. Some work in administrative capacities, and many engage in research activities related to medical genetics and clinical genetics. As genetic services proliferate, genetic counselors will play an increasing role on the staff of medical genetics clinics.

In 1975 the American Society of Human Genetics adopted the following definition of genetic counseling:

> *Genetic counseling is a communication process which deals with the human problems associated with the occurrence, or the risk of an occurrence, of a genetic disorder in the family. This process involves an attempt by one or more appropriately trained persons to help the individual or family to (1) comprehend the medical facts, including the diagnosis, probable course of the disorder, and the available management; (2) appreciate the way heredity contributes to the disorder, and the risk of recurrence in specified relatives; (3) understand the alternatives for dealing with the risk of occurrence; (4) choose the course of action which seems to them appropriate in view of their risk, their family goals, and their ethical and religious standards, and to act in accordance with that decision; and (5) to make the best possible adjustment to the disorder in an affected family member and/or the risk of recurrence of that disorder.*[1]

These operative principles include the belief that the decision to use genetic services should be voluntary. The prevailing philosophy is that information should be made available and tests offered when appropriate, but that the individual and their families should have the final word, unencumbered by pressure that a particular course of action is fiscally or socially or ethically responsible. However, many patients are referred for genetic services not at their own request but by a health care provider who has identified the need for such services. The primary caregiver can then facilitate the genetic counseling process by informing the patient about its availability and relevance, what it entails, and its possible benefits to the patient and his or her relatives (Box 10-1). This reduces the patient's fears about the session, lessens anxiety, and provides a sense of involvement in health care decisions.

### Patient Education

A central component of genetic counseling is patient education. The genetic counselor should discuss the following with the patient:

1. Features, natural history, and range of variability of the condition in question
2. Relationship between the development of the condition and genetic and non-genetic factors
3. Diagnosis and management options
4. Occurrence or recurrence risks
5. Social, financial, and psychological implications (positive and negative) for the patient and family
6. Available resources to help cope with the condition's challenges
7. Risk reduction and prevention strategies

Patient education is not complete unless the counselor provides complete disclosure of information that allows the patient to make an informed decision about what actions to take. Selective omission of relevant information in disclosure to patients fails to respect the patient's autonomy and ability to make a fully informed decision. Debate still surrounds what is "relevant" to particular patients, and it is doubtful that every available test (such as carrier testing for cystic fibrosis) needs to be offered and discussed with every patient. It is also questioned whether the genetic counselor should address issues that are not related to the reason for the referral (Figure 10-1). Despite the amount and complexity of the infor-

---

## BOX 10-1 GENETIC COUNSELING: THE PROCESS

- Construct a family history or pedigree with entry of all medical problems.
- Analyze the family history for genetic and/or birth defect risk.
- Assess and interpret the risk for occurrence (or recurrence) of genetic conditions in the family.
- Discuss the nature of the condition(s), including the contribution of heredity.
- Discuss the options available to reduce recurrence risk(s), including available testing.
- Present risks and benefits of each option, with careful attention to patient comprehension.
- Assist in selecting the option appropriate for an individual or family.
- Provide supportive counseling and/or referral to community resources when appropriate.
- Coordinate tests performed, when indicated.
- Write a summary letter documenting the counseling session, outlining the plan of care, and send it to the patient and/or referring physician.

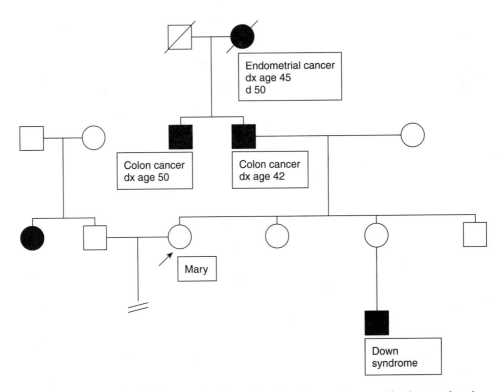

**FIGURE 10-1**   Mary's primary care physician referred her for genetic counseling because her sister had a son with Down syndrome. Mary was concerned about her risk of having a child with Down syndrome. The genetic counselor took a detailed family history, as shown. The counselor identified a susceptibility to colon cancer, specifically, hereditary nonpolyposis colon cancer (HNPCC). Should the counselor, in addition to discussing Mary's risk of having a child with Down syndrome, also address the risk of HNPCC in the family, even though this was not the intent of the referral? *dx,* Diagnosed; *d,* died.

mation conveyed, counselors strive to disclose information relevant to the decision-making process in ways that allow the patient to interpret and act.

As in other communications between practitioners and patients, most counselors exercise clinical judgment in determining which information is likely to be important and helpful to a patient's decision-making process or adjustment to a diagnosis. Their goal is to present this information clearly, accurately, and without bias so as not to encourage a particular course of action. This *nondirective approach* is the defining feature of genetic counseling (see Chapter 11). Occasionally, however, the directiveness that most primary caregivers use to promote their patient's health is applicable to genetic counseling as well. In cancer risk counseling, for example, health-related behaviors such as mammography, breast self-examinations, and colonoscopy are explicitly encouraged or recommended. In general, genetic counselors should engage in an interactive process in which patients are not only educated about their risk, but also helped with the complex tasks of exploring issues related to their condition. Counseling about these matters is intended to facilitate patients' decisions about reproduction, testing, or management that are consistent with their own belief system.

### Patient Autonomy and Privacy

Genetic counselors are trained to present complicated information in a manner that promotes patient autonomy. They assist patients through a process known as *anticipatory guidance,* helping them to envision how alternative events or courses of action are likely to affect them and their family members. To be effective in this process, genetic counselors must be attuned to the patient's cultural, social, economic, and educational experiences. They must pay particular attention to body language and affective responses and be able adjust to the patient's understanding of information.

One of the most sensitive and complicated challenges to genetic counselors involves respect for patient confidentiality and protection of privacy. Information about an individual's family history, carrier status, diagnosis, or risk of disease is potentially stigmatizing and may lead to discrimination by employers and insurance companies despite state and federal measures to protect patients. In addition, knowing a person's genetic makeup can sometimes provide important information about the genetic risk of relatives who may be unwilling to learn or share this information.[2] The use of computerized databanks and DNA banking facilities has exacerbated the problem of how to ensure the privacy of genetic information. Better legislative measures are needed to safeguard against misuse of genetic information.

As genetic research unearths new information and knowledge, new ethical, medical, social, and legal problems will also arise. Genetic counselors can help patients and their families to anticipate some of these problems and deal with them effectively.

## THE PROCESS OF GENETIC COUNSELING

Patients who seek genetic counseling may be young, elderly, male or female, pregnant or considering starting a family, affected with a disease, at increased risk for a disease, or interested in learning how genetics may influence their health (Box 10-2). Some genetic counseling sessions are simple and require only one visit. At other times, several sessions are needed to gather additional information, update the family, or deal with ongoing medical and psychosocial problems. The first step in a genetic counseling session is to determine why the individual is seeking genetic counseling and to identify what information is desired. Usually only one or two family members, typically a spouse or close family member, attend a counseling session. For genetic counselors the entire family must be considered, not just the person affected or potentially affected with a genetic disease.

### The Pedigree and Testing

Obtaining an accurate pedigree is an important part of genetic counseling. This facilitates diagnosis of a genetic disease, determination of risk of developing a genetic disease, and de-

## BOX 10-2 INDIVIDUALS AND COUPLES WHO MAY BENEFIT FROM GENETIC COUNSELING

- Persons or families with a history of cleft lip or palate, congenital heart defects, spina bifida, short stature, or other physical birth defects
- Persons or families with genetic disorders such as Down syndrome, Huntington disease, cystic fibrosis, muscular dystrophy, phenylketonuria, hemophilia, early-onset breast and ovarian cancer, and other inherited disorders
- Persons or families affected with mental retardation, hearing or visual impairments, learning disabilities, or other conditions that could be genetic
- Persons or families with a history of certain cardiac, cancer, psychiatric, or neurogenetic adult disorders
- Persons with a history of multiple miscarriages, stillbirths, or early infant deaths involving multiple congenital anomalies
- Women age 34 and older who are pregnant or are planning pregnancy
- Pregnant women at high risk because of abnormal maternal serum alpha fetoprotein or ultrasound screening tests
- Pregnant women concerned about the effects of exposure to medication, drugs, chemicals, infectious agents, radiation, or certain work conditions (subspecialty of teratology)
- Persons in specific ethnic groups or geographic areas with a higher incidence of certain disorders, such as Tay-Sachs disease, sickle cell disease, or thalassemias

termination of the risk of having a child with a genetic disease. Use of traditional symbols noting gender, biological relationships, pregnancy outcomes, and disease status allows other clinicians to interpret the family history.[3] Minimally, the pedigree includes first-degree relatives (parents, children, siblings), second-degree relatives (aunts, uncles, grandparents, nieces, nephews), and third-degree relatives (first cousins). The counselor may ask questions about more distant relatives (great-aunts, great-uncles, second cousins) when necessary. Besides depicting familial relationships, a pedigree also contains vital medical information, such as birthdate, age of death, cause of death, health problems, and results of genetic tests. Procuring the medical records of affected relatives can ensure that the verbally reported information is accurate.[4]

Occasionally a pedigree reveals information that was previously unknown by some family members, such as when paternity is misattributed or individuals are identified as carriers for specific genetic diseases. Patients' perception that insurance companies may use information from the pedigree to deny health or life insurance to an at-risk person is usually exaggerated. Until legislation and public policies are in place to safeguard this sensitive information, however, extreme care must be taken to maintain confidentiality.[5,6]

When the pedigree is completed and verified, medical tests may be offered to appropriate individuals. These may be specialized genetic tests such as karyotyping (to study chromosomes) or molecular genetic testing (to detect gene mutations). The tests may also be more general, such as a radiography, ultrasound, urinalysis, skin biopsy, or physical examination. Insurance companies do not always cover the cost of the medical testing, making it difficult or impossible for some relatives to have a complete genetic evaluation. After medical tests are completed and records collected, the genetic counselor may be able to make a diagnosis, or just as importantly, determine that a person does not have or is not at risk for a genetic disease. The pedigree can also be used to estimate the risk of developing the condition or having a child with the condition in other family members.

### Supportive Counseling

Genetic counseling involves more than just communicating complex medical information to families. The most compelling and challenging goal of the profession is to help families cope with the emotional, psychological, medical, social, and economic consequences of genetic disease. Learning about personal genetic or reproductive risk is likely to invoke powerful emotional responses that must be acknowledged and dealt with so that the information can be assimilated and acted on. Different patients react in different and unexpected ways when they learn their genetic risk status. Some take the information in stride, whereas others react with anger, shock, denial, grief, depression, confusion, or guilt.

The role of the genetic counselor is to facilitate coping with the many ramifications of hereditary conditions and genetic testing. Patients with severe psychosocial problems are referred to psychiatrists, social workers, or other clinicians, as appropriate. Many counselors help families having problems with insurance companies or employers who lack understanding of the medical implications of genetic testing. While providing supportive counseling to their patients, counselors serve as patient advocates by referring individuals and families to community or state support services.

## THE FUTURE OF GENETIC COUNSELING

The escalating impact of genetics on medical care by generalists is undeniable. Patients will come to expect medical recommendations that match their genetic profile. The genetic counseling process will increasingly be recognized and utilized as an integral part of the medical interaction. This may be an alarming prospect for hospital specialists and general practitioners who are unprepared to meet the challenges posed by advances in genetics. To meet these challenges, the extended genetic counseling session practiced in major medical centers must transform into an understanding of the theory and practice of genetic counseling by primary caregivers as well as professional genetic counselors. Through a revitalized curriculum capable of wide application, medical students must be prepared to provide the benefits of advances in genetics to all their potential patients. Trained genetic counselors can assist them in this process.

As the future of genetics unfolds, primary care practitioners face the daunting task of keeping abreast of relevant advances in genetics and applying this to their everyday practice while maximizing respect for patient autonomy, privacy, and confidentiality. The power of this knowledge about genetics must be harnessed to increase patients' awareness of their genetic inheritance so that genetic counseling becomes part of routine care. This will not happen unless clinician educators find ways to fill in the gaps in knowledge of genetics, as evident in a study of physicians' interpretations of the implications of APC testing for their patients (Box 10-3).

## BOX 10-3 IMPORTANCE OF CORRECT GENETIC INTERPRETATION

**Background**

The use of commercially available tests for genes linked to familial cancer has resulted in concern about the impact on patients. Familial adenomatous polyposis (FAP) is an autosomal dominant disease caused by a germline mutation of the adenomatous polyposis coli (APC) gene that causes colorectal cancer if prophylactic colectomy is not performed. A group from Johns Hopkins evaluated the clinical use of commercial APC gene testing.

**Methods**

They assessed indications for APC gene testing, determined whether informed consent was obtained and genetic counseling offered before testing, and interpreted the results through telephone interviews with physicians and genetic counselors in a nationwide sample of 177 patients from 125 families.

**Results**

Of the 177 patients tested, 83% had clinical features of FAP or were at risk for the disease, both valid indications for being tested. The appropriate strategy for presymptomatic testing was used in 79.4% (50 of 63 patients). Only 18.6% received genetic counseling before the test, and only 16.9% provided written informed consent. In 31.6% of cases the physicians misinterpreted the test results. Among the patients with unconventional indications for testing, the rate of positive results was only 2.3%.

**Conclusions**

Patients who underwent genetic tests for FAP often received inadequate counseling and would have been given incorrectly interpreted results. Physicians should be prepared to offer genetic counseling if they order genetic tests.

Modified from Giardiello FM, Brensinger JD, Petersen GM, et al: *N Engl J Med* 336(12):823-827, 1997.

## SUMMARY

The need for genetic information will soon be too pervasive to be optional for general practitioners and too ethically and emotionally charged to be provided without appropriate preparation.[7] Those with the skills necessary for effective genetic counseling in medical genetics clinics are best equipped to assist practitioners to function with similar effectiveness in the primary care setting.

## REFERENCES

1. American Society of Human Genetics Ad Hoc Committee on Genetic Counseling: Genetic counseling, *Am J Hum Genet* 27:240-242, 1975.

2. Holtzman NA, Watson MS: Promoting safe and effective genetic testing in the United States: final report of the Task Force on Genetic Testing, 1997.

3. Bennett RL, Steinhaus KA, Uhrich SB, et al: Recommendations for standardized human pedigree nomenclature, *Am J Hum Genet* 56:745-752, 1995.

4. Love R, Evans AM, Josten DM: The accuracy of patient reports of a family history of cancer, *J Chron Dis* 38:289-293, 1995.

5. Hudson KL, Rothenberg KH, Andrews LB, et al: Genetic discrimination and health insurance: an urgent need for reform, *Science* 270:341-352, 1995.

6. Rothenberg KH: Genetic discrimination and health insurance: a call for legislative action, *J Am Med Womens Assoc* 52:43-44, 1997.

7. Giardiello FM, Brensinger JD, Petersen GM, et al: The use and interpretation of commercial *APC* gene testing for familial adenomatous polyposis, *N Engl J Med* 336(12):823-827, 1997.

# CHAPTER 11

# Role of the Nurse in Clinical Genetics

*Lynn A. Jansen*

*Nondirectiveness* has been the dominant technique in genetic counseling for the past 30 years.[1] Nurses and other health care providers have widely endorsed this technique as the best way to protect patient autonomy during the decision-making process. Memories of oppressive social-engineering schemes also motivated strong support for the idea that genetic counselors should act as neutral advisors in their efforts to educate patients about the meaning and use of genetic information.

Despite its widespread appeal, however, doubts have recently been raised about the nondirective model.[2] Rapid advances in genetics have made it possible for clients to gain detailed genetic information about themselves. This information, in turn, increasingly has broad health implications for the relatives of clients as well as for society in general.[3] As a result, some critics of the nondirective approach now argue that too strict a commitment to it could result in harm to innocent third parties.[4]

These doubts clearly pose an important challenge to the nondirective model. Still, it is not clear what model should replace it if the nondirective approach is indeed deemed unsatisfactory. This chapter proposes an alternative approach to genetic counseling that is not strictly nondirective or directive. This *deliberative model* applies to all health care providers engaged in genetic counseling, with special implications for the nurse in this process. Nurses define themselves professionally as *patient advocates*.[5] The deliberative model fits well with this professional self-understanding.

## NURSING AND NONDIRECTIVENESS

New genetic technologies have increased the demand for genetic services. Genetic counseling is an attractive option for persons who desire susceptibility screening for late-onset diseases such as diabetes, coronary artery disease, Huntington disease, and certain cancers.[6] This increased demand for genetic information has created a need for highly trained professionals to deliver genetic counseling.[7] Nurses have begun to fill this need by assuming responsibility for the management of patients with genetic disorders. In particular, advanced practice nurses now function as members of multidisciplinary genetic counseling teams.[8] In this capacity, they develop treatment plans and provide counseling to patients and their families.

By responding to the increased demand for these services, highly trained nurses in genetic counseling fulfill an important practical need, but this involvement raises some difficult questions. Do nurses have any distinctive contribution to make to genetic counseling? What in their professional training and experience makes nurses valuable members of genetic counseling teams?

The answers to these questions depend on what disposition nurses adopt in the context of genetic counseling. These questions have different answers depending on whether nurses approach this role as patient advocates, a perspective that now defines their professional self-image, or through the nondirective model, which defines the professional self-image of the genetic counselor.

As patient advocates, nurses "have a prima facie obligation to act in ways that will protect and enhance the interests and rights of their patients."[9] This obligation directs nurses to assume a proactive role in educating patients and empowering them to make informed autonomous decisions.[10] The nurse's role as educator is not merely to provide medical information to patients, but also to help them understand and assess its significance for their lives. Importantly, when nurses function as patient advocates, they take an active interest in their patients' decisions and try to help them reach the best decisions.[11]

In contrast, the nondirective approach enjoins genetic counselors to adopt the morally neutral disposition of a technical expert.[2] The emphasis on moral neutrality requires the counselor to respect a strict fact/value division of labor between counselor and client.[12] According to this strict division of labor, the task of the genetic counselor is to ensure that the client has a clear understanding of all the relevant scientific facts concerning the "nature of the [client's] disorder, its severity and prognosis and whether or not there is effective therapy."[13] Conversely, the task of the client is to interpret this information in accord with his or her own values. On this understanding, the client's values are the only ones brought to bear on the decision-making process.[12] The counselor should respect the decision-making authority of clients by not attempting to "direct" them to any particular decision.

Therefore an incompatibility, or at least a tension, exists between these two perspectives. As patient advocate, the nurse strives to guide patients toward making the decision that she or he believes is in the patient's best interest. The demands of the nondirective technique require the nurse to adopt a more neutral stance when advising patients about genetic information.

Genetic counselors who defend the nondirective model may believe that nondirective genetic counseling protects and promotes clients' best interests. They may "believe that counselors will be most effective at communicating and conveying information if they listen carefully to those who seek their help and avoid directly challenging or confronting their clients."[2] This is not always true, however, and a genuine tension can develop between these two perspectives.

If the nondirective approach is the best technique for genetic counseling, the resolution of this tension requires nurses to adopt a different perspective when acting as genetic counselors than when serving in other professional capacities. This will make it more difficult to identify any distinctive contribution of nurses to genetic counseling. If, on the other hand, the nondirective approach is rejected in favor of some other technique, a stronger case may be possible for the role of nurses on genetic counseling teams. That is, the nurse's involvement may be viewed as serving a substantive function. For this reason, to understand the specific contribution nurses can and should make to genetic counseling, we must consider whether the nondirective model is the best approach.

## NONDIRECTIVE TECHNIQUE

The following three claims are frequently advanced in defense of nondirectiveness in genetic counseling:

1. The nondirective approach is necessary to respect client autonomy.
2. The evaluative significance of genetic information is strictly personal.
3. Directive genetic counseling could violate client privacy interests.

Proponents of the first claim defend a view of autonomy that emphasizes the right of clients to make choices free from outside interference.[4] On this view, genetic counselors respect the autonomy of their clients by presenting them with information in a clear and neutral manner and by leaving them free to interpret this information according to their own values.

Proponents of the second claim argue that the evaluative significance of genetic facts is strictly personal, since the client's values are the client's concern and are not subject to correction by the genetic counselor.[7] This argument rests on the assumption that the client's values are incorrigible.[14] Any decision the client reaches on the basis of these values cannot be faulted for being incorrect. On this assumption there is no reason to engage in rational discussion of the client's values with the aim of improving or correcting them. The only reason for such discussion would be to help clients clarify their values in light of the genetic information provided.

Proponents of the third claim argue that in some contexts, directive genetic counseling could violate the client's privacy interests. This concern is most evident when genetic counseling concerns reproductive issues.[6] Social, moral, and legal convictions about reproductive freedom and privacy have led some to think that genetic counselors must adopt the nondirective model.[3,15]

Clearly, these three claims raise valid concerns. Infringements of client autonomy, the imposition of the counselor's values on the client, and violations of client privacy should be avoided by the genetic counselor. However, these valid concerns would provide a reason to adopt the nondirective approach only if this was the only effective safeguard against such abuses. As seen with the deliberative model of genetic counseling, this is not the case.

### Challenges

Despite the claims in its favor, the nondirective technique has been questioned by recent developments in genetic technology. These developments strongly suggest that the conception of autonomy assumed in defense of nondirectiveness is too thin to meet the ethical demands of the new genetics. This conception of autonomy does not account for the ways in which genetic counselors are ethically required to help their clients deliberate effectively about genetic information.

Consider, for example, the difficulty of making autonomous decisions when one is confronted with complex information. In such a context, access to complete and accurate information may be necessary to autonomous decision making, but it is not sufficient. One must also be able to interpret this information and assess its impact on one's well-being. As genetic technologies progress and as genetic information becomes more complex, the assumption that clients can evaluate information independently becomes less plausible.[4] This is especially true with predictive genetic testing for adult-onset disorders. Research on decision making in this context suggests that clients often encounter difficulty understanding how the information bears on the medical options open to them, and they frequently solicit the counselor's opinion.[16] Clients also may consider other outside sources equally important for sound decision making. In some contexts, therefore, clients may reasonably "prefer to exercise their autonomy by controlling the method by which decisions are made, rather than controlling the ultimate decision."[17] Under such circumstances, respect for autonomy may require the genetic counselor to give prescriptive advice or offer normative recommendations about how the client should weigh the risks and benefits associated with the available options.[2]

The possible uses of advanced recombinant DNA technologies also challenge the evaluative significance of genetic information being strictly personal. These technologies permit genetic testing for a variety of genetic diseases, from coronary artery disease to cancer. The facts revealed are not only about the client but concern others as well. Suppose a client discovers through presymptomatic testing that he has a gene mutation for Huntington disease. The presence of this mutation strongly suggests that other family members may also be at risk for this disease.[18] If the client does not want to contact his relatives about this information, the genetic counselor is put in a difficult position. Should she attempt to persuade the client to consider informing his relatives of their increased risk, or should she maintain a commitment to moral neutrality? The nondirective technique clearly limits her role to informing the client of the genetic information. Because others could also benefit from this information, however, the client's decision about how to use the information is not strictly a personal affair.

A strong commitment to the nondirective model can put the counselor in an ethically tenuous position. As genetic information becomes relevant to a wider range of persons, the assumption that the client's preferences and values are incorrigible becomes increasingly less plausible. Counselors who encounter such situations often believe they have an obligation to move beyond simply informing the client. Whether or not they are right to believe this, the claim that the client's values could not be mistaken seems wrong. The idea actually is not plausible even when the genetic information concerns only the client. People often make mistakes in reasoning and fail to give sufficient weight to all the considerations that affect the choices before them. No reason exists to think that this ceases to be true when people make decisions based on genetic information they have received. This does not suggest that the counselor's values should override those of the client, but only that it is a mistake to assume that the values of clients cannot be improved through rational deliberation.

# DELIBERATIVE TECHNIQUE

The previous considerations suggest that the nondirective technique is not well suited for dealing with the problems created by the new genetics. This challenge rings hollow, however, as long as it remains unclear what alternative model of genetic counseling should replace the nondirective approach. Many will continue to support nondirectiveness in genetic counseling because they do not see a better alternative. As noted, directive genetic counseling has negative connotations, including a failure to respect the autonomy and privacy of clients. If the choice involves directiveness or nondirectiveness in genetic counseling, nondirectiveness will prevail.

This choice is misconceived, however, because there are other options. In particular, the counselor-client relationship can be conceived as a *deliberative relationship* in which both parties have a responsibility to engage in rational discussion with the purpose of discovering the best decision that the client should make in light of the genetic information that is revealed. This deliberative technique of genetic counseling cannot be described as directive or nondirective. It shares properties of both techniques. As in the directive approach, it holds that counselors should discuss evaluative considerations as well as factual information with their clients. As with the nondirective model, it holds that counselors must respect the autonomy of their clients and must therefore not simply impose their evaluative views on them.

The deliberative approach also fits well with the nurse's professional self-understanding. Rather than ask nurses to put aside the perspective of patient advocate when they engage in genetic counseling, it draws on the distinctive skills and experiences associated with nursing as a profession. If it can be shown to be a good model for genetic counseling, the earlier concerns about nurses' contribution can be addressed.

Evaluation of the deliberative model must answer the following questions:

1. What is the content of the deliberation that it recommends?
2. How does deliberative genetic counseling protect client autonomy?
3. Why is this kind of deliberation valuable?

## Deliberative Content and Stances

Deliberation between the genetic counselor and the client should begin when the counselor first encounters the client in the clinic and should extend to when the client is ready to make a decision about the genetic information disclosed. The counselor should assume the role of *deliberative partner* and discuss with the client the relevant genetic facts and consequences of alternative decisions. Partnership between counselor and client is emphasized because effective deliberation presupposes a dynamic of reciprocity in which both the counselor and the client have something to learn.

The deliberation between counselor and client should extend to the values of the client as well as to the relevant medical facts. The counselor should challenge clients to think about their reasons for the decisions being considered. The counselor should not be judgmental, but the counselor should consider that the client's values can be improved by rational discussion. Since this idea defines the difference between the deliberative model and the nondirective model, it is helpful to clarify the types of deliberation used. A counselor can take four stances with respect to the values and preferences of a client: (1) nonevaluative, (2) values clarification, (3) deliberative, and (4) judgmental (Table 11-1).

The *nonevaluative stance,* as discussed, requires the counselor to avoid discussing the client's values. The *values clarification stance* permits the counselor to discuss values with the client, but only for the limited purpose of helping the client to understand his own values. This stance is compatible with the idea that the client's values are incorrigible, since it assumes only that the client may not fully understand her own values. It does not assume that these values could be mistaken. Both the nonevaluative and the values clarification stances are associated with the nondirective model.

In sharp contrast with these two stances, the *deliberative stance* assumes that clients' values could be mistaken and thus could be improved by rational discussion. The counselor challenges clients to reflect on their values and consider their reasons for the decisions being considered. The counselor also discusses relevant evaluative considerations that clients are overlooking.

It is important not to confuse the deliberative stance with the *judgmental stance.* Judgmental genetic counselors assume their views are correct. They view their task as bringing the client's decisions into line with their own values. Therefore, since rational deliberation with the client is unnecessary, genetic counseling becomes an exercise in directing the client toward the "correct" decisions. Proponents of the nondirective technique frequently assume that the only alternative is directive genetic counseling. Distinguishing the deliberative

### TABLE 11-1

## Four Stances of Genetic Counseling

|  | Nonevaluative | Values Clarification | Deliberative | Judgmental |
|---|---|---|---|---|
| Counselor's responsibility | Provide client with all relevant factual information | Provide client with all relevant factual information; assist client in interpreting and understanding values | Provide client with all relevant information; assist client in thinking critically about values that bear on decision | Provide client with all relevant information; guide client toward correct decision as defined by counselor |
| Conception of client autonomy | Thin | Thin | Thick | Hostile |
| Client's values | Subjective and incorrigible | Subjective and incorrigible | Revisable and subject to correction and improvement | Objective and defined by counselor |

stance from the judgmental stance shows why this is a mistake. Genetic counselors can engage in rational discussion with their clients about the content of their clients' values without adopting the judgmental stance characteristic of directive genetic counseling.

### Client Autonomy

Even with the content of its deliberation clarified, the deliberative model may still seem paternalistic. Since some worry that client autonomy would be jeopardized if counselors adopted the deliberative stance, the decision-making phase must be distinguished from the deliberative phase of the genetic counseling process. In the deliberative phase the counselor and the client rationally discuss the facts and values that affect the choices open to the client. At some point, however, deliberation must end. In the best of circumstances, deliberation ends in consensus: counselor and client agree on the best course of action for the client. Sometimes, rational discussion fails to lead to consensus. According to the deliberative technique, the client has the authority to make the decision that he or she believes is best. In this way the deliberative approach safeguards client autonomy.

### Value of Deliberative Approach

Two primary values are promoted by rational deliberation: client autonomy and improved client decision making. The deliberative model not only safeguards client autonomy but actively promotes it. When clients are faced with difficult and complex information, rational deliberation can enable them to discover what they really want to do. The deliberative model embodies a "thicker" conception of autonomy than that seen with the nondirective approach. With the deliberative technique, "autonomy requires that individuals critically assess their own values and preferences; determine whether they are desirable; affirm, upon reflection, these values as the ones that should justify their actions; and then be free to initiate action to realize the values."[19] Autonomous decision making clearly requires more than nonjudgmental noninterference. It requires the critical scrutiny of the decision maker's values and preferences. By promoting this kind of critical scrutiny, deliberative genetic counseling promotes client autonomy.

Equally important, rational deliberation serves the value of improved client decision making. Rational deliberation does not guarantee that the client will make the correct or best decision, but it does increase the likelihood. Rational deliberation between counselor and client makes it more likely that all the relevant considerations—evaluative and nonevaluative—will be considered and that the client will think carefully about these considerations in his or her decision making.

## NURSING AND DELIBERATIVE COUNSELING

For the reasons discussed, the deliberative model is superior to nondirective genetic counseling. This conclusion applies to all health care providers involved in genetic counseling, but it has special importance for the nurse. Some disagree about the proper interpretation of nurses' professional identity as patient advocates, but most agree that it requires nurses to take an active role in advancing the best interests of their patients.[20] This ideal also requires nurses to act in ways that promote the autonomy of their patients. The nondirective technique of genetic counseling creates a tension with this ideal. In some contexts, particularly those involving new genetic technologies, nondirective genetic counseling will neither advance the best interests of clients nor promote their autonomy.

Deliberative genetic counseling also allows identification the distinctive contribution of nurses to genetic counseling teams. With their training and experience, advanced practice nurses are particularly well suited to serve as deliberative genetic counselors. This is true for two reasons. First, "nurses are often, in a physical and relational sense of the term, closer to individual patients than doctors."[9] Nurses often care for patients for extended periods and thus are more likely than physicians (or other members of the health care team) to develop insights into their patients' needs and values. This closeness to the patient encourages the development of a specific disposition in nurses. More so than other health care professionals, nurses are inclined to view patients as "whole persons."[9] This disposition would be valuable to genetic counselors. If the deliberative model is accepted, the counselor will need to engage in dialogue with the client about particular values and preferences.

Second, given their institutional role in the contemporary hospital, nurses must develop skill in collaborating with physicians, patients, and family members. This has led some to characterize nurses as "natural mediators."[21] To the extent that nurses' background and experience provide them with skill in mediating conflicts, nurses would likely contribute to the success of deliberative genetic counseling. Deliberative genetic counseling is best carried out in multidisciplinary teams of health care professionals that include physicians, social workers, geneticists, and nurses. If genetic counselors are to discuss values as well as nonevaluative facts with their clients, conflict will more likely arise between different team members, making participation by genetic counselors who can mediate conflicts more important.

Deliberative genetic counseling would establish an important role for advanced practice nurses on genetic counseling teams. Unlike the nondirective approach, which requires nurses to put aside their professional disposition and their distinctive professional skills when they become genetic counselors, the deliberative model allows them to draw freely on these skills. In so doing, the quality of genetic counseling would improve.

## SUMMARY

New genetic technologies have created significant opportunities for advanced practice nurses to participate in genetic counseling teams. To understand the contribution that nurses can make to genetic counseling, we must rethink the role of the genetic counselor. A new model for genetic counseling, the deliberative approach, responds to the challenges posed by new genetic tests and increases the value of including nurses on genetic counseling teams. Successful deliberative genetic counseling requires skills that nurses are likely to possess, given their training and professional experience. To the extent, therefore, that the deliberative model is accepted, the recent involvement of nurses on genetic counseling teams is a positive development and not merely a practical response to the increased demand for genetic counseling.

# REFERENCES

1. Sorenson JR: Genetic counseling: values that have mattered. In Bartels DM, LeRoy BS, Caplan AL, editors: *Prescribing our future: ethical challenges in genetic counseling,* Hawthorne, NY, 1993, Aldine de Gruyter.

2. Caplan AL: Neutrality is not morality: the ethics of genetic counseling. In Bartels DM, LeRoy BS, Caplan AL, editors: *Prescribing our future: ethical challenges in genetic counseling,* Hawthorne, NY, 1993, Aldine de Gruyter.

3. Harris R: The new genetics: a challenge to traditional medicine, *J R Coll Physicians Lond* 25(2):134-140, 1991.

4. Yarborough M, Scott JA, Dixon LK: The role of beneficence in clinical genetics: non-directive genetic counseling reconsidered, *Theor Med* 10:139-149, 1989.

5. Winslow GR: From loyalty to advocacy: a new metaphor for nursing, *Hastings Center Report,* June 1984, pp 32-40.

6. Fraser FC: Current issues in medical genetics, *Am J Hum Genet* 26:636-659, 1974.

7. Fine B: The evolution of nondirectiveness in genetic counseling and implications of the Human Genome Project. In Bartels DM, LeRoy BS, Caplan AL, editors: *Prescribing our future: ethical challenges in genetic counseling,* Hawthorne, NY, 1993, Aldine de Gruyter.

8. Lea HD, Jenkins JF, Francomano CA: *Genetics in clinical practice: new directions for nursing and health care,* Boston, 1998, Jones & Bartlett.

9. Kuhse H: *Caring: nurses, women and ethics,* Oxford, 1997, Blackwell.

10. Ryden MB: An approach to ethical decision making, *Nurs Outlook* 26:705-706, 1978.

11. Nelson ML: Advocacy in nursing: how has it evolved and what are its implications for practice? *Nurs Outlook* 36:136-141, 1988.

12. Gervais KG: Objectivity, value neutrality and nondirectiveness in genetic counseling. In Bartels DM, LeRoy BS, Caplan AL, editors: *Prescribing our future: ethical challenges in genetic counseling,* Hawthorne, NY, 1993, Aldine de Gruyter.

13. Williams A: Genetic counseling: a nurse's perspective. In Clarke A, editor: *Genetic counseling: practice and principles,* New York, 1994, Routledge.

14. Brock D: *Life and death: philosophical essays in biomedical ethics,* Cambridge, 1995, Cambridge University Press.

15. Pergament E: A clinical geneticist perspective of the patient-physician relationship. In Rothstein MA, editor: *Genetic secrets: protecting privacy and confidentiality in the genetic era,* New Haven, Conn, 1997, Yale University Press.

16. Kessler S: The psychological foundations of genetic counseling. In *Genetic counseling: psychological dimensions,* London, 1979, Academic Press.

17. Mahowald MB, Verp MS, Anderson RR: Genetic counseling: clinical and ethical challenges, *Annu Rev Genet* 32:547-559, 1998.

18. Mahowald MB: *Genes, women, equality,* New York, 2000, Oxford University Press.

19. Emmanuel L, Emmanuel E: Four models of the doctor-patient relationship, *JAMA* 267(16):2221-2226, 1992.

20. Watt E: An exploration of the way in which the concept of patient-advocacy is perceived by registered nurses working in an acute care hospital, *Int J Nurs Pract* 3:119-127, 1997.

21. Mallik M: Advocacy in nursing: perceptions and attitudes of nursing elite in the United Kingdom, *J Adv Nurs* 28(5)1001-1011, 1998.

# PART III

# SPECIFIC ISSUES FOR PRIMARY CAREGIVERS

# CHAPTER 12

# Ethical Issues in Obstetric Genetics

*Cathleen M. Harris*

*Marion S. Verp*

Obstetrics has raised more ethical and social issues than other areas of medicine, as illustrated by the ongoing debate about abortion and by the complex issues of assisted reproduction. Genetic analysis of early embryos is now possible in conjunction with in vitro fertilization through preimplantation genetic diagnosis (see Chapter 5). This union of reproductive and genetic technologies has created ethical dilemmas previously present in separate domains. With accelerated genetic testing and treatment options, these issues will increase in number and complexity.

This chapter addresses some of the ethical issues raised in the obstetric setting by advances in genetics. The goal is to facilitate care for pregnant or potentially pregnant patients. The recommendations offered later have not been formally reviewed or officially endorsed by organizations such as the American College of Obstetrics and Gynecology or the Institute of Medicine, but they are consistent with guidelines developed by those groups.[1-4]

## PRENATAL GENETIC DIAGNOSIS AND WOMEN'S AUTONOMY

The availability of prenatal diagnosis and therapy may increase a pregnant woman's autonomy and enhance reproductive decision making by allowing her to make informed choices about her pregnancy. When offered in the context of genetic counseling, prenatal diagnosis is intended to help individuals achieve their reproductive goals. Since prenatal genetic testing provides women with the choice of whether or not to bear children with abnormalities, it enhances autonomy.[5]

Paradoxically, however, a pregnant woman's autonomy may be jeopardized by the availability of prenatal diagnosis. This could occur when a woman feels compelled to accept testing. For some women, merely receiving the offer of genetic testing could imply that a provider endorses and recommends such an approach. The availability of new genetic tests for an increasing number of conditions may pressure women to undergo testing for genetic problems and possibly to abort affected fetuses. Coercion to participate in genetic testing may come from a variety of sources, including "researchers interested in the information that genetic testing generates, clinicians whose incomes are based on procedures performed, and technology companies that profit from providing genetic analyses."[6] Additional influences on women's reproductive decision making include family, insurance agencies, and society. All these could also represent threats to women's autonomy. Fortunately, laws have generally upheld women's autonomy as taking precedent in situations of conflict.

### Nondirective Counseling

Nonetheless, the growing amount of genetic information available to clients makes some women feel overwhelmed and burdened by their choices. With the advent of new genetic tests, the validity of nondirectiveness in genetic counseling, a central tenet of the profession, has been reexamined. Some believe that nondirectiveness contradicts the general methods and goals of public health programs, that is, identifying persons in high-risk groups and effecting behavior change.[7] True nondirectiveness is probably unattainable. In some circumstances, however, genetic counselors are intentionally directive in their advice, particularly when a woman's behavior is likely to influence the health outcome. Examples include recommending folic acid supplementation to reduce the risk of neural tube defects or following a prescribed diet for pregnant women with phenylketonuria. Nondirectiveness remains appropriate, however, when reproductive decisions are involved.

With the increasing volume and complexity of genetic information, women will consult their providers and genetic counselors more often for guidance. It may not be detrimental for counselors to respond to clients' queries and offer directive advice in certain cases. The advice may not be paternalistic even if it is directive, "so long as it does not constitute imposition on the client's capacity to make her own decision."[6]

Nondirective counseling empowers counselees with the capacity and ability to make their own decisions; it enhances a counselee's self-determining capacities. With directiveness, the counselor takes responsibility for the counselee's actions and decisions, and the directive carries the weight of the counselor's expertise. Nondirective approaches may be best used to clarify a counselee's thinking, needs, and desires. Directive counseling can then confirm the counselee's direction.[8] Such an integrated approach to genetic counseling may become more acceptable and appropriate.

## NEW GENETICS AND "MATERNAL-FETAL CONFLICT"

The concept of the fetus as a patient has become part of clinical practice as a result of prenatal diagnosis. Prenatal diagnosis was initially criticized as being merely a "search and destroy" mission, because the only option available to women with affected fetuses was abortion or delivery. The recent potential for successful treatment of unborn patients is a result of new genetic tests and other technologies such as ultrasonography.

Therefore the appropriateness of prenatal diagnosis and therapy relates to the moral status of the fetus, embryo, or preembryo. If fetuses, embryos, and preembryos have no status as persons, society has no obligation to offer treatment to them for genetic diseases. Because embryos and fetuses have a new genotype, however, and some will become children and adults, the "preborn" should be given full moral status as persons who have a right to life. In this case, society is obliged to offer therapy to fetuses affected with genetic diseases. A third possibility is that society considers preembryos, embryos, or fetuses as potential persons. As such, they should be regarded with dignity and their rights should be respected, but these rights do not supersede those of others. Many consider this egalitarian definition of developing humans to be acceptable. Even with this compromise, however, no consensus exists on the stage of development at which the status of potential or full human should be conferred. Chervenak and McCullough[9] suggest that the moral status of the previable fetus "can be established only by the pregnant woman's autonomous decision to confer the status of being a patient." This definition would seem to apply equally well to an embryo or a fetus, but it is less clear how the distinction applies to preembryos.

Many who work in the field of prenatal diagnosis and therapy seem comfortable with the assumption that the "preborn" do not have full moral status but are potential persons. Thus, attempting to treat disease in this population is a reasonable goal. However, most fetal conditions or malformations do not threaten maternal health. In fact, interventions that have potential benefit for the fetus (or embryo) are often a risk to the pregnant woman. Therefore she must be willing to accept significant risks and discomfort from testing procedures and treatments intended to help her offspring. These considerations are not changed by the new genetics.

Incorporating the advances in genetics into prenatal diagnosis and therapy is not likely to change the way society views fetuses. This paradigm shift has already occurred, and society has conferred on some fetuses the status of patients. Rather than a change in the nature of "maternal-fetal conflict," a change in the frequency of these scenarios is more likely. More diseases are potentially amenable to in utero diagnosis and treatment as a result of the new genetics. Therefore more women may need to balance the best interests of their offspring with their own health. (An intervention that does not involve the previous reasoning is the prospect of treatment of preimplantation embryos with germline gene alteration. At present, such therapies are proscribed.)

## PRIVACY OF GENETIC INFORMATION

Genetic information has been regarded as a privileged type of health information because it relates to one's genetic identity, it predicts one's future health, and it is relevant to other family members. Through new technology, genetic makeup can be examined as distinct from physical characteristics. Individuals may want to keep their genetic information private because it can be used to stigmatize and discriminate against them; it may also be embarrassing. In particular, prenatal screening increases the amount and type of genetic information included in a woman's medical files. If such information were revealed, it could harm a patient's reputation and increase family conflict.[10] Thus, keeping genetic records private is critically important if prenatal diagnosis programs are to gain wider public acceptance.

With the incorporation of new genetic tests into clinical medicine, adults will undergo multiple genetic tests, possibly revealing that they are carriers of mutations for single-gene disorders or susceptibility genes for common diseases. This information has a significant impact on the individual, offspring, and other family members. Problems of confidentiality include issues of full disclosure to women and their relatives at risk and disclosure to employers or insurers.

Two common clinical scenarios illustrate the ethical dilemmas with regard to disclosure of information to patients and their relatives. First, prenatal genetic testing occasionally leads to unexpected findings of misattributed paternity. Most geneticists indicate that they would communicate this information to the woman but would not volunteer this information to her partner. This approach does not address possible conflicts between family members' interests and inevitably leaves the counselor to subordinate the partner's right to know to the woman's right to privacy—an uncomfortable position for everyone.

Second, a counselee's confidentiality can be threatened if serious harm would occur to a third party because of inherited gene mutations. Physicians are legally permitted but not legally required to disclose genetic information to relatives against a patient's wishes. There is precedent for such breaches of confidentiality of health information. Public health departments have used partner notification programs for reportable sexually transmitted diseases to alert persons exposed to infections, with the rationale that it is acceptable to compromise an individual's privacy in the interest of the population's health.

An ethical argument for testing and disclosure of genetic testing for partners or blood relatives is that they could be at risk of developing a genetic disorder or having children with a genetic disorder. It is arguable, however, whether genetic disorders should be considered public health risks. Again, geneticists tend not to advocate disclosure to relatives in such cases, but there is clearly no consensus on this matter. From a philosophical standpoint, providers and genetics counselors need to decide whether their client is the individual or the family.[7]

With regard to disclosure to employers and insurers, employers and insurance companies may want to exclude individuals whose future health care bills are expected to be costly. This phenomenon initially began among adults with genetic disorders but has already started to occur with prenatal diagnosis. For example, some insurers have refused to pay medical costs for children with cystic fibrosis born to couples who had prenatal diagnosis and who chose to carry an affected child to term.[7] Women must be allowed to access genetic services while preserving their right to refuse genetic screening (for carrier testing or for prenatal genetic diagnosis) and preventing their choice from being used to discriminate against them or their offspring.

## PRENATAL DIAGNOSIS WITHOUT MEDICAL INDICATIONS

Traditionally, prenatal genetic testing has dealt with diagnosing conditions incompatible with life or seriously disabling. With new genetic testing, clinicians will be able to test fetuses for less serious disorders and even for specific characteristics. Providers and genetic counselors will likely face conflicts about being nondirective regarding testing for "low-burden" disorders or particular characteristics.

Over time, however, advances in medical care, societal norms, and expectations often change what society considers serious versus mild disease. For example, Down syndrome was considered a serious disorder because of reduced life expectancy and need for institutionalization, but today many families accept the responsibility of raising a child with Down syndrome because of a shift in society's perceptions of persons with Down syndrome.[11] Many geneticists consider it paternalistic to withhold testing for mildly severe diseases. More than ever, providers need to understand the factors that influence their beliefs and those of their patients.

To have "more perfect" babies, some women will seek prenatal diagnosis without clear medical indications. As prenatal diagnosis becomes safer for the fetus and as noninvasive methods are developed, such as analyzing fetal cells in maternal blood, demands for prenatal diagnosis of milder disorders are likely to increase. Again, withholding this testing from a woman may be criticized as unnecessary and paternalistic. Nonetheless, tension is likely to increase between offering testing for mild disorders and dealing with the consequences of possible pregnancy terminations for fetuses with nonlethal abnormalities or undesired characteristics.[7]

In this regard, sex selection is the most controversial use of prenatal diagnosis. Sex selection can be performed by chorionic villus sampling, amniocentesis, or ultrasound and through preimplantation diagnosis. Most ethicists conclude that sex selection for whatever purpose, even "balancing" the children in a family, works to the overall disadvantage of women because it reinforces gender stereotyping. In many parts of the world, however, including the United States, physicians do not consider sex selection a social problem. Some see it as an extension of parental free choice, just as parents can choose the number and spacing of their children.[7] Selection of male or female fetuses may be justified on medical grounds, such as the case of inherited X-linked disorders, and may be morally defensible in other situations, provided the intentions and results are not sexist.[6]

## ACCESS TO GENETICS SERVICES

Most would agree that women should have equal access to whatever genetic services exist, regardless of their ability to pay. However, equal access to genetic services for low-income women and women of color has not been attained. Women with high levels of education and high socioeconomic status are more likely to use genetic services than women with low levels of income or education. Most women using genetic services are white, well educated, and middle to upper class. Access to prenatal diagnosis is related to access to health care in general. Thousands of families continue to be uninsured, and many providers will not accept Medicaid from women seeking prenatal care. Although women may receive prenatal care at federally funded clinics, new patients often have to wait a long time. Long waiting periods can prohibit women from accessing genetics services, particularly when they seek care late in pregnancy. Further, Medicaid funding for prenatal diagnosis and abortion services varies considerably among states, and these services are not covered in some states.

Aside from financial concerns, sociocultural barriers block utilization of genetic services. Language barriers may prevent some minority women from receiving genetic services. Cultural factors can shape women's attitudes toward prenatal genetic services.

Low-income women and women of color may not hold the same views as the dominant culture and the medical profession. For example, prenatal testing may have little value for women who for religious reasons would not terminate a pregnancy or who are unable to pay for an abortion if they would decide to terminate an affected fetus.[12]

There is a widening gap in the technologies accessible to affluent women versus indigent women. New genetic tests are marketed shortly after mutations for diseases are found, but the tests are available only to those who can pay for them. Poor women are likely to have access to such new tests only if their participation is useful to researchers.[6] One author suggests that the number of children with genetic conditions born to minority and low-income women could increase due to these types of disparities. Conversely, in the future, poor people might be coerced to abort because they are perceived to create an economic burden on society by having a disabled child.[10]

## SUMMARY

An underlying assumption in the development of molecular techniques for prenatal genetic diagnosis has been that physicians someday would be able to prevent the negative consequences of genetic disease by diagnosing and treating human embryos or fetuses before irreversible changes lead to disability. Before the advances in genetics, options available to parents at increased risk of having a child with a genetic disease included (1) choosing not to have children, (2) adopting a child, (3) becoming pregnant and hoping the child is unaffected, or (4) undergoing prenatal diagnosis using conventional cytogenetics, with or without abortion of an affected fetus. With the new genetic technology, however, parents will have much more information about the health of their fetuses. They also have more options for diagnosis and treatment, such as preimplantation diagnosis, which potentially circumvents the issue of abortion, or prenatal therapy for conditions amenable to treatment.

The ethical dilemmas surrounding prenatal genetic testing are not alleviated by the incorporation of the new genetic tests into clinical practice. More options may lead to more dilemmas. Issues of maternal autonomy, privacy, and equal access to services will increase. At this time, there is no universally accepted approach to dealing with ethical problems in prenatal diagnosis and therapy. The new genetic technology is incorporated into clinical medicine to empower patients and physicians to make informed decisions about their health and to develop rational strategies for minimizing or preventing disease. This is similar to the original goals of prenatal diagnosis and therapy. Clinicians must take an active role to ensure that women and their offspring are not controlled, coerced, or discriminated against on the basis of their choices.

## RECOMMENDATIONS

- Genetic screening during pregnancy should remain strictly voluntary, but all pregnant women or women contemplating pregnancy should be offered genetic counseling and screening services.
- Counseling regarding reproductive decisions should continue to be nondirective because of the many different value systems regarding pregnancy, abortion, and prenatal therapy.

Directiveness in genetic counseling may be acceptable when a woman's behavior has a clear impact on the outcome.
- Prenatal genetic test results should remain confidential, unless serious harm to a third party would occur.
- Women and children should not be subject to discrimination based on their genotypes.
- Prenatal diagnosis should not be performed without a clear genetic indication—either a suspected genetic condition or a child from a high-risk family. Conversely, genetic services need not always be withheld from women seeking genetic diagnosis for mild disorders or other traits.
- Pregnant women should not be compelled to participate in prenatal treatment for a fetal condition, especially when treatments place her at some health risk.
- Equal access to genetic services should be provided for all pregnant women; this requires significant changes in the health care system.

# REFERENCES

1. American College of Obstetricians and Gynecologists: Prenatal detection of neural tube defects, ACOG Technical Bulletin No 99, Washington, DC, 1986, ACOG.

2. American College of Obstetricians and Gynecologists: Genetic technologies, ACOG Technical Bulletin No 208, Washington, DC, 1995, ACOG.

3. American College of Obstetricians and Gynecologists: Maternal multiple marker screening, ACOG Educational Bulletin No 228, Washington, DC, 1996, ACOG.

4. Andrews LB, Fullarton JE, Holtzman NA, Motulsky AG, editors: *Assessing genetic risks: implications for health and social policy,* Institute of Medicine Committee on Assessing Genetic Risks, Washington, DC, 1994, National Academy Press.

5. Gates EA: Prenatal genetic testing: does it benefit pregnant women? In Rothenberg KH, Thomson EJ, editors: *Women and prenatal testing: facing the challenges of genetic technology,* Columbus, 1994, Ohio State University Press.

6. Mahowald MB: *Genes, women, equality,* New York, 2000, Oxford University Press.

7. Wertz DC: Ethical and legal implications of the new genetics: issues for discussion, *Soc Sci Med* 35(4):495-505, 1992.

8. Kessler S: Psychological aspects of genetic counseling. VII. Thoughts on directiveness, *J Genet Counsel* 1(1):9-17, 1992.

9. Chervenak FA, McCullough LB: Ethical implications for early pregnancy of the fetus as a patient: a basic ethical concept in fetal medicine, *Early Pregnancy* 1(4):253-257, 1995.

10. Nsiah-Jefferson L: Reproductive genetic services for low-income women and women of color. In Rothenberg KH, Thomson EJ, editors: *Women and prenatal testing: facing the challenges of genetic technology,* Columbus, 1994, Ohio State University Press.

11. Fine B: The evolution of nondirectiveness in genetic counseling and implications of the Human Genome Project. In Bartels DM, LeRoy BS, Caplan AL, editors: *Prescribing our future: ethical challenges in genetic counseling,* Hawthorne, NY, 1993, Aldine de Gruyter.

12. Mahowald MB, Levinson D, Cassel C, et al: The new genetics and women, *Milbank Q* 74(2):239-283, 1996.

# CHAPTER 13

# Ethical Issues
# in Pediatric Genetics

*Lainie Friedman Ross*
*Margaret R. Moon*

Clinical genetics is an integral part of pediatrics. Genetic diseases are common in childhood: as many as 53 per 1000 children and young adults can be expected to have diseases with an important genetic component.[1] This rate increases to 79 per 1000 if congenital anomalies are included. In addition, 12% to 40% of all pediatric hospitalizations are caused by genetic diseases and birth defects.[2-4] Despite its importance in primary care pediatrics, genetics has maintained its subspecialty status. Newborn screening for genetic diseases is the only aspect of genetics that has been incorporated as routine pediatric practice.[5]

The Human Genome Project (HGP) is expanding knowledge of the genetic basis of disease at an incredible rate, with new technology making widespread genetic testing feasible. Because there are not enough geneticists or genetic counselors to provide adequate counseling, primary care physicians will need to increase their knowledge about genetics and become the frontline providers of some of these services.[6] However, many primary care pediatricians are not sufficiently prepared to provide genetic counseling.[7-10] Even beyond the necessary medical knowledge, new genetic technology raises ethical and social policy concerns that further challenge the primary care physician.[11,12]

This chapter helps prepare pediatricians to respond to the ethical and policy challenges resulting from new genetic advances. Recent developments in genetics do not necessarily create new ethical concerns, but they highlight how social, political, and economic factors influence the implementation, use, and regulation of new biotechnologies. Current policies and consensus statements regarding genetic testing of children help provide pediatricians with a framework to interpret genetic testing in their own practice. Ethical issues are raised in three clinical scenarios: (1) diagnostic genetic testing, (2) population-based genetic screening, and (3) carrier identification.

---

This chapter is modified from Ross LF, Moon MR: Ethical issues in genetic testing of children, *Arch Pediatr Adolesc Med* 154:873-879, 2000.

## ETHICS OVERVIEW

To date, the HGP's greatest successes are in gene discovery and the development of commercial genetic tests; gene therapy is still in an early experimental stage. Genetic testing of children can occur for many reasons and in various contexts, each of which raises a myriad of ethical questions, particularly with respect to consent and confidentiality.

Traditionally in pediatric medicine, parents are presumed to be best suited to make decisions for their children. Various arguments support parental control over medical decision making for minor children.[13-15] First, parents are presumed to have the child's best interests at heart because they naturally care deeply for their children and because they are in a position to know the child best. Second, for parents to fulfill the responsibilities of child-rearing, they need significant leeway. This includes control over decisions about medical care, provided the parents and their decisions are neither abusive nor neglectful. This parental discretion is appropriate because the financial and emotional consequences of these decisions primarily affect the parents and the child. Third, society has an interest in supporting the family as the primary childrearing institution, which requires that families be afforded a wide degree of privacy and freedom from government intrusion.

One constraint on parental control is the evolving understanding of children's autonomy and their role in the informed consent process. Historically, health care providers downplayed the child's capacity for decision making, but the current attitude is to give greater weight to this capacity[16,17] and future autonomy.[18] Providers rely on parents to make decisions for their children while remaining open to possible input from the child. However, parental autonomy is not and should not be absolute. The American Academy of Pediatrics (AAP) argues that in some situations, parents should not be empowered to consent on their child's behalf; in other situations the child's dissent should be binding.[16] Although the AAP does not make specific reference to genetic services, in some genetics cases the parents' and child's interests may be in conflict. Evaluating parental requests requires finding the appropriate balance between the child's needs and interests and those of the family.[19-22]

In genetics, however, knowledge about one family member may have great significance for other members. To view decisions about genetic testing in the context of a single patient ignores the relationships and obligations of individuals to those with whom they are genetically related, because genetic information often applies to families as much as to individuals.[23,24] Confidentiality of genetic information requires clarification: confidentiality for whom and from whom? This is even more complex in pediatrics because of the role of the parents in the consent process[25] (see Chapter 14).

## TESTING HIGH-RISK CHILDREN

Children who are symptomatic or a member of a high-risk family may be tested for heritable genetic traits and diseases. Genetic testing is least controversial when a patient has some identifiable symptom or some specific risk factor that is best diagnosed through genetic testing. The use of genetic testing for confirming clinical diagnoses is indistinguishable from using other therapeutic medical tests. The differential diagnosis of a child born with weak muscle tone and a large tongue include (1) the genetic condition of Down syndrome and (2) the nongenetic condition of hypothyroidism; the former is tested by chromosomal analysis; the latter by endocrine function. The differential diagnosis of a child who has failure to thrive and chronic recurrent upper respiratory infections includes cystic fibrosis (CF), an autosomal recessive genetic condition, and acquired immunodeficiency syndrome (AIDS), a nongenetic condition. In the symptomatic child, human immunodeficiency virus (HIV) may be determined by Western blot or polymerase chain reaction (PCR) testing, depending on the child's age and maternal antibody status. CF can be diagnosed by measuring sweat chloride or by genetic mutational analysis. None of these tests is medically controversial in a symptomatic child if adequate consent is obtained.

If a patient has an extra chromosome 21 or two CF mutations, the clinician can conclude that the patient has Down syndrome or CF, respectively; the genetic tests confirm the clinical diagnoses. These genetic tests are not controversial when performed postnatally to provide appropriate clinical services for the affected child and family.

## Populations at Risk

In contrast, presymptomatic genetic testing is used to identify disease in a healthy person known to be at risk. Such testing identifies the genes for retinoblastoma or Huntington disease (HD). Both are autosomal dominant conditions, meaning that a 50% probability exists that an offspring of an affected adult (symptomatic or presymptomatic) will inherit the gene. Both conditions are virtually 100% penetrant, which means that all individuals with the gene will become symptomatic.

In hereditary retinoblastoma, most children present in the first year of life.[26] About 40% of retinoblastoma cases are familial, related to a mutation of a tumor suppressor gene on chromosome 13. Identification allows targeted surveillance by frequent ophthalmologic examinations to minimize disease morbidity and mortality. The genetic test prevents unnecessary harm because it targets at-risk children in at-risk families. Children found to be positive for the gene are followed with frequent ophthalmologic testing (often under general anesthesia) in an attempt to detect the disease early, and children who test negative for the gene can avoid frequent examinations. Without the test, all children in an at-risk family would require frequent examinations. The genetic test optimizes treatment by enabling clinicians to focus on truly at-risk children and to avoid stigma and unnecessary medicalization of low-risk children from high-risk families.

In contrast, childhood onset of HD accounts for less than 5% of all affected individuals.[27] The value of testing children is to minimize uncertainty, allow them to incorporate their positive or negative status as part of their self-concept, and allow better lifetime planning. The risks to the child who tests positive are the psychosocial effects on relationships and interactions within the family, at school, and with potential employers. The child who tests negative may also experience serious psychosocial sequelae, ranging from survivor guilt to the possible social ostracization that occurs when a child is perceived as different from siblings and parents.[28,29]

In retinoblastoma and HD the tests are targeted to populations known to be at risk. The difference, however, is that preventive measures and treatments are available for children with retinoblastoma, but neither preventive measures nor treatments can minimize the morbidity of HD. Most genetic conditions are similar to HD in that they are currently untreatable, and diagnostic testing often offers no clear medical benefit to the patient. This does not mean that testing is necessarily harmful; rather the calculation of benefit and risk will focus on psychosocial factors.

Retinoblastoma and HD are atypical genetic diseases in that they are almost 100% penetrant. Most genes and associated genetic tests only identify an increased susceptibility, and their expression is widely variable, even within the same family. The probabilistic nature of genetic information adds further complexity to the ethical issues, in part because physicians and patients have difficulty understanding uncertainty and using such information in the decision-making process.[8-10,30] BRCA1 testing for inheritable breast cancer exemplifies the point. A positive test for the BRCA1 gene identifies an increased risk of developing breast or ovarian cancer before age 65. In women of Ashkenazi Jewish ancestry with a positive family history, the probability can be as high as 85%.[31] Presymptomatic genetic diagnosis can offer some medical benefit for adult women, who can choose to undergo prophylactic mastectomy and oophorectomy, thereby reducing their chances of disease.[32] Currently, however, no preventive measures are appropriate for children or adolescents. Individuals who undergo testing for BRCA1 and BRCA2 must understand that the gene is neither necessary nor sufficient for the development of breast cancer. BRCA1 and BRCA2 account for less than 10% of all breast cancers.[31] Even if an individual has one of these inherited genetic predispositions, the BRCA1 mutation is only the first step in the development of breast or ovarian cancer. A "second hit," probably nongenetic, is required for a tumor to develop.[33-35] The nature of the second hit is not well specified, but a significant number of women with the BRCA1 mutation avoid it.

Individuals who are not members of high-risk families may also test positive for BRCA1 and BRCA2. Although they also have an increased risk of breast cancer compared with the general population, the risk is lower than for members of high-risk families.[31,36] Parents may want to test their children for these genes because of family history, heightened awareness through an ill friend, or a community educational program. These parents need to know that presymptomatic genetic testing in low-risk families is often difficult to interpret. False-positive screening results may create a lasting burden of worry, and false-negative screening results may provide undue reassurance. Parents who request genetic testing of children for BRCA need extensive counseling about the test and the results, which only provide information about increased or decreased disease susceptibility. A positive test does not predict whether the disease will affect a particular individual, at what age it might present, how aggressive the cancer might be, or whether it will be responsive to standard chemotherapy.

### Risks and Benefits

For parents to interpret the risks and benefits of a particular genetic test, they need to understand the differences among (1) genetic testing in a child who is symptomatic, (2) genetic testing for a virtually 100% penetrant gene that has not yet expressed itself, and (3) genetic testing to determine increased susceptibility to a particular disease. The calculation of risks and benefits must include the test's technological quality, predictive value, reliability, and validity. Genetic technology is developing rapidly and being introduced into the clinical setting quite early, such that the actual quality of a test cannot be taken for granted and must be factored into decision making.[7,37,38]

The first step in helping parents to calculate the risks and benefits is to delineate any medical benefits of genetic testing. Genetic testing that determines the cause of a child's symptoms has obvious medical benefits if treatments are available. Even if treatments are not available, the diagnosis can serve to prevent unnecessary additional workup. Genetic testing that diagnoses a presymptomatic child or a child with a genetic predisposition also has medical benefits when preventive or therapeutic measures are available at an early stage. Most other genetic testing, however, has no medical benefits. Even genetic testing that offers medical benefits is associated with medical risks created by false-negative and false-positive results.[7,39]

The next step is to consider the emotional and psychosocial benefits and risks, for which empirical data are inadequate and difficult to obtain. These issues are further complicated by the long time lag between genetic testing and diagnosis in childhood versus disease presentation in adulthood. Psychosocial benefits may include the following[28,29]:

1.   Family uncertainty about the future can be reduced.
2.   Planning for the future can be more practical.
3.   Parental expectations for the child's future can be more "realistic."

Potential psychosocial risks include the following[28,29]:

1.   Stigmatization may be associated with genetic abnormality, even in the absence of phenotypic abnormality.
2.   Parent-child bonding may be inhibited.
3.   Normal family relationships may be disrupted by guilt on the part of parents or on behalf of the unaffected siblings (survivor guilt).
4.   A variation of the "vulnerable child syndrome" may develop.
5.   Parental expectations may be modified, often subconsciously.

Data are limited about how parents quantify the risks and benefits of presymptomatic and susceptibility testing in their children or how these children develop in contrast with their peers who were not diagnosed in childhood.

Other risks that must be incorporated into decisions about genetic testing include discrimination related to genotypic abnormalities, even if the condition is not 100% penetrant, and the long-term privacy of genetic information. Although scientists are only in the early stages of understanding the genotype-phenotype correlation and the interaction of various genotypes with the environment, this has not stopped different institutions from using this information in a discriminatory manner.[40-42]

Given that a risk-benefit analysis of most genetic tests will not yield an easy or obvious decision, pediatricians must learn to help their families navigate this decision-making process. Figure 13-1 summarizes a basic algorithm for decisions about genetic testing for children with known risk factors or symptoms. Genetic tests performed on children with symptoms or known risk factors that have immediate medical benefit to the child are ethically noncontroversial, despite the potential for psychosocial disruption. As medical benefits become less available, genetic testing becomes more controversial. The decision on whether to test a child, however, should also consider the psychosocial benefits and risks of testing for the child and the family. Although the values of the family are paramount, the pediatrician can help the family by ensuring that they examine all scenarios.

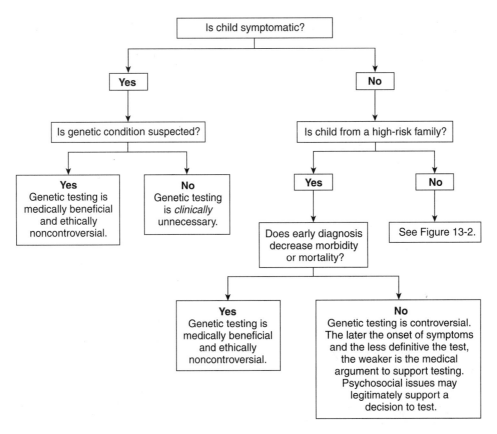

FIGURE 13-1   Genetic testing in high-risk children. Child has symptoms or is from a high-risk family.

## Psychosocial Component

The importance of the psychosocial analysis must not be underestimated. In many ways, the medical benefit of genetic testing in pediatrics is the simple question. More important and more difficult to know is the immediate and long-term impact of testing on the child and family. Some would argue that physicians should refuse all requests for genetic tests that do not offer immediate medical benefit. The psychosocial benefit of a test, however, even a test that has little or no medical benefit, may be decisive for a particular family. Pediatricians need to work with families to ensure that they understand what the test does and does not offer and that they consider all consequences and repercussions such information may have on the child during childhood and in adulthood, as well as on the family unit. Although physicians may discourage parents from pursuing genetic information that offers no medical benefit, parents, not clinicians, must ultimately decide what is in the child's best interest. This includes weighing medical and nonmedical factors, many of which the pediatricians may not be cognizant, for this particular family in their particular circumstances.

## GENETIC SCREENING

Genetic screening, in contrast to genetic testing, refers to testing entire populations for disease, usually without regard to particular risk factors. Population-based screening of children is most often done in the newborn period but may be done at other stages. Newborn screening is performed for a variety of medical conditions, both genetic and nongenetic. For example, thyroid disease, a nonmendelian condition, is included in all newborn state screens.[5] The National Institutes of Health (NIH) and the AAP recommend universal newborn screening for hearing loss in children, which may or may not be genetic in origin.[43,44] Beyond the newborn period, pediatricians should screen targeted populations of children for lead poisoning[45,46] and tuberculosis.[47]

Newborn screening is integral to pediatrics. The list of genetic diseases varies by state, but screening for phenylketonuria, hemoglobinopathies, and galactosemia are nearly universal in the United States.[5] In 1994 the Institute of Medicine (IOM) recommended that population-based newborn screening programs fulfill the following three criteria:

1. There is a clear indication of benefit to the newborn.
2. A system is in place to confirm the diagnosis.
3. Treatment and follow-up are available for affected newborns.

Additional criteria to justify screening entire populations include the following[11]:

1. The condition is frequent and severe enough to be a public health concern.
2. The condition causes a known spectrum of symptoms.
3. The screening test is simple and reliable, with low false-positive and false-negative rates.

Medical data show that newborn screening for most of the conditions included in state screens is beneficial in reducing morbidity and mortality. In that regard, we support such testing, although we are opposed to the current policy that mandates such testing without parental consent. We support parental consent because it gives authority to the parents, who are the appropriate surrogate decision makers for their children.[39,48] Through the consent process, the parents would be informed about the conditions for which testing is offered, why follow-up may be necessary, and why follow-up should be done early. Currently, parental consent is only sought in Maryland, where fewer than one parent in 1000 refuses testing for their newborn.[49] Although this means an affected child may not be screened, the probability is much lower than the chance of missing an affected child because of a false-negative test or an inadequate or lost specimen.[50]

An even more serious challenge for the future, however, is to evaluate all new proposals for population-based screening programs and not to institutionalize programs that do not meet at least the IOM criteria. Historically, newborn screens have not fulfilled these criteria at implementation. For example, when newborn screening for sickle cell disease was first initiated, there was no known benefit to presymptomatic diagnosis.[11] Now that penicillin prophylaxis has been shown to reduce morbidity and mortality, newborn screening for sickle cell disease is a paradigm case of justifiable universal screening,[51] but this does not justify its earlier implementation. Even today, governments continue to test for conditions for which newborn testing has no benefit. For example, two states screen for CF even though the data do not show that early initiation of therapy changes the course of disease.[52,53] In some countries, children are tested for Duchenne muscular dystrophy even though there are no known early treatments.[54] The justification is to educate couples about their future reproductive risks. Early diagnosis can benefit the affected child because it will avoid unnecessary workup when symptoms develop. Early diagnosis may place the child at risk, however, because the parents may now view their healthy-appearing child as ill or even doomed and may bond poorly or otherwise neglect the child. The expansion of mandatory newborn testing to these conditions is not warranted because the risks to the child and family may outweigh the benefits.

On the other hand, some genetic conditions may not warrant universal screening because the cost is too great or the cost/benefit analysis does not justify it. However, genetic testing for these conditions should still be offered. If identifiable groups may be at an increased risk, and if early diagnosis can decrease morbidity and mortality, such as with maple syrup urine disease in the Amish population or Gaucher disease in the Ashkenazi Jewish population, the medical benefits may support screening in these targeted populations. Even in low-risk communities, parental requests for specific genetic testing of their newborn may be justifiable. Parental anxiety alone may justify genetic testing, particularly when the condition is treatable. Parents who seek broad-spectrum testing of their newborn, however, need to be counseled that even the exclusion of many genetic and nongenetic conditions does not guarantee a healthy child.

Recommendations for universal screening are summarized in Figure 13-2. Even when universal screening cannot be justified from a medical cost/benefit analysis, screening targeted populations or testing particular children may still be ethically permissible. Again, the final determination will depend on the psychosocial benefit/risk calculation that is made by the parents with appropriate counseling.

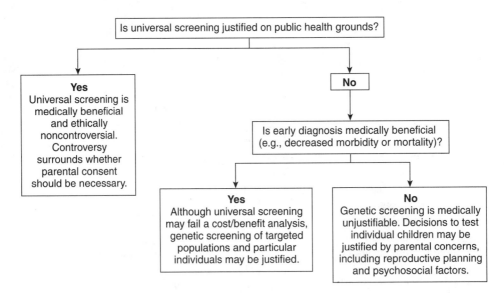

FIGURE 13-2   Genetic screening and testing in low-risk children. Child is asymptomatic and from a low-risk family.

## IDENTIFICATION OF CARRIER STATUS

All individuals carry several recessive genes that would prove lethal if a fetus received a double dose.[55] Other recessive genes are not lethal in the homozygous state but cause serious diseases. Carriers of recessive genes are often asymptomatic and unaware that they carry particular genes. For most recessive genetic traits, being a carrier confers no known medical morbidity. As such, tests to identify carrier status are not intended to provide a medical benefit to the patient but to provide information for reproductive decisions.

Carrier testing is most often done in the prenatal setting. Sometimes, however, carrier status is determined incidentally. For example, every child with a quantifiable amount of hemoglobin S on newborn screening in the United States is brought back for retesting. Hemoglobin electrophoresis determines whether they are homozygous for hemoglobin S (sickle cell anemia) or whether they are heterozygous (sickle cell trait). Currently, parents in the United States are told if their child is found to be a carrier. The IOM recommends that parents not be told their child's trait status, since the information has no clinical relevance but only reproductive relevance, for which the child has a right to privacy and a right not to know.[11] We disagree with the IOM's recommendation in that it implies the state has more right to information about a child than the child's parents. Parents need appropriate counseling to understand the distinction between clinical and reproductive relevance of this information so they do not erroneously treat their child as "diseased" and so they can counsel their child effectively. Longitudinal research is needed to determine the impact of such knowledge on children and adolescents and their families over the life cycle so that any policy changes can be based on empirical analysis of harms and benefits.

Even more controversial than informing parents of trait status when the information is determined incidentally is whether parents electively can request to test their children for carrier status. Often the interest is prompted by the diagnosis of a sibling or other relative with the disease.[56] Figure 13-3 outlines the possible scenarios and the framework with which to respond.

The arguments in favor of honoring the parents' requests are the following:

1.  Being informed of carrier status in childhood may make it easier to accept that status and incorporate it into the child's personal identity.[57]
2.  It may be useful for other family members.
3.  Parents, not the state, are in a better position to decide if the benefits of knowledge outweigh the risks for a particular child.[25]

The main arguments for refusing a parental request for carrier state testing are the following:

1.  It frustrates the child's right *not* to know as an adult.
2.  It fails to respect the child's right to confidential reproductive knowledge.
3.  It may adversely affect the child's self-concept.
4.  It may expose the child to unwarranted genetic discrimination.

There is also concern that parental misunderstanding of test results may result in treating the carrier child as an ill or potentially ill child.[57]

Although we neither encourage nor recommend carrier testing of children solely for informational purposes, we also do not universally prohibit such testing. Rather, we are will-

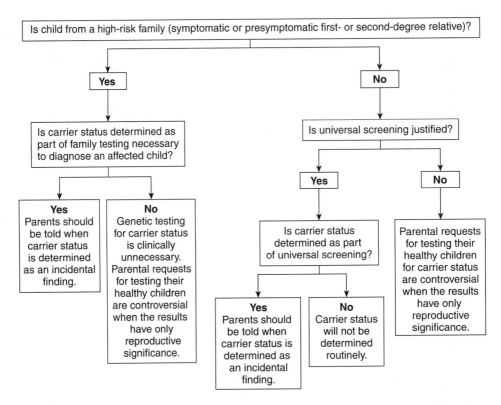

FIGURE 13-3 Genetic testing for carrier status. Autosomal recessive or sex-linked conditions in which carrier status confers no risk or minimal risk of morbidity or mortality but is important for reproductive decisions.

ing to respect parental requests, after appropriate counseling, on the grounds that they known what is best for the child and the family. Again, longitudinal research on the impact of such knowledge over the life cycle is important. Pediatricians need this information to help counsel families who request carrier testing of their children. We would reconsider our position if research found that knowledge of carrier status causes more harm than benefit for most children over the life cycle.

## SUMMARY

Genetic testing may be targeted or universal in statewide screening programs. Testing may uncover disease risk for which treatments may or may not exist or reveal information that has only reproductive relevance. Testing may yield results of varying predictive value.

Genetic testing is complicated because knowledge about one family member may have significant impact on other family members. This is further complicated in pediatrics because the decisions may have lifelong repercussions for the individual who did not consent to this testing. Further research on the psychosocial and ethical implications of genetic information is needed to ensure that policies are designed to meet patients' needs as individuals and as members of families, communities, and society. In addition, primary care pediatricians need to become familiar with the scientific and psychosocial data regarding genetic services to better serve children and their families.

1. Baird PA, Anderson TW, Newcombe HB, Lowry RB: Genetic disorders in children and young adults: a population study, *Am J Hum Genet* 42(5):677-693, 1988.

2. Hall JG, Powers EK, McIlvaine RT, Ean VH: The frequency and financial burden of genetic disease in a pediatric hospital, *Am J Med Genet* 1:417-436, 1978.

3. Scriver CR, Neal JL, Saginur R, Clow A: The frequency of genetic disease and congenital malformation among patients in a pediatric hospital, *Can Med Assoc J* 108: 1111-1115, 1973.

4. Yoon PW, Olney RS, Khoury MJ, et al: Contributions of birth defects and genetic diseases to pediatric hospitalizations: a population-based study, *Arch Pediatr Adolesc Med* 151:1096-1103, 1997.

5. American Academy of Pediatrics, Committee on Genetics: Newborn screening fact sheet, *Pediatrics* 98:473-501, 1996.

6. Holtzman NA: Primary care physicians as providers of frontline genetic services, *Fetal Diagn Ther* 8(suppl 1):213-219, 1993.

7. Holtzman NA: *Proceed with caution: predicting genetic risks in the recombinant DNA era,* Baltimore, 1989, Johns Hopkins University Press.

8. Hofman KJ, Tambor ES, Chase GA, et al: Physicians knowledge of genetics and genetic tests, *Acad Med* 68:625-632, 1993.

9. Giardiello FM, Brensinger JD, Petersen GM, et al: The use and interpretation of commercial APC gene testing for familial adenomatous polyposis, *N Engl J Med* 336: 823-827, 1997.

10. Rowley P et al: Cystic fibrosis carrier screening: knowledge and attitudes of prenatal care providers, *Am J Prev Med* 9:261-266, 1993.

11. Andrews L, Fullarton J, Holtzman N, Motulsky G, editors: *Assessing genetic risks: implications for health and social policy,* Washington, DC, 1994, National Academy Press.

12. Marteau T, Richards M, editors: *The troubled helix: social and psychological implications of the new human genetics,* Cambridge, 1996, Cambridge University Press.

13. Buchanan A, Brock D: *Deciding for others: the ethics of surrogate decision making,* Cambridge, 1990, Cambridge University Press.

14. Blustein J: *Parents and children: the ethics of the family,* New York, 1982, Oxford University Press.

15. Ross LF: *Parents, children, and health care decision making,* Oxford, UK, 1998, Oxford University Press.

16. American Academy of Pediatrics, Committee on Bioethics: Informed consent, parental permission, and assent in pediatric practice, *Pediatrics* 95:314-317, 1995.

17. Alderson P, Montgomery J: *Health care choices: making decisions with children,* London, 1996, Institute for Public Policy Research.

18. Feinberg J: *The child's right to an open future.* In Aiken W, LaFollette H: *Whose child? Children's rights, parental authority, and state power,* Totowa, NJ, 1980, Littlefield, Adams.

19. Sharpe NF: Presymptomatic testing for Huntington's disease: is there a duty to test those under the age of eighteen years? *Am J Med Genet* 46:250-253, 1993.

20. Patenaude AF: The genetic testing of children for cancer susceptibility: ethical, legal and social issues, *Behav Sci Law* 14:393-410, 1996.

21. Cohen CB: Wrestling with the future: should we test children for adult-onset genetic conditions? *Kennedy Inst Ethics J* 8:111-130, 1998.

22. Davis DS: Genetic dilemmas and the child's right to an open future, *Rutgers Law J* 28:549-592, 1997.

23. American Society of Human Genetics, Social Issues Subcommittee on Familial Disclosure: ASHG Statement: professional disclosure of familial genetic information, *Am J Hum Genet* 62:474-483, 1998.

24. Deftos LJ: The evolving duty to disclose the presence of genetic disease to relatives, *Acad Med* 73:962-968, 1998.

25. Ross LF: Genetic testing of children: who should consent? In Burley J, Harris J, editors: *A companion to genetics: ethics and the genetic revolution,* Oxford, 2001, Blackwell.

26. Birch JM: Genes and cancer, *Arch Dis Child* 80:1-3, 1999.

27. Baraitser M: Huntington's chorea. In Baraitser M, editor: *The genetics of neurological disorders,* Oxford, 1990, Oxford Medical Publications.

28. American Society of Human Genetics Board of Directors, American College of Medical Genetics Board of Directors: Points to consider: ethical, legal and psychological implications of genetic testing in children and adolescents, *Am J Hum Genet* 57:1233-1241, 1995.

29. Report of a Working Party of the Clinical Genetics Society (UK): The genetic testing of children, *J Med Genet* 31:785-797, 1994.

30. Davison C: Predictive genetics: the cultural implications of supplying probable futures. In Marteau T, Richards M, editors: *The troubled helix: social and psychological implications of the new human genetics,* Cambridge, 1996, Cambridge University Press.

31. Burke W, Daly M, Garber J, et al: Consensus statement: recommendations for follow-up care of individuals with an inherited predisposition to cancer. II. BRCA1 and **BRCA2,** *JAMA* 277:997-1003, 1997.

32. Hartmann LC, Schaid DJ, Woods JE, et al: Efficacy of bilateral prophylactic mastectomy in women with a family history of breast cancer, *N Engl J Med* 340:77-84, 1999.

33. Armitage P, Doll R: A two-stage theory of carcinogenesis in relation to the age distribution of human cancer, *Br J Cancer* 11:161-169, 1957.

34. Ashley DJB: The two "hit" and multiple "hit" theories of carcinogenesis, *Br J Cancer,* 23:313-328, 1969.

35. Knudson AG: Hereditary cancer: two hits revisited, *J Cancer Res Clin Oncol* 122:135-140, 1996.

36. Malone KE, Daling JR, Thompson JD, et al: BRCA1 mutations and breast cancer in the general population, *JAMA* 279:922-929, 1998.

37. Task Force on Genetic Testing: *Promoting safe and effective genetic testing in the United States,* Baltimore, 1998, Johns Hopkins University Press.

38. Holtzman NA, Murphy PD, Watson MS, Barr PA: Predictive genetic testing: from basic research to clinical practice, *Science* 278(5338):602-605, 1997.

39. Paul D: Contesting consent: the challenge to compulsory neonatal screening for PKU, *Perspect Biol Med* 42:207-219, 1999.

40. Billings P et al: Discrimination as a consequence of genetic testing, *Am J Hum Genet* 40:476-482, 1992.

41. Duster T: *Backdoor to eugenics,* New York, 1990, Routledge.

42. Draper E: *Risky business: genetic testing and exclusionary practices in the hazardous workplace,* New York, 1991, Cambridge University Press.

43. NIH Consensus Statement: Early identification of hearing impairment in infants and young children, 1993.

44. American Academy of Pediatrics: Joint Committee on Infant Hearing 1994 position statement, *Pediatrics* 95:152-156, 1995.

45. American Academy of Pediatrics: Lead poisoning from screening to primary prevention, *Pediatrics* 92:176-183, 1993.

46. Centers for Disease Control and Prevention: Preventing lead poisoning in young children, Atlanta, 1991, US Department of Health and Human Services.

47. American Academy of Pediatrics, Committee on Infectious Diseases: Update on tuberculosis skin testing of children, *Pediatrics* 97(2):282-284, 1996.

48. Annas GJ: Mandatory PKU screening: the other side of the looking glass, *Am J Public Health* 72:1401-1403, 1982.

49. Faden R, Chwalow J, Holtzman NA, Horn SD: A survey to evaluate parental consent as public policy for neonatal screening, *Am J Public Health* 72:1350, 1982.

50. Holtzman NA, Leonard CO, Farfel MR: Issues in antenatal and neonatal screening and surveillance for hereditary and congenital disorders, *Annu Rev Public Health* 2:219-251, 1981.

51. Consensus Conference: Newborn screening for sickle cell disease and other hemoglobinopathies, *JAMA* 258:1205-1209, 1987.

52. NIH Consensus Statement: Genetic testing for cystic fibrosis, 1997.

53. Wald NJ, Morris JK: Neonatal screening for cystic fibrosis, *BMJ* 316:404-405, 1998.

54. Bradley DM, Parsons EP, Clarke AJ: Experience with screening newborns for Duchenne muscular dystrophy in Wales, *BMJ* 306:357-360, 1993.

55. Lee JK et al: Number of lethal equivalents in human populations: how good are the previous estimates? *Heredity* 77:209-216, 1996.

56. Balfour-Lynn I, Madge S, Dinwiddie R: Testing carrier status in siblings of patients with cystic fibrosis, *Arch Dis Child* 72:167-168, 1995.

57. Fanos JH: Developmental tasks of childhood and adolescence: implications for genetic testing, *Am J Med Genet* 71:22-28, 1997.

58. Bowman JE: Genetics and African Americans, *Seton Hall Law Review* 27:919-937, 1997.

# CHAPTER 14

# Genetic Services for Children: Who Should Consent?

*Lainie Friedman Ross*

Informed consent is at the foundation of clinical ethics and the physician-patient relationship. Informed consent is a process in which physicians provide medical information and discuss its significance so that patients can make decisions that best reflect their own values. Informed consent is important at both the diagnostic stage and the therapeutic stage. It includes discussing the risks and benefits of the proposed procedures or therapies and the alternatives, including nonaction. The consent process is a continuing dialogue, but the final decision belongs to the patient.

Informed consent and the physician-patient relationship are more complicated in genetics. The traditional confidential nature of the relationship is challenged by genetics because an individual's diagnosis is not isolated but reflects disease probability or risk factors in siblings, parents, children, and other blood relatives. This raises consent issues because information about one individual may inadvertently provide information about other family members, including those who may not want to know. Informed consent for genetic services is further complicated because results often signify disease predilection but not definitive diagnoses. Even when testing provides a definitive diagnosis, treatments may be only experimental. Also, many physicians do not understand genetics and are poor at counseling in genetics, and both patients and physicians have a difficult time grasping probabilities.[1-4]

Informed consent and the physician-patient relationship are also more complicated in pediatrics, where the physician-patient dyad is a triad that includes the physician, the child, and the parents. Traditionally, parents make decisions for their children, although currently there are movements around the world to increase the child's voice, particularly the older child.[5,6] Some argue that mature children (adolescents) should be allowed to make their own decisions without their parents' permission and even without their awareness.[7,8]

This chapter is modified from Ross LF: Genetic testing of children: who should consent? In Burley J, Harris J, editors: *A companion to genetics: ethics and the genetic revolution,* Oxford, 2001, Blackwell.

Whether this autonomy should be expanded to genetic services depends on what role children have in health care decisions and whether decision making in genetics is comparable to other health care decisions.

## NEWBORN SCREENING: MANDATORY TESTING VERSUS INFORMED CONSENT

Consent for genetic testing of children has been overridden in the United States in newborn screening programs, which are universally state-mandated in 49 of the 50 states. Although each state has a different panel of tests, the most common tests are for phenylketonuria (PKU), hypothyroidism, hemoglobinopathies (including sickle cell disease), congenital adrenal hyperplasia (CAH), and galactosemia.[9] Maryland had state-mandated screening but repealed it in 1976 for a statute and regulations requiring informed parental consent.[10]

The conditions listed are autosomal recessive (except hypothyroidism, which is sporadic), meaning that an affected child has two asymptomatic parents who carry this recessive allele, and the affected child is homozygous recessive. Each condition meets the criteria for screening: it represents an important health problem with an accepted treatment that, if begun early, can prevent many or all of the negative sequelae. The screening test is simple and inexpensive, and the follow-up testing is highly accurate. The cost of case finding, diagnosis, and treatment is economically balanced in relation to possible expenditures on total medical care.[11,12]

The major benefit of mandatory screening is to ensure that all infants are screened in order to treat affected newborns (true positives) quickly and accurately and to reassure parents of those who do not have the disease (true negatives). To accrue the benefits of testing, affected infants must be given appropriate and timely treatment, although not all states that mandate screening pay for follow-up or treatment.[13,14]

The major danger of mandatory screening is that historically, testing has become institutionalized before an adequate understanding of the test's capabilities and limits. In 1963, for example, Massachusetts adopted a mandatory PKU screening program even though a collaborative project to study the effects of dietary restriction on the physical, cognitive, and psychosocial development of PKU did not begin until 1967. Many other states implemented mandatory PKU statutes before it was known that some children with elevated levels of phenylalanine did not respond to a phenylalanine-free diet, or that some benign causes of elevated levels of phenylalanine did not require treatment.[15] The result was that some healthy children were placed on these diets, which led to malnourishment or worse.[16,17]

Virtually all parents, when asked, consent to testing. In Maryland, where testing is voluntary, fewer than one parent in 1000 refuses testing for their newborns,[18] much less than the chance of missing a PKU infant because of a false-negative test, and less than the number of children not tested due to lost and improperly obtained specimens.[13] Universal testing of newborns for the conditions listed earlier is possible either by mandatory or voluntary consent methods because parents want to do what is best for their children. For most parents, this means diagnosing early-onset conditions *early,* when safe and effective treatments are available.

The following arguments support parental consent for newborn screening, even if virtually all parents would consent:

1.   Consent is a requirement for diagnostic and therapeutic interventions because the examination or testing of individuals without their consent is battery or assault. Parents serve as the surrogates for their newborns, who cannot give their own consent.
2.   Obtaining parental consent for newborn screening is a symbol of respect for the family. Families are the primary source of childrearing, and families, not the state, will bear the greatest costs if an affected child is not screened and diagnosis is delayed.
3.   Obtaining consent serves a valuable educative role. By requiring consent, parents must be educated about the purpose and limitations of screening, which may give them incentive to follow up on abnormal screening results. Knowledge of negative test results may be reassuring to parents, particularly those with personal knowledge of conditions being tested.

The major arguments against requiring parental consent for newborn screening are as follows[19,20]:

1.   Obtaining consent is time-consuming.
2.   Even when consent is obtained, the data suggest that the consent is perfunctory and not informed.

Neither objection justifies circumventing the consent process. Obtaining consent takes time. This is true for all diagnostic tests, not only newborn tests. Parents need information and time to make well-informed decisions for their children. Perfunctory and uninformed consent is not proof that consent is unnecessary, but a sign that physicians are not fulfilling their role in the consent process.

## ROLE OF CHILDREN IN INFORMED CONSENT PROCESS

Beyond the nursery, parental consent is sought for all health care decisions, although there is a movement to give older children sole decision-making authority. When children (and adults) give informed consent, the consent (1) is informed (made knowingly), (2) is competent (made intelligently), and (3) is voluntary. Despite these requirements, most health care decisions do not fulfill the three components of informed consent.[21]

Intuitively it might seem that the main difference between children and adults is their ability to understand diagnostic or treatment alternatives and the consequences of each. The empirical data are insufficient, however, to show whether consent by adults is significantly different (presumably better) than consent by competent children. The few studies that do compare adolescent and adult decision making have not shown marked differences in process or content.[22]

Even if adolescents can knowingly and intelligently come to a rational decision, however, two reasons suggest they will not act on this ability. First, adolescents may fail to act competently because they acquiesce to parents or caregivers. Young adolescents are highly submissive to authority and are likely to conform to social norms and expectations.[22] Although peer conformity and deferential response have significantly diminished by age 15 years, parental influence remains strong.[21,23]

Second, adolescents may fail to act competently because choosing to do the right action also requires them to act accordingly. Despite their knowledge regarding motor vehicle safety, adolescents account for a disproportionate number of fatal accidents. Despite knowing about the transmission of acquired immunodeficiency syndrome (AIDS) and other sexually transmitted diseases (STDs), adolescents are becoming a high-risk group for STDs, including AIDS.[24] Scherer and Reppucci[23] argue that most of the studies do not capture such differences because the studies depict hypothetical situations, which may not accurately reflect the differences that would be revealed in "a more naturalistic setting."

The scant empirical data suggest that by age 12, 14, or 16, depending on the study and theory, there may not be a clear rationale to characterize children as a class as incompetent or as incapable of giving informed consent. If competency is all that is necessary for health care autonomy, adolescents should be given health care autonomy. This also would hold true for genetic services, unless particular facts about genetic services make adolescents particularly vulnerable.

The moral argument against giving adolescents full autonomy to consent to genetic services is based on the general claim that competency is necessary but not sufficient for health care autonomy.[25] The following two arguments support the continued participation of parents in their children's health care decisions:

1. Parents provide children with a protected period in which to develop "enabling virtues"—habits, including self-control, that advance their lifetime autonomy and opportunities[26]—rather than rely on a mere threshold level of competency.
2. Parents provide children with the opportunities to gain world experience, the lack of which distorts the capacity for sound judgment.[27]

Parental participation is also supported by the pragmatic argument that parents are responsible for the moral, physical, and emotional well-being of their children, and this requires them to ensure for their child's medical well-being as well.

The parents' role may even be stronger in the context of genetics because treatment and prevention may not be available, the results may be ambiguous, and the value of testing may depend on how one interprets and integrates the psychosocial implications of the results. Data are scant, although theoretically it would seem that even mature adolescents are at a disadvantage due to their lack of world experience and focus on short-term considerations rather than long-term or overall impact.[28] This does not argue against a role for children in the decision-making process, although it may argue against giving them independent autonomy. Even when the child's decision is not binding, medical tests and treatments should be explained to help them understand what is being done to them and at least to gain their cooperation.[29]

## EARLY-ONSET GENETIC CONDITIONS

Testing young children (children who do not have decision-making capacity) for early-onset conditions includes two very different categories: (1) conditions such as retinoblastoma and familial adenomatous polyposis, for which early diagnosis and treatment save lives, and (2) conditions such as Duchenne muscular dystrophy and cystic fibrosis (CF), for which early diagnosis and treatment do not affect the disease course. The value of presymptomatic testing in the first category is to prevent serious morbidity and mortality. Children in at-risk families should be tested or should undergo frequent surveillance examinations. Failure to do so is neglectful because it places children at unnecessary and imminent risk. It is assumed that parents are the child's appropriate decision makers, although if parents refuse testing or diagnostic workups, physicians may be compelled to seek state permission to override their refusal.

In the second category the value of presymptomatic diagnosis is to (1) avoid delay in diagnosis when early symptoms are nonspecific, (2) target surveillance screening more accurately, (3) allow parents to prepare for a child who will have special needs, and (4) assist parents in their own reproductive planning. Psychological benefits may include reducing family uncertainty about the future and allowing for more practical planning. Particularly for families with another affected child, a negative result serves to reassure parents that nonspecific symptoms are not signs of impending disease. On the other hand, early diagnosis may create a vulnerable child, may adversely affect parent-child bonding and the child's self-esteem, and may make it difficult to obtain appropriate health insurance for the child and even healthy siblings.[30] Parental expectations for the future also may be unnecessarily limited.

The risk-benefit balance of presymptomatic testing will depend on the values and needs of each family. Physicians need to be aware of the possibility for presymptomatic diagnosis and must be prepared to counsel families about the risks and benefits of testing. Some parents may value such information, particularly if they know an affected biological relative; other parents may choose to remain uninformed unless (until) the child develops symptoms, so as to avoid treating the child as vulnerable before the child becomes ill. Since presymptomatic testing has not been shown to improve morbidity or mortality, it goes beyond the definition of what states can morally mandate. Some states do mandate testing for CF, however, and some countries test newborns for Duchenne muscular dystrophy.

Physicians should be nondirective in their dialogue and respect a decision to test as well as a decision not to test.[31] If testing is deferred, the physician should note the patient's risk factors and be vigilant in clinical practice in case the child develops related symptoms.

## LATE-ONSET GENETIC CONDITIONS

Testing children for late-onset conditions is highly controversial and has been the focus of much of the debate on consent for genetic services in pediatrics.[32-34] These conditions can be divided into two categories: (1) conditions such as Huntington disease (HD), for which presymptomatic testing virtually guarantees the development of or freedom from the disease, but for which there are no known treatments to modify or prevent the course of illness, and (2) the majority of conditions, for which genetic testing reveals only a probability or predilection for a particular condition, such as BRCA1 and BRCA2 genes, which account for 5% of breast cancer. Patients who test positive for these genes may elect prophylactic mastectomy as a young adult, although even this does not guarantee that they will not develop breast cancer.

Before genetic testing became available, studies found that most individuals in families affected with HD, for example, would want to know their risk status, even if nothing could be offered to change the course of their illness.[35,36] As testing became available, however, the number of at-risk individuals who sought testing was much lower than predicted. To date, less than 15% of individuals at risk for HD have been tested.[37-39]

When such predictive testing is done in adults, the recipients receive pretest and posttest counseling. For some, knowing is important in making career and reproductive decisions and in reducing anxiety about the unknown. For many, uncertainty allows them to retain hope that they are unaffected. Recipients of both positive and negative results may have surprising psychological reactions to their test results. Although one might expect those who test positive to have depression, distress, or increased anxiety, some patients find the result liberating because they can now make realistic plans about the future. Many who test negative experience great relief, but some experience survivor guilt. These reactions cannot be predicted.[40]

In the early years of testing, particularly when HD testing required linkage analysis, the desire not to know was deemed to trump the desire to know, and individuals whose family members refused to participate in linkage analysis could not be tested. Now that the specific gene has been located, direct genetic testing is available. Individuals are counseled about the possible negative impact on family members, but an informed request is usually honored.

Should children be tested for late-onset diseases, particularly conditions for which no treatment exists? If parents can choose to have their children tested, the children lose the right *not* to know as adults, and many patients *do* choose not to know. On the other hand, an outright ban prohibits adults from having the right to have known since childhood, which may interfere with their ability to plan for their future with any certainty.

Empirical data about the psychological impact of testing children are lacking. Despite the lack of evidence, virtually all geneticists and specialists argue against providing such services,[16,30,31,41,42] although such testing occurs.[43] If treatment or early lifestyle choices during childhood had an impact on the probability or severity of illness, position statements would need to be reevaluated.

General pediatricians are more divided about whether parents should have the right to have their children tested for these conditions.[31] In some cases, reasons may exist why families will benefit (or at least believe they will benefit) from such knowledge. The potential benefits of testing children for late-onset diseases are that it may (1) foster openness within the family, (2) allow the child to adjust to genetic destiny, (3) reduce the anxiety associated with not knowing, and (4) identify children who will need genetic counseling before childbearing. A positive result, however, may (1) adversely affect the parent-child relationship, (2) distort the family's perception of the child, (3) lead to unnecessarily limited expectations of the child, (4) adversely affect the child's self-esteem, and (5) lead to discrimination in education, employment, or insurance. Many families label or scapegoat one or more children as positive and treat the child differently than siblings, even without testing.[44] A negative test, in contrast, may bring great relief, although it also may distort family relationships if some children test negative and others positive.

The issue then becomes whether families have the right to decide what is best for them or whether this should be imposed by professionals.[45] Generally, when the balance between benefits and harms of a medical option are unknown, decision making is left to the family.

It is expected that parents will act to promote their child's best interest, although many ethicists realize that parents often need to balance an individual child's interest with the needs and interests of the family.[29,34]

What role should the child play in this decision? Some argue that testing should be deferred until the child can at least assent, which is often defined as school-age (6 or 7 years); others would defer testing until adolescence, when the child can give an informed consent. Most ethicists would hold the child's dissent as binding when such testing does not offer clear and direct medical benefits.[32] I support a policy of discouraging parental requests for children of all ages. At minimum, I would try to convince parents to defer testing until their child can participate in the decision-making process, at which time the child's dissent should be binding. I would not prohibit testing of the young child, however, because some families may decide that the benefits outweigh the risks.

Should the adolescent be able to make these decisions independently? Even if one supports confidential health care for children, genetic services may be different because (1) they potentially provide a great deal of information about one's parents (including nonbiological parentage), and (2) they have significant short-term and long-term psychosocial implications that children are neither emotionally nor cognitively fully able to grasp.[46] Given the serious psychosocial risks of genetic testing for late-onset diseases, particularly those for which no current treatment can modify the course, I would not support a policy that allowed adolescents to seek such care confidentially.

## CARRIER STATUS

All individuals carry several recessive genes that would prove lethal if a child were born homozygous recessive. Similarly, all individuals carry recessive genes that can result in significant health conditions for their homozygous recessive progeny. Usually, carriers are asymptomatic and unaware. Although carrier status may be integral for reproductive decision making, it is rarely relevant to an individual's medical well-being. In general, therefore, it is unnecessary to test children for carrier status.

Whether parents have the right to know the carrier status of their children raises two issues. First, in some newborn screening programs, such as testing for sickle cell anemia, screening identifies carriers as well as those affected with the disease. The follow-up test distinguishes children with disease and children with trait. The Institute of Medicine (IOM) of the National Academy of Science has argued against informing parents of their child's carrier status, although most screening programs currently do inform parents.[16] In part the rationale is pragmatic: parents asked to bring their child for follow-up testing should know the reason. There is also a moral argument to inform parents: to withhold trait status from parents implies that the state, not the parents, are the guardians or the owner of such information on behalf of the child. Based on the latter argument, I support the present policy in which parents are told about carrier status if it is determined as an incidental finding.

Another argument in favor of disclosing trait status is that carrier status may have important implications for the child's parents. If parents do not know that they carry such alleles, learning that a child is a carrier can serve as a warning that future children may be at risk. It may result in each parent being tested for carrier status.

The IOM specifically rejected use of the child's test result as a means for providing reproductive information to parents. Their argument is based on a flawed understanding of the Kantian dictum: "Act in such a way that you treat humanity, whether in your own person or in the person of another, always at the same time as an end and never simply as a means."[47] The categorical imperative does not prohibit the use of persons as means, it prohibits the use of persons *solely* as a means. Testing for sickle cell anemia is done because early prophylaxis with penicillin is known to decrease morbidity and mortality.[9] In the process of determining disease status, the child may be found to be a carrier, which has reproductive implications for the child's parents and for the child later in life. As such, the primary goal is to promote the child's well-being; only secondarily does the child serve as a means by which the parents learn of their potential reproductive genetic risks.

The second type of case in which carrier status information is broached relates to parents who request carrier testing for their child on a "want-to-know" basis. Often the interest is prompted by the diagnosis of a child's relative with the disease. Other reasons include parental requests in response to an educational outreach program in communities at risk or parents' desire to counsel their children regarding responsible procreation as they reach reproductive age.

Should such testing be deferred until the child is able to participate in medical decisions and can be counseled directly about testing? The main arguments for refusing a parental request are as follows:

1. It frustrates the child's right not to know as an adult.
2. It fails to respect the child's right to confidential reproductive knowledge.
3. It may adversely impact the child's self-concept.

There is also concern that parental misunderstanding of test results will lead to treating the child with trait as an ill or potentially ill child.[46] The arguments in favor of honoring the parents' requests are as follows:

1. Being informed of carrier status in childhood may be easier to accept and incorporate into one's personal identity.
2. It may be useful for other family members.
3. Parents, not the state, are in a better position to decide if the benefits of knowledge outweigh the risks for a particular child.

Who within the family should make the decision to test a child for carrier status? As with testing for late-onset conditions, which serves no immediate medical benefit, I support a policy of discouraging parental requests. Parents should defer testing until their child can participate in the decision-making process, at which time the child's dissent should be binding. Again, I would not prohibit testing of the young child, since in some cases, families may decide that the benefits outweigh the risks.

Should adolescents be able to learn of their status independently? Given the potential for serious psychological stress and misunderstanding of genetics[48] and the public's poor understanding of genetics,[49] such testing is best done with parental involvement. As such, I do not advocate state-supported programs that test adolescents in high schools without parental consent.[50] Nevertheless, if an adolescent or a partner seeks testing because of pregnancy and refuses to involve the parents, I would provide these services.

## GENETIC RESEARCH

It is hoped that gene therapy will be an important modality in the treatment and prevention of disease. Such therapy may work by replacing defective genes, adding normal copies of genes to defective cells, or adding genes that introduce a new function into cells. Two major problems are (1) developing a vector to carry the manipulated genetic material to its target and (2) regulating the newly inserted genetic material.

Gene therapy can be targeted either to somatic (nonreproductive) cells or germline (reproductive) cells, which will be passed on to the person's children. To date, the only successful gene therapy has been in somatic cells of children with adenosine deaminase deficiency, a form of severe combined immunodeficiency.[51] Currently, investigation into human germline therapy is proscribed.

Gene therapy is currently experimental. In 1977 the United States National Commission for the Protection of Human Subjects of Biomedical and Behavioral Research[52] concluded that, when possible, experimental research should begin with studies in animals and adults before involving children. In the United Kingdom the Institute of Medical Ethics working group on the ethics of clinical research investigation in children came to similar conclusions.[53] However, many genetic conditions are lethal in childhood or lead to significant morbidities. Thus it may be necessary to begin gene therapy trials with children as the first subjects. These studies will require stringent ethical review, particularly how to test innovative gene therapy in conditions with an alternative therapy. For example, sickle cell disease is primarily treated symptomatically but can be cured by bone marrow transplantation.[54] Because transplantation has significant risks, it is used only in high-risk patients.[55] In the future, gene therapy might be the treatment of choice, but the known and serious risks of bone marrow transplantation must be compared with the unknown risks of gene therapy.

Whose consent should be necessary for enrolling children as subjects of genetic research? In part, the answer will depend on whether the genetic research has therapeutic intent. In the United States, when research involves the potential for direct therapeutic benefit, parental permission is necessary, and the child's assent is desirable but may be overridden. The National Commission's regulations[52] were the basis for federal regulations (1978, revised in 1983 and 1991), which require only parental permission for therapeutic research.[56] Similar policy recommendations exist in the United Kingdom for children younger than 14 years.[57-60] The working group on ethics differed from the National Commission, however, in stating that consent and the refusal to consent to therapeutic research by children older than 14 should be binding.[53]

When research is nontherapeutic, such as research to develop new predictive genetic tests, whether children should participate depends on the degree of risk. Genetic research often requires a blood sample or at most a tissue sample, the procurement of which has minimal physical risks. From a psychosocial perspective, however, the risks are substantial and include the potential to alter family relationships or to cause discrimination and stigmatization if the results are divulged. Since the research is nontherapeutic, a preference should exist for using adult subjects. If children do serve as subjects, both the U.S. and U.K. policies recommend that the child's assent should be obtained and that the child's dissent should be binding.

Despite the emerging perspective that children should be given a greater role in health care decision making, a recent survey of consent forms for genetic research does not reflect this. Rather, Weir and Horton[61] found that many consent forms modified for adolescents were "confusing or unclear" and did not "reflect the current or the developing ethical and legal standards." They also found that of 70 consent documents dealing with genetic research in children, only one consent form mentioned the psychosocial risks, and did so by minimizing its potential impact.

In research the informed consent process leads to serious inequities; the process serves as a social filter in that better-educated and wealthier individuals are more likely to refuse to participate and are underrepresented in most research.[62] The problem is perpetuated in pediatrics because parents who volunteer their children are less educated and underrepresented in the professional and managerial occupations compared with their nonvolunteering counterparts.[63] Assuming that these trends will hold for genetic research in children, the skewed subject selection may lead to public outcries because of its potential for exploitation of vulnerable subclasses of children. Further public distrust may develop when it is realized that most genetic research is done with a commercial partner and that the subjects and their families relinquish their rights to profit from the research.[64]

Genetic research using human subjects, including children, is important. As with all research on children, however, subjects and their parents need to understand the personal risks that the research imposes on children, often not for their own benefit, but for the benefit of future generations. The consent process must ensure that child subjects and their parents are being recruited fairly and that they are given enough information to give voluntary and informed consent.

## SUMMARY

Genetics is a rapidly evolving field. It has great potential for changing how we see ourselves, how health is understood, and how medicine is practiced. It also has great potential for being misused or abused, particularly while our knowledge is incomplete. As such, informed consent for genetic services is critical. This is particularly true in pediatrics, where errors may lead to long-term morbidity or lifelong social stigmatization.

## REFERENCES

1. Geller G, Holtzman NA: Implications of the Human Genome Initiative for the primary care physician, *Bioethics* 5:318-325, 1991.
2. Hofman KJ, Tambor ES, Chase GA, et al: Physicians' knowledge of genetics and genetic tests, *Acad Med* 68:625-632, 1993.
3. Giardiello FM, Brensinger JD, Petersen GM, et al: The use and interpretation of commercial APC gene testing for familial adenomatous polyposis, *N Engl J Med* 336:823-827, 1997.
4. Andrews LB: Compromised consent: deficiencies in the consent process for genetic testing, *J Am Med Women Assoc* 52:39-44, 1997.
5. American Academy of Pediatrics, Committee on Bioethics: Informed consent, parental permission, and assent in pediatric practice, *Pediatrics* 95:314-317, 1995.
6. Alderson P, Montgomery J: *Health care choices: making decisions with children,* London, 1996, Institute for Public Policy Research.

7. Holt J: *Escape from childhood,* New York, 1974, Dutton.

8. Cohen H: *Equal rights for children,* Totowa, NJ, 1980, Rowman & Littlefield.

9. American Academy of Pediatrics, Committee on Genetics: Newborn screening fact sheets, *Pediatrics* 98(3):474-493, 1996.

10. Holtzman NA: Public participation in genetic policymaking: the Maryland Commission on Hereditary Disorders. In Milunsky A, Annas GJ, editors: *Genetics and the law,* New York, 1984, Plenum.

11. Wilson JMG, Jungner F: *Principles and practice of screening for disease,* Geneva, 1968, World Health Organization.

12. Faden R, Kass NE, Powers M: Warrants for screening programs: public health, legal and ethical frameworks. In Faden R, Geller G, Powers M, editors: *AIDS, women, and the next generation,* New York, 1991, Oxford University Press.

13. Holtzman NA, Leonard CO, Farfel MR: Issues in antenatal and neonatal screening and surveillance for hereditary and congenital disorders, *Annu Rev Public Health* 2:238, 1981.

14. Clayton EW: Issues in state newborn screening programs, *Pediatrics* 90:642, 1992.

15. Acuff KL, Faden RR: A history of prenatal and newborn screening programs: lessons for the future. In Faden R, Geller G, Powers M, editors: *AIDS, women, and the next generation,* New York, 1991, Oxford University Press.

16. Andrews LB, Fullarton JE, Holtzman NA, Motulsky AG, editors: *Assessing genetic risks: implications for health and social policy,* Washington, DC, 1994, National Academy Press.

17. Holtzman N: Dietary treatment of inborn errors of metabolism, *Annu Rev Med* 21:335-356, 1970.

18. Faden R, Chwalow J, Holtzman NA, Horn SD: A survey to evaluate parental consent as public policy for neonatal screening, *Am J Public Health* 72:1350, 1982.

19. Holtzman NA, Faden R, Chwalow AJ, Horn SD: Effect of informed parental consent on mothers' knowledge of newborn screening, *Pediatrics* 72:807-812, 1983.

20. Statham H, Green J, Snowdon C: Mother's consent to screening newborn babies for disease, *BMJ* 306:858-859, 1993 (letter).

21. Grisso T, Vierling L: Minor's consent to treatment: a developmental perspective, *Profession Psychol* 9:415, 1978.

22. Gardner W, Scherer D, Tester M: Asserting scientific authority: cognitive development and adolescent legal rights, *Am Psychol* 44:897-899, 1989.

23. Scherer DG, Reppucci ND: Adolescents' capacities to provide voluntary informed consent: the effects of parental influence and medical dilemmas, *Law Hum Behav* 12:125, 1988.

24. DiClemente R: Preventing HIV/AIDS among adolescents: schools as agents of behavior change, *JAMA* 270:760-762, 1993.

25. Ross LF: Health care autonomy for minors: is it in their best interest? *Hastings Center Report* 27:41-45, 1997.

26. Purdy LM: *In their best interest? The case against equal rights for children,* New York, 1992, Cornell University Press.

27. Gaylin W: Competence: no longer all or none. In Gaylin W, Macklin R, editors: *Who speaks for the child: the problems of proxy consent,* New York, 1982, Plenum.

28. Michie S: Predictive genetic testing in children. In Marteau T, Richards M, editors: *The troubled helix: social and psychological implications of the new human genetics,* Cambridge, 1996, Cambridge University Press.

29. Ross LF: *Children, families, and health care decision making,* Oxford, 1998, Oxford University Press.

30. The American Society of Human Genetics Board of Directors, American College of Medical Genetics Board of Directors: Points to consider: ethical, legal and psychological implications of genetic testing in children and adolescents, *Am J Hum Genet* 57:1233-1241, 1995.

31. Report of a Working Party of the Clinical Genetics Society (UK): The genetic testing of children, *J Med Genet* 31:785-797, 1994.

32. Wertz DC, Fanos JH, Reilly PR: Genetic testing for children and adolescents: who decides? *JAMA* 272:875-881, 1994.

33. Hoffmann DE, Wulfsberg EA: Testing children for genetic predispositions: is it in their best interest? *J Law Med Ethics* 23: 331-344, 1995.

34. Clayton EW: Genetic testing in children, *J Med Philos* 22:233-251, 1997.

35. Schoenfeld M, Myers RH, Berkman B, Clark E: Potential impact of a predictive test on the gene frequency of Huntington's disease, *Am J Med Genet* 18:423-429, 1984.

36. Meissen GJ, Berchek RL: Intended use of predictive testing by those at risk for Huntington's disease, *Am J Med Genet* 26:283-293, 1987.

37. Craufurd D, Dodge A, Kerzin-Storrar L, Harris R: Uptake of pre-symptomatic testing for Huntington's disease, *Lancet* ii:603-605, 1989.

38. Bloch M, Adam S, et al: Predictive testing for Huntington's disease in Canada: the experience of those receiving an increased risk, *Am J Med Genet* 42:499-507, 1992.

39. Benjamin CM, Adam S, Wiggins S, et al: Proceed with care: direct predictive testing for Huntington disease, *Am J Hum Genet* 55:606-617, 1994.

40. Marteau TM, Croyle RT: Psychological responses to genetic testing, *BMJ* 316:693-696, 1998.

41. Guidelines for molecular genetics predictive test in Huntington's disease, *Neurology* 44:1533-1536, 1994.

42. National Kidney Foundation, Scientific Advisory Board: Gene testing in autosomal dominant polycystic kidney disease: results of National Kidney Foundation workshop, *Am J Kidney Dis* 13:85-87, 1989.

43. Wertz DC, Reilly PR: Laboratory policies and practices for the genetic testing of children: a survey of the Helix Network, *Am J Hum Genet* 61:163-168, 1997.

44. Kessler S: Preselection: a family coping strategy in Huntington's disease, *Am J Med Genet* 31:617-621, 1988.

45. Sharpe NF: Presymptomatic testing for Huntington disease: is there a duty to test those under the age of eighteen years? *Am J Med Genet* 46:250-253, 1993.

46. Fanos JH: Developmental tasks of childhood and adolescence: implications for genetic testing, *Am J Med Genet* 71:22-28, 1997.

47. Kant I: *Grounding for the metaphysics of morals* (1785). Translated by JW Ellington, Indianapolis, 1981, Hackett.

48. Ponder M, Lee J, Green J, Richards M: Family history and perceived vulnerability to some common diseases: a study of young people and their parents, *J Med Genet* 33:485-492, 1996.

49. Durant J, Hansen A, Bauer M: Public understanding of the new genetics. In Marteau T, Richards M, editors: *The troubled helix: social and psychological implications of the new human genetics,* Cambridge, 1996, Cambridge University Press.

50. Clow CL, Scriver CR: The adolescent copes with genetic screening: a study of Tay-Sachs screening among high-school students, *Prog Clin Biol Res* 18:381-393, 1977.

51. Blaese RM: Development of gene therapy for immunodeficiency: adenosine deaminase deficiency, *Pediatr Res* 33(suppl 1):S49-S55, 1992.

52. National Commission for the Protection of Human Subjects of Biomedical and Behavioral Research: *Research involving children: report and recommendations,* DHEW Pub No (OS) 77-0004, Washington, DC, 1977, US Government Printing Office.

53. Nicholson RH, editor: *Medical research with children: ethics, law, and practice,* Oxford, 1986, Oxford University Press.

54. Kodish E, Lantos J, Siegler M, et al: Bone marrow transplantation in sickle cell disease: the trade-off between early mortality and quality of life, *Clin Res* 38:694-700, 1990.

55. Walters MC, Patience M, Leisenring W, et al: Bone marrow transplantation for sickle cell disease, *N Engl J Med* 335:369-376, 1996.

56. US Department of Health and Human Services: Additional protections for children involved as subjects in research, *Federal Register* 48(46):9819, 1983.

57. Medical Research Council, Working Party on Research on Children: *The ethical conduct of research on children,* London, 1991, The Council.

58. Royal College of Physicians: *Supervision of the ethics of clinical research investigations in institutions,* London, 1973, The College.

59. Department of Health and Social Security: *Supervision of the ethics of clinical research investigations and fetal research,* London, 1975, The Department.

60. British Paediatric Association: *Guidelines for the ethical conduct of medical research involving children,* London, 1992, The Association.

61. Weir RF, Horton JR: Genetic research, adolescents, and informed consent, *Theor Med* 16:347-373, 1995.

62. Silverman WA: The myth of informed consent in daily practice and in clinical trials, *J Med Ethics* 15:6-11, 1989.

63. Harth SC, Johnstone RR, Thong YH: The psychological profile of parents who volunteer their children for clinical research: a controlled study, *J Med Ethics* 18:86-93, 1992.

64. Nelson D, Weiss R: Hasty decisions in the race to a cure? Gene therapy study proceeded despite safety, ethics concerns, *Washington Post,* Nov 21, 1999, p A1.

# CHAPTER 15

# Genetic Screening in General Internal Medicine

*Jason H. T. Karlawish*
*William H. Peranteau*

In addition to the diagnosis and treatment of patients with disease, the practice of internal medicine increasingly involves screening asymptomatic and apparently healthy persons for risk factors for disease. The histories of hypertension, osteoporosis, and cholesterol screening document the risk-oriented and preventive approaches of internal medicine.

New genetic testing promises that internists of the future will have the means to render a genetic risk profile of their patients.[1] Someday, during a routine clinic visit, after a simple blood draw, internists will be able to order genetic tests that quantify the chance that a person will develop disorders such as Alzheimer disease, non-insulin-dependent diabetes, and familial hypercholesterolemia. Adapting the terminology that describes packaged tests for serum electrolytes and enzymes as a "chem screen," this package of tests might be called a "gene screen."

Will a gene screen provide people with a precise balance sheet that details their health risk profile? Such a balance sheet could be achieved today; along with new genetic testing, health care systems and technologies permit internists to gather and synthesize large volumes of health risk information. Population-based medicine and information technologies could allow internists to translate a person's genetic, environmental, and personal habit information into a final calculation of health risks.[2,3] For example, persons at risk for adult-onset diabetes would be told to watch their weight and persons at risk for certain cancers advised to have periodic screening tests.

Although a gene screen may lead to a more effective and individualized practice of preventive medicine, it will present significant challenges to the internist. Screening tests, genetic or otherwise, are the focus of significant and contentious debates in internal medicine.[4-8] For example, whether a man over age 50 should be tested for his level of prostate-specific antigen (PSA) as a screen for prostate cancer is a question that divides the profession. Until consensus exists, practicing internists are advised to review with each of their patients various statistical representations of risk and benefits.[9] One internist concluded that this solution to one problem only creates another, as follows:

> *In clinical practice, time is crucial . . . explain[ing] the PSA screening controversy to patients takes time, and PSA screening is not the only gray area in terms of cancer detection . . . . I am left with a long list of recommendations and precious little time.*[10]

A gene screen may worsen this problem of limited time because it introduces additional clinical challenges. This chapter facilitates the acquisition of essential knowledge and skills to use genetic screening in general medical care.

Currently, nearly all common genetic diseases (150 to 200) and a large number of rare genetic diseases (600 to 800) have been traced back to one or more genes. Researchers have identified 1500 to 2000 genes that are associated with genetic diseases.[11] The Human Genome Project will soon complete the sequencing of the entire human genome.[12] More genes will be added to those already associated with various diseases.

The potential benefits of this scientific prosperity place an expectation of genetic services on general internists. Health care professionals certified in genetic counseling and medical genetics are unlikely to assume this role because their numbers have not kept pace with the increase in discovery of disease-related genes and the possible clinical applications of these discoveries.[13] The mismatch between demand for "genetic health care" and the supply from medical geneticists and genetic counselors means that primary care physicians will have to practice some kinds of genetic testing and intervention. Unfortunately, most primary care physicians have not had a single hour of instruction in genetics.[14] Before they introduce a genetic test into their clinical practice, physicians should have skills in the following:

1. Understanding the qualities of a useful genetic test
2. Deciding who is an appropriate candidate for a genetic test
3. Interpreting the results of a genetic test
4. Interacting with a patient when providing the option and the results of a genetic test

## QUALITIES OF USEFUL GENETIC TEST

The successful application of a genetic test requires knowing the key qualities that describe the test's resulting information and the positive test's suggested interventions.

### Is This a Predictive or a Predispositional Test?

This distinction is important because it describes the degree of certainty that a positive test entails for persons at risk for specific diseases. A *predictive genetic test* is for a gene that ultimately results in the presence of a disease in the individual, such as Huntington chorea, provided the person lives long enough for the phenotype to be expressed. Mendelian diseases are a classic example of these kinds of disorders. Although the presence of a gene in a predictive genetic test foreshadows the associated disease, the presence of a gene does not determine the time of onset or severity of the disease.

In contrast to predictive testing, a *predispositional genetic test* is for a gene associated with an increased incidence, or risk, of a disease. These "complex genetic diseases" include many of the common diseases that general internists diagnose and treat, such as diabetes, coronary artery disease, and Alzheimer disease. As in predictive genetic testing, the presence of the gene does not generally indicate the time of onset or severity of the disease, but predispositional genetic testing introduces an additional clinically important uncertainty. The individual may never develop the disease, since such a gene only indicates the predisposition or risk of a disease.

## What Are the Chances of a False-Negative Test?

Mendelian diseases and common complex diseases share features that can introduce uncertainty into a negative test result.[15] Not all disease-causing genotypes will be detected, since many diseases can result from several different inherited mutations at one gene locus (allelic diversity) or several loci (genetic or locus heterogeneity), and not all these mutations can usually be detected. This appears to be the case with many common diseases such as hypertension, for which not a single gene, but multiple genes, are likely to be implicated. Thus the provider must be aware of false negatives and have an effective method to communicate this to a patient.

## Will This Test Lead to a Clinically Useful Intervention?

This question is not unique to a genetic test and should be asked of any screening or diagnostic test. The experience of the U.S. Preventive Services Task Force shows that the evidence-based claim that a test is "useful" involves controversies in trade-offs in health outcomes and judgments about the harms and benefits of a screening test.[16] Health care policymakers and the general public sharply disagree about how to address these trade-offs and judgments.[4] Genetic tests are no exception to these disagreements. The general internist who adopts a genetic test as part of a "gene screen" has a duty to patients to ensure (1) consensus exists that the endpoints used to establish the test's benefit are sensible, (2) the balance of benefits to risks is favorable, and (3) the intervention does not involve controversial trade-offs for the patient.

Disagreements about usefulness can occur because claims of effectiveness may be based on health outcomes such as mortality without accounting for morbidity or on an intermediate endpoint such as bone mineral density or cholesterol levels. Even when agreement exists on endpoints to measure, controversy may exist regarding how to balance competing endpoints. For example, is a significant difference in a primary endpoint, such as reduction in nonfatal heart attack, outweighed by a significant difference in a secondary endpoint, such as increase in hemorrhagic stroke? Answering this question requires methods such as a decision analysis to determine whether or not the intervention maximizes utility. Attributing different weights to these harms and benefits can lead to conflicting judgments about the test's usefulness. In genetic testing, these judgments can be all the more challenging because the potential "harms" of the test include stigmatization and discrimination as a result of having a positive test.

## APPROPRIATE CANDIDATES FOR SPECIFIC GENETIC TEST

After understanding the qualities of a useful genetic test, the general internist must decide who should be offered the test. Family history and past medical history begin to describe a patient's risk of a genetic disease and thus the need for a test. Family histories are most useful when the mode of inheritance of a disease is X linked or autosomal dominant; they are less useful when assessing the risk of an autosomal recessive disease. After eliciting the history, the general internist can then use a genetic test to identify specific disease-related alleles in people with positive histories. This information defines the patient in need of an intervention that meets the qualities described earlier.[13]

If a family history is not available to provide guidance on whether to offer a genetic test, the physician should weigh the potential benefits of the intervention that follows a positive test. If the disease can be prevented or more effectively treated in its presymptomatic stage, and if the test has been shown to be effective in population-wide screening, the test should be offered regardless of the patient's family history. Such tests can be packaged into a "gene screen."

## GENETIC TEST RESULTS

Having identified useful genetic tests and the patients who should receive them, a general internist needs to have the skills to interpret test results. Genetic tests are no different than many nongenetic tests in clinical practice and are not perfect predictors. Their results require interpretation. The probability that a disease will occur when a test is positive or not occur when negative is not 100%. A general internist must be aware of the characteristics of the tests being ordered, including their sensitivities, specificities, and positive and negative predictive values.

Several useful heuristics provide a general framework for interpreting the results of a genetic test. A positive finding is most likely to be a correct prediction of eventual disease if (1) the disorder is mendelian, (2) the test is being performed in a high-risk family, and (3) the test identifies a mutation known to occur in the patient's affected relatives.[17] Similarly, a negative finding is most likely to be a correct prediction that the patient will remain free of a disease if (1) the disorder is mendelian, (2) the test is being performed in a high-risk family, and (3) the test identifies the absence of a mutation shared by the patient's affected relatives. In all other circumstances the meaning of a positive or negative test result with respect to the future acquisition of a disease is less certain and will be expressed by the test's characteristics. This uncertainty requires an internist to have the skills to communicate effectively with a patient about genetic testing.

## COMMUNICATION WITH PATIENTS

The general internist's fund of genetic knowledge, ability to determine which patients would benefit most from a genetic test, and ability to interpret findings correctly are instrumental in deciding which tests to apply in clinical practice. Also important is the primary care physician's ability to interact with a patient when providing the option and the results of a genetic test. This ability includes appreciating what patient factors influence decision making and knowing when to refer a patient to a genetic counselor.

The patient's willingness and desire to take a genetic test are instrumental to the test's use. Patients are more willing to take a test if they perceive effective methods to treat or prevent a disorder. For example, only 10% of patients who are offered predictive genetic testing for Huntington disease, a disease with no effective treatment, have the test. In contrast, approximately 80% of patients offered genetic testing for familial adenomatous polyposis, a disease for which there is effective treatment, accept it.[18] Willingness to have a test also depends on how a test is offered. Invitation by letter to take a genetic test has lower response rates than offering the test in person. Performing the test immediately after offering the test in person also increases a patient's willingness.[18]

In addition to a patient's perception of the effectiveness of interventions, reducing uncertainty[18] and tolerating the test's imperfection[17] are the most common reasons patients undergo a predictive genetic test. Thus a physician should elicit a patient's perceived risk of disease and tolerance for uncertainty. Questions might include the following:

- How much are you bothered by the uncertainty of whether you have the gene?
- What do you think about the test's uncertainties?
- Do you think you are at risk for the disease?

A patient who chooses to have genetic testing may experience psychological morbidity as a result of the test. People who discover they carry a mutation that predisposes them to a disorder tend to be more distressed than those whose test results are negative. However, an individual who has a negative test may experience distress as a form of survivor guilt. In both instances the distress is generally within a normal range.[18]

A person's pretest mood also influences the response to a genetic test. For example, individuals who were distressed before undergoing genetic testing for Huntington disease are likely to experience an adverse psychological outcome after testing.[19] When a test identifies a serious disease for which no intervention or only a burdensome intervention is available, the physician should assess the patient's mood. Even mild cases of depression or anxiety may warrant treatment before proceeding with a test.

Independent of the result, other factors are important in understanding and predicting an individual's response to genetic testing. Pretest expectations may play a prominent role. If individuals have a family history suggestive of familial polyposis, they may be aware that they are at risk and may have a pretest expectation that the genetic test will be positive. Such expectations may explain why those who are aware of their risk experience less distress than those who do not believe they are at risk. Women are more likely than men to experience negative feelings after genetic testing; for both sexes, however, social supports and psychological resources affect the individual's response to a genetic test.[18]

A physician may influence patients' willingness to have a genetic test and their reaction to its results. Offering and performing a test during the same office visit result in the greatest use of the test. In conditions with effective treatment, a high rate of testing may be the most important goal, so this approach may be the most appropriate. When no effective treatment is available, however, general internists may refer the patient to a genetic counselor with special training and certification. The more a genetic counseling model governs the approach to a patient, the more clinic time and access to counseling will be needed. In such a model the plan to link tests in a screening package is less acceptable.

What qualities of a genetic test determine that its clinical application requires the skills of a genetic counselor? The more the genetic information and its implications adhere to accepted notions of health and standards of diagnosis and treatment, the more that information may be well managed by a general internist. In contrast, the more the information fits within the category of personal and nonmedical issues, such as whether a couple chooses to have a child with Down syndrome, the more that information should be managed according to nondirective genetic counseling.

This guideline conforms with the Institute of Medicine's recommendations that (1) tests can be linked with similar tests in regard to how health care professionals present such a package, and (2) "the goal of nondirective counseling, so crucial in genetic services pertaining to reproductive planning, may not always be appropriate when primary prevention or effective treatments are available."[20] This guideline also addresses internists' concern about available time in the clinic to implement screening tests. Nondirective presentation requires more counseling time. When a person's counseling needs exceed the abilities or time available to a general internist, referral to a genetic counselor is appropriate.

## SUMMARY

Someday, internists will employ genetic tests as part of their routine clinical practice, including a "gene screen" for late-onset genetic disorders. The development and implementation of a gene screen should not be an exclusively professional matter. Internists and society together need to address important issues as candidate tests move from research into practice. With each test, broad consensus should establish that each test is effective. Furthermore, if internists are to use the test, they should understand the qualities of a useful genetic test and have the skills to decide who is an appropriate candidate for a specific genetic test and to communicate with a patient when providing the option and the results of a genetic test. Failure to address any of these issues will likely lead to controversial recommendations, intensifying the concern about insufficient time in the clinic to implement genetic tests.

## REFERENCES

1. Hilts P: Love of numbers leads to chromosome 17, *New York Times,* 1996, pp B5-B6.
2. Harris JJ: Disease management: new wine in new bottles? *Ann Intern Med* 124:838-842, 1996.
3. Epstein R, Sherwood L: From outcomes research to disease management: a guide for the perplexed, *Ann Intern Med* 124:832-837, 1996.
4. Ubel P et al: Cost-effectiveness analysis in the setting of budget constraints—is it equitable? *N Engl J Med* 334:1174-1177, 1996.
5. Pauker S: Deciding about screening, *Ann Intern Med* 118:901-902, 1993 (editorial).
6. Davidoff F: Evangelists and snails redux: the case of cholesterol screening, *Ann Intern Med* 124:513-514, 1996 (editorial).
7. Garber A, Brown W, Hulley S: Clinical guideline. Part 2. Cholesterol screening in asymptomatic adults, revisited, *Ann Intern Med* 124:518-531, 1996.
8. LaRosa J: Cholesterol agnostics, *Ann Intern Med* 124:505-508, 1996.

9.  Woolf S: Screening for prostate cancer with prostate specific antigen: an examination of the evidence, *N Engl J Med* 333:1401-1405, 1995.

10. Hensel W: Screening for prostate cancer, *N Engl J Med* 334:667, 1996 (letter).

11. Bobrow M: Foreword, *Lancet* 354(suppl 1), 1999.

12. Collins FS et al: New goals for the U.S. Human Genome Project: 1998-2003, *Science* 282:682-689, 1998.

13. Holtzman NA, Watson MS, editors: *Promoting safe and effective genetic testing in the United States,* Baltimore, 1998, Johns Hopkins University Press.

14. Collins F: Shattuck Lecture—Medical and societal consequences of the human genome project, *N Engl J Med* 341:28-37, 1999.

15. Holtzman N, Shapiro D: Genetic testing and public policy, *BMJ* 316:852-856, 1998.

16. Woolf S et al: Developing evidence-based practice guidelines: lessons learned by the U.S. Preventive Services Task Force, *Annu Rev Public Health* 17:511-538, 1996.

17. Holtzman N: Molecular genetics in clinical practice XI: bringing genetic tests into the clinic, *Hosp Pract* 32:107-128, 1998.

18. Marteau T, Croyle R: Psychological responses to genetic testing, *BMJ* 316:693-696, 1998.

19. Decrvyenaere M et al: Prediction of psychological functioning one year after the predictive test for Huntington's disease and impact of the test result on reproductive decision making, *J Hum Genet* 33:737-743, 1996.

20. Andrews L et al, editors: *Assessing genetic risks: implications for health and social policy,* Washington, DC, 1994, National Academy Press.

# CHAPTER 16

# Genetic Testing as a Family Affair

*Robert J. Moss*
*Shelly A. Cummings*
*Mary B. Mahowald*

Primary care physicians must understand the broad implications of the Human Genome Project, that is, the unraveling of 3 billion base pairs or the 50,000 to 100,000 genes that make up the human genetic constitution.[1] DNA-based testing already has the potential to provide presymptomatic diagnosis for a number of single-gene disorders and to discern predisposition to many other genetically influenced diseases.[2] A panel of screening tests to identify numerous genes will likely be offered in the near future, not unlike the chemistry screening panels of today. How will primary care physicians assimilate, integrate, and apply all this information about the genetic makeup of patients? How will they obtain a truly informed consent from patients for testing, when the amount of genetic information is so enormous and its implications often so uncertain? When a patient decides to undergo testing, what are the consequences, intended or not, for other family members and future generations?

Despite the recommendation of professional organizations that genetic testing for cancer susceptibility be confined to research protocols, such testing has already been introduced into clinical practice.[3] Along with this testing, evidence indicates that not all patients have the opportunity of pretest genetic counseling or a formal process of informed consent. In a recent survey of practitioners in the United States, 28% of those who offered genetic tests for breast cancer reported that their patients did not have access to a genetic counselor despite laboratory requirements for such counseling.[4] A confidential inquiry into counseling for genetic disorders by nongeneticists in the United Kingdom found that practitioners frequently overlooked the need for counseling and fewer than half of patients were referred to a geneticist.[5] A prospective study of genetic testing for familial adenomatous polyposis (FAP), one of the few conditions potentially treatable by high-risk surveillance and prophylactic colectomy, examined these issues further. Fewer than 20% of individuals received pretest genetic counseling or gave written informed consent for testing, and approximately one third of the time, physicians misinterpreted the meaning of test results.[6]

The new era of genetics also gives rise to a unique subset of medical-ethical dilemmas, many previously unexplored. These dilemmas include conflicts between the patient's interests and those of other family members and between the right to be tested and informed of test results and the right to refuse testing and disclosure of results. Because genetic information is personal and familial, relatives of a person tested may have a right to learn that person's test results if the information is relevant to their own health and could not be obtained in other ways. "A shared biologic risk creates special interests and moral obligations and these may outweigh an individual's wishes for access to genetic information."[7]

This chapter begins with several cases that highlight this potential dilemma, then discusses the role of the family in decision making and examines the differences between genetic tests and other medical tests. Because of the special nature of genetic testing, family decision making is often not only desirable but unavoidable. Studies of genetic testing for specific conditions and consequences of such testing are considered next. Then the cases are reexamined, with questions to facilitate discussion of genetic testing with patients and family members. The chapter concludes with central points to consider in the process of obtaining consent to genetic testing as a family affair.

## CASE EXAMPLES

### Huntington Disease

The proband, a 69-year-old man with symptoms of Huntington disease (HD), had a direct DNA test, which was positive. He has monozygous twin sons in their 30s, an attorney and a medical researcher. Each twin was asked whether he wished to participate in genetic counseling and testing to determine his risk for HD. Twin #1 made an appointment to meet with the geneticist but refused to register at the front desk. He wanted no paper trail of his risk status and asked if he could be counseled without any record of the visit. The physician refused but told him that her notes would be brief and would reflect only that a confidential discussion was held. When twin #1's wife asked if the visit could be recorded under her patient account number, the physician agreed. This alternative was not acceptable to twin #1, however, who left without being seen after deciding that he did not want to know his future risk status. Twin #2 met with the geneticist but left undecided. He was considering testing even if his brother would not agree.

### Breast-Ovarian Cancer

The patient is a 35-year-old woman with two teenage daughters. The patient's mother had bilateral breast cancer at age 34, was successfully treated, and currently has no evidence of disease recurrence. A strong family history for breast and ovarian cancer in the patient's family is documented in three generations. The patient is very distressed about this history and believes that she is at significant risk for developing breast or ovarian cancer. She is also concerned about her daughters' risks. The patient is considering a bilateral mastectomy and possibly an oophorectomy to reduce her cancer risk. Her decision could be facilitated by knowledge of whether she carries a mutation in one of the cancer susceptibility genes, BRCA1 or BRCA2. Due to the complexity of these genes, testing for them is more informative when it can be compared with test results in a family member who has had the disease. Her mother is her only living affected relative, and she will not agree to be tested. The proband still has the option of undergoing genetic testing, which may be covered by insurance because of her strong family history. Prophylactic surgery would probably be covered by insurance if she tests positive regardless of whether her mother is tested.

### Familial Adenomatous Polyposis

A middle-aged man was tested and found to have an alteration in the adenomatous polyposis coli (APC) gene, which causes FAP, an autosomal dominant condition. He refused to tell his adult children that he had the altered gene. Concerned about the relevance of this information to the children, the physician wonders whether he has any legal, moral, or professional obligations to them.

## ROLE OF THE FAMILY IN MEDICAL DECISION MAKING

Primary care practitioners increasingly find themselves trying to balance the moral claims of one patient against those of other patients. By acknowledging the rights of other patients, physicians move from a medical ethic recently dominated by the principal of autonomy toward one that promotes the principle of justice. Several authors, however, have argued that the principle of justice does not go far enough in addressing the nonmedical interests of those intimately involved with the patient, such as the family.[8-13] They suggest that families also have legitimate claims in medical-ethical decision making and that their interests must be balanced against the rights of the individual patient. They question whether family members may legitimately be asked to sacrifice their own interests to ensure optimal care of the patient. Presumably, even if family members are asked to promote the patient's interests at the expense of their own, they may legitimately refuse to do so at times. Different people may have competing interests that need to be considered, as follows:

> *Many individuals other than the patient possess moral interests that demand respect; and autonomy of the patient is but one factor among many real moral claims. Accommodation rather than autonomy should determine an ethically appropriate arrangement. Accommodation requires mediating between the patient's desires and the reality of available services and the real competing interests of others.*[13]

Focusing exclusively on the patient's autonomy ignores that patients "are social beings intertwined with the lives of others." Hardwig[12] thus advises clinicians who might otherwise fail to consider the relationships or responsibilities of patients: "You cannot detach the lives of patients from other lives that are close to them. When you are close, you no longer have a life entirely your own. . . . Patients also must weigh medical need against the non-medical benefits and burdens of treatment to self and family."

In 1993 the American Medical Association's Council on Scientific Affairs[14] advocated for a model that considers the caregiver and the patient as a single unit of care. The council not only legitimized the role of the family caregiver, but also dramatically changed traditional thinking about the patient-physician relationship. An estimated. 2.2 million family members and friends provide health care and other instrumental assistance to about 1.3 million frail elderly persons, saving the formal health system billions of dollars annually. Approximately half of seniors cared for by family members require assistance in five or more activities of daily living. The average caregiving workload can vary between 4 and 8 hours per day, lasting 1 to 4 years.[14]

Family caregivers deserve to be involved in decisions for patients because their caregiving is often a threat to their own health. The risks they face include high rates of depression, lower rates of preventive health practices for themselves, and increased susceptibility to alterations in the immune system.[14] Beyond such specific risk factors, caregiving has been shown to be an independent factor for mortality.[15]

The social impact of caregiving on family members is marked as well. When someone is seriously ill, for example, Covinsky and colleagues[16] found that 20% of the time, a family member had to quit work or make another major life change to provide care for the patient. Loss of most or all of the family savings was reported by 31% of families, with 29% reporting the loss of a major source of income. Many families had to make changes in life plans by moving to a less expensive home, delaying education, or putting off medical care for others. Medically and socially, the burden of caregiving for a family member can be even greater than the burden of illness or disability borne by the patient. "In many cases family members have a greater interest than the patient in which treatment option is being exercised and should be able to override the patient."[12]

The role for the family in medical-ethical decision making has generally been unexplored. Using a semistructured interview with patients and families, however, Reust and Mattingly[10] attempted to clarify the process by describing three potential roles that family members play in medical decision making, as follows:

1. In a supportive role, families help the patient think through the relevant medical options and provide emotional support.
2. In a patient advocate role, families ask questions of the health care team, communicate information, and ensure that the patient receives all necessary care.
3. In a caregiver role, families not only provide care but are affected in various ways by its provision.

The authors confirmed that patients do consider how their illness disrupts daily routines for family members as well as for themselves.[10] The general practitioner, who often sees the impact of caregiving on family members, legitimizes the family's role in medical-ethical decision making, helping resolve ethical dilemmas more equitably. When the decision making involves genetic information, the importance of family involvement is even greater.

## DIFFERENCES BETWEEN GENETIC TESTS AND OTHER MEDICAL TESTS

Arguments for involvement of the family in decision making are stronger in the context of genetics than in other areas of health care because of the special character of knowledge about genes or heredity. Genetic tests may be contrasted with other medical tests in several ways. The first difference is that although genetic testing may result in a definitive diagnosis, providing an assessment of individual risk, it does not indicate the status of a person's health as it reclassifies the individual from healthy to at-risk status. The degree of risk may depend on the specific mutation identified. Testing provides predictive but not precise information about the time of onset, rate of progression, severity, and disease manifestations. Variable expressivity, incomplete penetrance, and genetic heterogeneity reduce the ability of a genetic test to predict future disease accurately. Also, for many diseases, multiple genes may interact with environmental factors to impact disease occurrence.[17-21]

A second difference is the therapeutic gap between the ability to test for susceptibility to a genetic disease and the limited ability to reduce mortality and morbidity of a particular condition. Even if the level of prediction is high, there is often no proven strategy of prevention, early detection, or treatment for the identified genetic disease. There is even less information about the risk of secondary malignancies when screening for cancer susceptibility genes with regard to prevention or treatment. It therefore becomes exceedingly difficult to know how to integrate genetic information into the care of patients who are identified at high risk for acquiring the disease.[17-19,21]

Third, genetic testing can be considered experimental in nature because the full risks and benefits of testing are often unknown to the individual at testing. Except for prenatal diagnosis, the principal consequences of genetic testing appear to be psychological and social rather than physical. These consequences have been studied for a limited number of conditions. For most genetic diseases, no clinical standards exist to determine when testing for high-risk status is appropriate. Predictive testing is not without hazards, often creating difficult choices for the individual and family.

Fourth, the physician who provides genetic testing to one patient often recognizes its implications on other family members for whom the physician may be responsible.[22] Through the testing of one patient, family members often learn (whether or not they may want to know) that they are predisposed to a condition that can be inherited and passed on to other family members as well as future generations. Recently, for example, a New Jersey appeals court heard a case of a woman with FAP who sued the estate of her deceased father's deceased physician for not warning relatives of their risk 20 years earlier. In England the House of Commons veered toward the other direction, stating that an individual's decision to withhold such information should be respected. The British Task Force on Genetic Testing seems to stress confidentiality more than the duty to warn, stating that providers should not communicate results to relatives except in extreme circumstances.[19]

Fifth, family members may be placed in the unfortunate position of being the primary caregiver for the patient with a genetic disease, while suffering the emotional and social consequences of being at risk for the disease themselves. Ultimately, they may be transformed from caregiver to patient.

Finally, genetic testing often requires direct family involvement. Typically, genetic diagnoses obtained from history taking need to be confirmed by testing first-degree and second-degree relatives.[23] Confirmed family histories are often used as major screening criteria for further testing. For a genetic test to be useful to an individual family member, other members have to be willing to provide their own genetic background and often a sample of their blood for analysis. Family involvement is most needed in linkage analysis and least needed in the direct DNA testing of a genetic disease with few common mutations.

## GENETIC TESTING FOR SPECIFIC CONDITIONS

To obtain truly informed consent to genetic testing, physicians need to understand why an individual would choose to undergo genetic screening. Presumably the reasons parallel those that influence other types of health-related behavior: (1) perceived susceptibility and severity of the condition under consideration, (2) perceived benefits of action to decrease susceptibility or severity of the condition, and (3) barriers or personal costs of the health action.[24] These factors differ for different genetic conditions.

### Huntington Disease

One condition for which considerable data exist regarding the desirability and impact of genetic tests on patients and family members is Huntington disease, or Huntington chorea. This is a severe, untreatable, late-onset neurodegenerative, autosomal dominant condition for which genetic testing has been available since 1993. Before the discovery of the HD gene, when those at risk for HD were asked whether they would undergo a predictive genetic test for it if such a test became available, 56% to 75% indicated they would do so. Surprisingly, less than 20% of at-risk individuals have actually entered a predictive testing program, and rates as low as 5% have been reported.[25]

About two thirds of respondents at risk for HD see predictive testing as an opportunity rather than a threat to them. Knowledge of their risk status may enhance personal autonomy by allowing affected individuals to plan better for the future and assist them in making decisions about procreation. Although time of onset remains uncertain, even a positive test may relieve the anxiety of not knowing whether an individual is affected or not. In general, the greater the genetic burden and the more treatable the condition, the greater is the participation in testing.[25-27]

Reasons why respondents did not want to undergo predictive testing for HD included the following:

- Lack of access to a testing center
- Lack of available treatment
- Concern about the presumed emotional and psychological consequences of knowing that they were at increased risk
- Satisfaction with their lives as currently lived
- Disinterest in knowing what might happen years ahead
- A sense that the certainty of acquiring HD would make their present lives unbearable

Limitations in the accuracy of a linked genetic test (before DNA testing was available for HD) and the need to test often unavailable family members were additional reasons for decisions against testing. Most respondents thought that pretest counseling should be mandatory and that testing should be withheld from persons who were psychologically unstable or threatening suicide.[25-27]

When a genetic test for HD was introduced, investigators asked what factors led individuals already risk-stratified by linkage analysis testing to undergo more sensitive DNA testing and whether the availability of a more sensitive test would lead to greater participation in predictive testing.[25] Approximately three fourths of those previously involved in linkage studies said they would participate in a program that involved a direct test for the mutation. Individuals who had not participated previously in the predictive testing program, either because the DNA markers used were not informative in their families or because no blood was available from crucial family members, were highly likely to choose this new opportunity. Less than half of those who previously refused testing said they would request the more accurate DNA tests, primarily because of the lack of any effective treatment for HD.[25]

Preferences for predictive DNA testing for HD also depended on the individual's perception of the current risk situation. Individuals already determined to be at low risk by indirect genetic linkage analysis avoided taking any further risk to change that. In contrast, individuals found to be at high risk by linkage analysis were more interested in further testing.[25]

**Breast-Ovarian Cancer**

Because of the greater prevalence of complex conditions, studies of genetic tests for susceptibility to them may be more relevant to primary caregivers than studies of single-gene, relatively rare disorders such as HD. For example, a prospective study of decisions to undergo BRCA1 testing in families with hereditary breast-ovarian cancer showed that 43% of the participants requested test results when offered. The most frequently anticipated benefit of testing was learning an offspring's risk status, and the greatest perceived risk was the fear of losing health insurance. Requests for results were more common in those with health insurance, in first-degree relatives with breast cancer, or in those with greater knowledge about BRCA testing.[28] In a study of breast cancer in a group of women less than 50 years of age, 72% indicated that they wanted to be tested for the BRCA1 gene. Three to 15 months later, however, only 49% of these women had contacted a genetic counselor, and only one half had been tested. The intention to be tested was associated with (1) the presence of breast cancer, (2) a greater perceived benefit of testing, (3) higher levels of concern about genetic risk in relatives, and (4) perception of lower personal risk or costs.[24]

**Prenatal Testing**

With regard to prenatal testing for single-gene disorders, studies of HD and cystic fibrosis (CF) testing are informative.

## HUNTINGTON DISEASE

In a 5-year study of prenatal testing for HD, 43% of predictive testing candidates indicated they would use prenatal testing if they or their spouses became pregnant. If the prenatal test revealed an increased risk to the fetus, 40% said they would terminate the pregnancy, 25% would complete the pregnancy, and 35% were uncertain. Despite these results, the actual demand for prenatal testing by eligible candidates was only 18%. The most frequently cited reason for declining prenatal testing was the hope that a cure would be found in time to benefit the child. Compared with those who declined testing, those who requested prenatal testing were just starting their families and were less likely to be practicing members of religious organizations.[29]

## CYSTIC FIBROSIS

When parents of children with CF were queried about their reproductive plans, the majority said they did not plan to have more children; 77% of the others said they would consider prenatal diagnosis in subsequent pregnancies. Of those who would consider testing, 28% indicated that they would undergo an abortion if the test were positive, 44% would carry to term, and 28% were undecided. The decision to use prenatal genetic testing was associated with the following three psychosocial factors[30]:

1. Respondent's willingness to undergo an abortion if the test were positive
2. Concerns about the impact of termination on other children
3. Severity of symptoms in the child or children already affected

### Hereditary Nonpolyposis Colorectal Cancer

Recent studies in hereditary nonpolyposis colorectal cancer (HNPCC) showed that before the availability of genetic testing, 83% of the general population and 82% of first-degree relatives of colon cancer patients were interested in testing. When testing became available, however, only 43% elected to participate in a counseling and testing program. Among women with depressive symptoms, rates of testing were reduced fourfold. The relationship between depression and test acceptance was stronger in women than in men, with lower levels of testing in those with less education.[31]

### Fragile X Syndrome

Most parents indicated that they would want their children at risk for fragile X syndrome to undergo carrier testing. They thought their children should have knowledge of their carrier status before sexual activity and should be allowed to marry with knowledge of their genetic risk. They did not believe that their children would be treated differently if they were identified as carriers. Mothers were more concerned than fathers about raising a child with knowledge of carrier status. The parents' right to have their children tested was associated with (1) the need to resolve the issue of carrier status, (2) concern about potential behavioral or educational problems, (3) a sense that such knowledge was relevant to decisions about marriage and sexual activity, and (4) the desire to provide anticipatory guidance to the child.[32]

### Familial Bipolar Disorder

Familial bipolar disorder (FBP) provides an example of possible genetic testing for psychiatric conditions. As with other complex diseases, FBP is associated with multiple genetic loci acting independently or in concert. After FBP was linked to chromosome 18, individuals with a bipolar disorder and their spouses were surveyed regarding their attitudes toward genetic testing. The majority said they would want testing in all domains, including prenatal, presymptomatic, and testing for minors. The greatest perceived benefit was to obtain treatment to prevent illness. Of patients diagnosed with FBP, 84% said they would take the test. Most spouses (85%) wanted to know their affected partner's test result. If they underwent prenatal testing and obtained positive results, 55% of those affected and 65% of their spouses would not abort; 55% would not be deterred from having children. With regard to marriage, 91% of those affected and 79% of their spouses probably or definitely would still have married each other.[33]

## POSTTEST SEQUELAE

Adverse consequences have been reported for individuals who undergo predictive testing and find themselves at high risk for a genetic disease. The HD predictive testing programs provide considerable data on the topic. The most serious potential response to being identified at high risk for HD is suicide. Many individuals reported that they had little or no consistent or reliable source of support. In one pretesting counseling program, approximately 2% to 6% of the participants were discovered to be at high risk for severe psychiatric response. When the respondents were asked before genetic testing about their reaction to a positive test result, 10% spontaneously said they would commit suicide, and more than half of these maintained this position even after pretest counseling. Approximately a third reported that they knew of or had an immediate relative who had been hospitalized for attempted suicide or other psychiatric reasons. However, no suicides or psychiatric hospitalizations have been reported subsequent to pretest or posttest counseling in the HD testing programs.[26,34-36]

Other sequelae of positive testing for HD also affect family members. These include profound anxiety and depression, resentment, dread of the future, broken relationships, alteration of body image, and a deep sense of loss of control. Concern about being a burden to or pitied by others often results in voluntary isolation. Although HD is uniquely devastating because of the severity of its symptoms, the definitiveness of the predictive test, and its incurability, some sequelae are applicable to other genetic tests. Different defensive postures and patterns of dealing with "bad news" are critical variables in helping individuals cope with their positive diagnoses.[26,34-36]

Many individuals fear the social consequences of their decision to undergo predictive testing. Uncertain about their rights to privacy and confidentiality, they worry about discrimination in the workplace or the difficulty of obtaining life or health insurance if others knew their risk status. In a survey of people with a known genetic condition in the family, 22% indicated that they had been refused health insurance coverage because of their genetic status, whether or not they were sick.[37] Legislation is gradually being introduced to reduce the incidence of genetic discrimination in employment and insurance coverage (see Chapter 19). In general, however, patients, family members, and practitioners need to act cautiously in considering this factor in decisions about genetic testing.

Several potential adverse consequences of prenatal testing are described for CF. If a woman plans to carry a pregnancy to term regardless of the results, prenatal testing becomes the equivalent of predictive genetic testing in childhood. Distortion in parent-child or sibling-sibling relationships may occur. For example, the parents may have lower expectations for the child, the child may have loss of self-esteem or self-worth, and siblings may experience survivor guilt.[30,38] Families have reported changes in feelings toward their infants after learning the diagnosis of CF. Although many (55%) consider themselves overprotective and more attached to affected children, 14% temporarily rejected them.[39]

At times, for the abnormality diagnosed prenatally, the implications and prognosis are unclear. Marital discord may occur because of different beliefs about prenatal diagnosis and termination of pregnancy. Such unresolved conflicts may affect couples' relationships far into the future.[26,29-30,40] Again, to date, no catastrophic psychological responses to prenatal testing, including emotional breakdowns or suicide, have been described in HD collaborative studies. However, some couples have felt compelled to use the test in every pregnancy after using it in the first one. Extensive counseling may be needed to free couples from feeling they must make the same choice they made in previous pregnancies. The psychological suffering that might result from the successive loss of repeated pregnancies has to be balanced against the possible relief of knowing that the current pregnancy is at low risk for having inherited the gene for HD.[29]

Prospective studies have not reported major adverse outcomes of predictive genetic testing for HD or breast cancer.[35] Mutation carriers identified through BRCA1 testing of families with hereditary breast-ovarian cancer showed no increase in their level of depressive symptoms or functional impairment 1 month after disclosure of the result. The potential for discrimination by insurance carriers was identified as the greatest barrier for testing. Approximately a third of these carriers reported planning a prophylactic oophorectomy and 15% a prophylactic mastectomy.[28]

Less is understood about the consequences of genetic testing for diseases that are polygenic or have an environmental component. At one institution, however, newborns were screened for increased genetic risks for type I diabetes. Levels of parenting stress in mothers notified of increased risk in their infants did not significantly change compared with those of mothers of low-risk infants.[41]

Predictive genetic testing has clear benefits for those found to be at low risk for some genetic diseases. For example, persons identified as low risk after predictive testing for HD reported lower rates of depression.[42] Similarly, studies of persons found to be noncarriers of a mutated BRCA1 gene also demonstrated improvements in psychosocial functioning.[28] However, approximately 10% of those initially at risk for HD had difficulty coping with their new low-risk status, often requiring professional intervention and counseling. Some had already made irreversible decisions in their life based on the belief that they would develop HD. When test results contradicted that expectation, coping with a previously unplanned future became difficult.[42] Also, their low-risk status did not necessarily empower these individuals to make new decisions about their lives, since their decisions had to be made from a new perspective of strength, health, and a full life span rather than disease, disability, and a short life span. Some with negative results experienced survivor guilt, continuing to worry about other family members. One spouse was unhappy with his wife's new low-risk status because he had retired and was looking forward to taking on the role of a caregiver for his wife.[42]

## CASE EXAMPLES REVISITED

Figures 16-1 to 16-3 highlight a significant ethical dilemma often experienced in the informed consent process for genetic testing. At times, an individual's right to determine his or her genetic status may be in direct conflict with family members' right *not* to know their status. In addition, an individual's right *not* to know his or her status may be in conflict

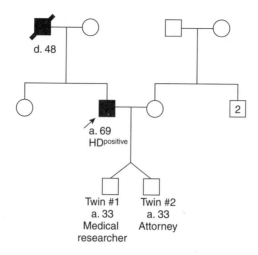

**FIGURE 16-1**   Huntington disease *(HD)* in twins. See text.

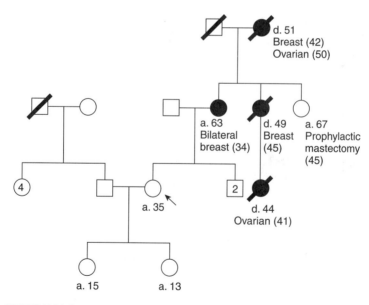

**FIGURE 16-2**   Breast and ovarian cancer risk in three generations. See text.

with the family's right to know. The initial decision to pursue testing involves more than the individual because its implications are both personal and familial. The common bond of shared genetic risk creates special moral obligations for both parties. Because the many risks and benefits to both parties overlap, a sharp distinction between the individual's rights and those of the family is not supportable. Involvement of family members in decisions about genetic testing is thus not only clinically optimal but also ethically justified.

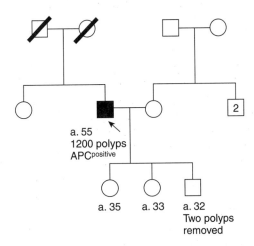

a. 55
1200 polyps
APCpositive

a. 35    a. 33    a. 32
Two polyps
removed

**FIGURE 16-3** Adenomatous polyposis coli *(APC)* gene and familial adenomatous polyposis. See text.

As already stated, however, little guidance is available on how to incorporate families into the process of obtaining informed consent for genetic testing.[43-45] Family members may want to participate in pretest genetic counseling together so that a family history can be confirmed and basic information provided about the relevant genetic disease and test. Because individuals can easily be overwhelmed by too much information, having other family members present may help clarify understanding. It may also reinforce the idea that risks for the disease are shared. The complex issues of confidentiality, potential discrimination, and other social consequences of decisions about genetic testing need to be explored as issues that family members have in common. Because individual family members may differ with regard to their risks and preferences, however, they should be offered the opportunity for individual counseling to address their personal concerns. They should also be encouraged to meet again among themselves to express their concerns about further testing to each other. The following questions serve as a guide to such discussions as well as those involving the general practitioner:

- Is the genetic disease in question a treatable, potentially treatable, or untreatable condition?
- How effective are the treatments?
- Are there mechanisms to prevent this disease once genetic status is known? If not, can the overall risk be reduced? If so, by how much?
- What interventions exist for risk reduction or treatment: to forego childbearing, to use gamete donation, to terminate an affected fetus, to be screened for the disease more frequently or at a younger age, to undergo prophylactic surgery?
- What are the burdens and benefits of testing to the individual and the family for this condition?
- Are the consequences only psychological or social, or do physical risks and benefits also exist?
- What does the test cost, and will it be covered for this patient or family?
- What kind of genetic test is available, and how definitive and accurate is the information?
- How necessary is the testing of other family members to identify the genetic mutation?

- Are there alternative means of quantifying the risk without genetic testing?
- What is the nature and number of mutations associated with this disease, the risk associated with the mutation type, and the expected severity of the disease?
- What are the religious, cultural, and ethnic values that may further influence family decision making?
- Do family members have common goals or reasons for genetic testing, and do these meet the personal needs of the individual? If not, how can individual differences be resolved?
- Is further counseling needed for the individual or the family?

The more preventable or treatable the genetic disease, the more compelling are the individual or family's rights to know their genetic status. The potential benefit of cure would seem to outweigh even the heaviest burden of knowing that one is at high risk for the disease. As a genetic condition becomes less treatable and preventable, however, the burdens to be weighed tend to be more psychological and social. The risks of knowing may then outweigh the benefits, and the right *not* to know or disclose one's genetic status may take precedence over the right to know or disclose it. Accordingly, the American Society of Clinical Oncology recommends testing (1) in families with well-defined hereditary syndromes only when a positive or negative test result would change medical care and (2) in hereditary syndromes when the medical benefit of carrier identification is presumed but not proved.[45] Genetic testing is higher for diseases with effective therapies or preventive measures, for example, 10% for HD versus 50% for BRCA1 screening and 80% for FAP.[36]

### Huntington Disease

Because HD is an autosomal dominant devastating disease with no effective treatment, the medical, psychological, and social risks to the individual as well as family members are significant (see Figure 16-1). By eliminating a paper trail, twin #1 in the case example apparently hopes to avoid social discrimination, which might otherwise occur through loss of his job or health insurance. Although we know little about the motivation of twin #2, it is likely that if he learns his risk status, twin #1 will also learn his status. The practitioner in this case should convene a family meeting at which the available information about HD and the implications of testing are discussed. A person who is not genetically related to either twin but is part of the family is the wife of twin #1. Her wishes and welfare, particularly with regard to childbearing, ought to weigh heavily in this discussion. Her moral right *to* know may even supersede her husband's right *not* to know. If reproductive decisions will not be affected by this information, however, and given the significant health and social risks to patients informed that they have the HD mutation, twin #2 probably has a moral obligation to protect the rights and interests of his brother by not obtaining the test for himself. In other words, if the risks to twin #1 outweigh the risk of not knowing to twin #2, twin #2 should yield in this case to his brother. If twin #2 persists in his request for testing, however, he has a legal right to obtain this information.

### Breast-Ovarian Cancer

Breast and ovarian cancer are potentially treatable conditions for which intensified surveillance strategies are effective (see Figure 16-2). Positive tests for mutations in the BRCA1 or BRCA2 gene indicate up to an 85% lifetime risk of developing breast cancer and up to 60% risk of developing ovarian cancer.[46,47] Prophylactic surgeries may reduce these risks considerably, but the extent of the reduction is unknown.[48-50] In the case example the mother probably has a moral obligation to be tested to facilitate a more informative result in her daughter's test. Again, a family meeting might identify the source of the mother's refusal and address it to the satisfaction of both parties. The mother's refusal may be motivated by fear or ignorance (both of which may be reduced through the provision of accurate information), by pressures from other family members, by tensions between mother and daughter, or by a sense of responsibility for having "passed on" a deleterious mutation. In the absence of the mother's agreement to be tested, however, neither the daughter nor the practitioner should pressure her in that regard. Because of her strong family history, however, the daughter's desire to be tested should be supported regardless of whether her mother provides blood for the genetic test. A positive genetic test of the daughter alone will give practitioners medical justification for performing prophylactic surgery if she so chooses; it will also provide insurance companies adequate grounds for covering the procedure.

### Familial Adenomatous Polyposis

FAP is a genetic condition that has a 100% chance of developing into a cancer that would be readily preventable through colectomy (see Figure 16-3).[6] In the case example the father would seem to have a compelling moral obligation to disclose his genetic status to his children to help prevent them from developing colon cancer. His children's right to know would outweigh his right to withhold this information.

## SUMMARY

Genetic screening affects not only the individual but potentially every member of the family now and in future generations. It is therefore important that physicians begin to view genetic issues within the broader context of the family.[51] Family members may play three roles in medical decision making: support system, advocate, and caregiver.[10] Because genetic information is familial as well as personal, a fourth role may occur in genetic testing—potential patient. This role arises because of the significant chance that the family caregiver may develop the same disease.

Although primary care practitioners do not play the fourth role with regard to patients, they are part of the patient's support system as advocates and caregivers. Physicians can facilitate the involvement of family members, who do fulfill the fourth role. Primary care physicians should consider the following points in recognition of consent to genetic testing as a family affair:

1. The person participating in the testing program should be encouraged to involve other family members.
2. Family counseling about genetic testing, as well as individual counseling, should be routinely offered and encouraged but should not be imposed.
3. Whether or not family members participate in genetic counseling or testing, the potential impact on them should be discussed with the patient.

4. Family members who are asked to donate blood for genetic testing should be fully informed about the potential consequences to them.

5. Social risks, such as insurance and employment discrimination, should be discussed with patients and with family members who participate in genetic counseling or testing.

## REFERENCES

1. Collins FS: Medical and societal consequences of the Human Genome Project, Shattuck Lecture, *N Engl J Med* 341(1):28-37, 1999.

2. Olopade OI: Genetics in clinical cancer care: the future is now, *N Engl J Med* 335 (19):1455-1456, 1996.

3. Kodish E, Wiesner GL, Mehiman M, Murray T: Genetic testing for cancer risk: how to reconcile the conflicts, *JAMA* 279(3): 179-181, 1998.

4. Cho MK, Sankar P, Wolpe PR, Godmilow L: Commercialization of BRCA1/2 testing: practitioner awareness and use of a new genetic test, *Am J Med Genet* 83:157-163, 1999.

5. CEGEN Steering Committee: Clinical governance and genetic medicine: specialist genetic centres and the confidential enquiry into counseling for genetic disorders by non-geneticists, *J Med Genet* 36:350-351, 1999.

6. Giardiello FM, Brensinger JD, Petersen GM, et al: The use and interpretation of commercial APC gene testing for familial adenomatous polyposis, *N Engl J Med* 336 (12):823-827, 1997.

7. Stephenson J: Ethics group drafts guidelines for control of genetic material and information, *JAMA* 279(3):184, 1998.

8. Kuczewski MG: Reconceiving the family: the process of consent in medical decision making, *Hastings Center Report,* March-April 1996, pp 30-37.

9. Jecker NS: The role of intimate others in medical decision making, *Gerontologist* 30(1):65-71, 1990.

10. Reust CE, Mattingly S: Family involvement in medical decision making, *Fam Med* 28(1):39-45, 1996.

11. Nelson JL: Taking families seriously, *Hastings Center Report,* July-August 1992, pp 6-12.

12. Hardwig J: What about the family, *Hastings Center Report,* March-April 1990, pp 5-10.

13. Collopy B, Dubler N, Zuckerman C: The ethics of home care: autonomy and accommodation, *Hastings Center Report,* March-April 1990, pp 1-16.

14. American Medical Association, Council on Scientific Affairs: Physicians and family caregivers: a model for partnership, *JAMA* 269(10):1282-1284, 1993.

15. Schulz R, Beach SR: Caregiving as a risk factor for mortality: the caregiver health effects study, *JAMA* 282(23):2215-2219, 1999.

16. Covinsky KE, Goldman L, Cook EF, et al: The impact of serious illness on patients' families, *JAMA* 272 (23):1839-1844, 1994.

17. Geller G, Botkin JR, Green MJ, et al: Genetic testing for susceptibility to adult-onset cancer: the process and content of informed consent, *JAMA* 277(18):1467-1474, 1997.

18. Halsted CH: Pitfalls of genetic testing, *N Engl J Med* 334(18):1192-1194, 1996.

19. Holtzman NA, Shapiro D: Genetic testing and public policy, *BMJ* 316:852-856, 1998.

20. Couch FJ, Hartman LC: BRCA1 testing: advances and retreats, *JAMA* 279(12):955-956, 1998.

21. Cotton P: Prognosis, diagnosis, or who knows? Time to learn what gene tests mean, *JAMA* 273(2):93-95, 1995.

22. Juengst ET: Genetic testing and the moral dynamics of family life, *Public Understanding Sci* 8(9):193-207, 1999.

23. Douglas FS, O'Dair LC, Robinson M, et al: The accuracy of diagnoses as reported in families with cancer: a retrospective study, *J Med Genet* 36:309-312, 1999.

24. Cappelli M, Surh L, Humphreys L, et al: Psychological and social determinants of women's decisions to undergo genetic counseling and testing for breast cancer, *Clin Genet* 55:419-430, 1999.

25. Babul R, Adam S, Kremer B, et al: Attitudes toward direct predictive testing for the HD gene: relevance for other adult-onset disorders, *JAMA* 270:2321-2325, 1993.

26. Kessler S, Field T, Worth L, Mosbarger H: Attitudes of persons at risk for HD toward predictive testing, *Am J Med Genet* 26:259-270, 1987.

27. Decruyenaere M, Evers-Kiebooms G, Van den Berghe H: Perceptions of predictive testing for Huntington's disease by young women, *J Med Genet* 30:557-561, 1993.

28. Lerman C, Narod S, et al: BRCA1 testing in families with hereditary breast-ovarian cancer: a prospective study of patient decision making and outcomes, *JAMA* 275 (24):1885-1892, 1996.

29. Adam S, Wiggins S, Whyte P, et al: Five year study of prenatal testing for HD: demand, attitudes, and psychological assessment, *J Med Genet* 30:549-556, 1993.

30. Wertz DC, Janes SR, Rosenfield JM, Erbe RW: Attitudes toward the prenatal diagnosis of cystic fibrosis: factors in decision making among affected families, *Am J Hum Genet* 50:1077-1085, 1992.

31. Lerman C, Hughes C, Trock BJ, et al: Genetic testing in families with hereditary nonpolyposis colon cancer, *JAMA* 281(17): 1618-1622, 1999.

32. McConkie-Rosell A, Spiridigliozzi GA, Rounds K, et al: Parental attitudes regarding carrier testing in children at risk for fragile X syndrome, *Am J Med Genet* 82: 206-211, 1999.

33. Trippitelli CL, Jamison DR, Folstein MF, et al: Pilot study on patients' and spouses' attitudes toward potential genetic testing for bipolar disorder, *Am J Psychiatry* 155: 899-904, 1998.

34. Bloch M, Adam S, Wiggins S, et al: Predictive testing for HD in Canada: the experience of those receiving an increased risk, *Am J Med Genet* 42:499-507, 1992.

35. Wiggins S, Whyte P, Huggins M, et al: The psychological consequences of predictive testing for HD, *N Engl J Med* 327:1401-1405, 1992.

36. Marteau TM, Croyle RT: Psychological responses to genetic testing, *BMJ* 316:693-696, 1998.

37. Hudson KL, Rothenberg KH, Andrews LB, et al: Genetic discrimination and health insurance: an urgent need for reform, *Science* 270:391, 1995.

38. Wertz DC, Fanos JH, Reilly PR: Genetic testing for children and adolescents: who decides? *JAMA* 272(11):875-881, 1994.

39. Al-Jader LN, Goodchild MC, Ryley DC, Harper PS: Attitudes of parents of cystic fibrosis children towards neonatal screening and antenatal diagnosis, *Clin Genet* 38:460-465, 1990.

40. Gates EA: The impact of prenatal genetic testing on quality of life in women, *Fetal Diagn Ther* 8(suppl 1):236-243, 1993.

41. Yu MS, Norris JM, Mitchell CM, et al: Impact of maternal parenting stress of receipt of genetic information regarding risk of diabetes in newborn infants, *Am J Med Genet* 86:219-226, 1999.

42. Huggins M, Bolch M, Wiggins S, et al: Predictive testing for HD in Canada: adverse effects and unexpected results in those receiving a decreased risk, *Am J Med Genet* 42:508-515, 1992.

43. National Society of Genetic Counselors: Predisposition genetic testing for late-onset disorders in adults, *JAMA* 278(15):1217-1220, 1997.

44. Elias S, Annas GJ: Generic consent for genetic screening, *N Engl J Med* 330(22): 1611-1613, 1994.

45. American Society of Clinical Oncology: Genetic testing for cancer susceptibility, *J Clin Oncol* 14(5):1730-1736, 1996.

46. Ford D, Easton DF, Bishop D, et al: Risks of cancer in BRCA1 mutation carriers, *Lancet* 343:692-695, 1994.

47. Struewing JP, Hartge P, et al: The risk of cancer associated with specific mutations of BRCA1 and BRCA2 among Ashkenazi Jews, *N Engl J Med* 336:1401-1408, 1997.

48. Rebbeck T, Levine A, Eisen A, et al: Breast cancer risk after bilateral prophylactic oophorectomy in BRCA1 mutation carriers, *J Natl Cancer Inst* 91(17):1475-1479, 1999.

49. Hartmann L, Schaid D, Woods J, et al: Efficacy of bilateral, prophylactic mastectomy in women with a family history of breast cancer, *N Engl J Med* 340(2):77-84, 1999.

50. Schrag D, Kuntz KM, Garber JE, Weeks JC: Decision analysis: effects of prophylactic mastectomy and oophorectomy on life expectancy among women with BRCA1 or BRCA2 mutations, *N Engl J Med* 336(20):1465-1471, 1997.

51. Hayes CV: Genetic testing for HD: a family issue, *N Engl J Med* 327(20):1449-1551, 1992.

# PART IV

# POLICY ISSUES FOR PRIMARY CAREGIVERS

# CHAPTER 17

# Commercialization of Predictive Genetic Testing

*Michael J. Malinowski*

Scientists are homing in on the 0.1% of the human genome that distinguishes us genetically (genetically, we are approximately 99.90+% the same) through the Human Genome Project (HGP). Although the HGP has focused on assembling a map of the human genome to serve as a shared research tool, its ultimate goal is to learn more about gene function and to improve the treatment and prevention of diseases through the development of effective tests and therapies.[1] Completion of the HGP coupled with use of information technology in genetic research suggests that extensive, clinically useful predictive genetic testing capabilities may be developed more quickly than many anticipated.[2,3]

Although this technology remains relatively removed from the delivery of primary care, the practice of medicine is poised at the transition from treatment to prevention. Increasingly, the medical community is debating *when* rather than *whether* a patient's DNA will enable health care providers to assess susceptibility to most common diseases, improve preventive care, and predict likely reactions (positive and adverse) to medications and other treatments.[4,5] Moreover, with the proliferation of genetic influences on human health, use of genetics in the delivery of medical care is shifting from specialists to primary care physicians.

This chapter provides basic information on regulation and commercialization of predictive genetic testing services to primary care practitioners. Two assumptions underlie this chapter. First, the present disconnection between predictive genetic testing and primary care is largely a consequence of the regulatory and legal environment surrounding this technology. Second, predictive genetic testing should be integrated into the health care delivery system incrementally, to correlate with emerging instances of clinical utility and to facilitate meaningful education for both the public and health care providers.

As used in this chapter, the term *predictive genetic testing* primarily relates to how a genetic test is used.[6] The purpose of the test must be to assess (1) the probability of onset of symptoms of a presently asymptomatic health condition or (2) a change in a health condition associated with a particular treatment or other environmental exposure. The changes in an individual's physical or mental state for which predictive genetic testing measures susceptibility are associated with the gene, genes, or genetic characteristics that are the focus of the test. This definition encompasses genetic tests used to determine responsiveness/non-responsiveness to a particular drug or other treatment; it thus includes tests that identify specific genetic characteristics, such as the presence or absence of particular proteins, to predict the impact of a specific treatment or other defined stimulus or exposure on a particular patient. For example, the definition would include the use of a genetic test to assess expression of the Her-2/neu gene to determine whether a 38-year-old woman whose mother and aunt died from breast cancer in their 30s should consider taking Herceptin as an additional preventive measure.[7]

The chapter describes emerging approaches to the use and commercialization of predictive genetic testing technology, including regulatory uncertainties and liability risks. It explores the possible role of regulation in contributing to the integration of predictive genetic testing capabilities into delivery of quality health care and introduces a proposal for regulatory reform.

## EMERGING APPROACHES TO COMMERCIALIZED TESTING

More than 5000 human health conditions have identified genetic components, and of those, more than 1000 have been mapped to specific chromosomal regions.[8-10] Many common health disorders, including cancers and cardiovascular disease, have genetic components now identified.[11] For example, women with certain mutations in the BRCA1 and BRCA2 genes may have a 56% lifetime risk of developing breast cancer and 16% lifetime risk of developing ovarian cancer, compared with risks of 12% (breast cancer) and less than 2% (ovarian cancer) in the general population.[12] At this time, more than 450 genetic tests could be used to predict susceptibility to diseases, but most are accessible only through research laboratories.[13]

In 1998 a predictive genetic test to determine overexpression of the Her-2 gene was introduced into the market as an accompaniment to Herceptin, an innovative drug for the estimated 35% of breast cancer patients who carry this genetic characteristic.[7] Herceptin represents an emerging class of more genuine biotechnological drugs, that is, drugs developed through knowledge of gene function, which work by altering disease pathways. General trends in pharmaceutical research and development suggest that Herceptin foreshadows a forthcoming generation of much more precise and potent drugs developed through and accompanied by genetic profiling.[14] Entire fields of science have emerged in conjunction with the HGP that are centered on identification of gene and protein function—*genomics* and *proteomics,* respectively. These fields include pharmacogenomics, pharmacogenetics, and bioinformatics.

*Pharmacogenomics* is the use of genomics or proteomics technology in drug development. *Pharmacogenetics* entails correlating often minute variations in an individual's DNA with response to medications, ranging from efficacious responsiveness to severe adverse reactions.[5,15] Some of these variations consist of single-nucleotide polymorphisms (SNPs), which affect a person's ability to metabolize drugs. At this time, hundreds of potentially medically relevant mutations have been pinpointed.[16-18] At least one company, Orchid Biocomputers (New Jersey), intends to introduce a website, Geneshield.com, that will enable subscribers to determine whether they have genetic characteristics identified as triggering side effects or reducing the efficacy of some widely used prescription drugs.[18]

Advances in *bioinformatics,* using powerful software to collate massive data libraries and compare the genetic profiles of tens of thousands of individuals in minutes, have dramatically accelerated identification of gene function. After a decade of using DNA sequencing technology to break the human genome down into its 3 billion base pairs, bioinformatics technologies are now enabling researchers to put vast amounts of information together to identify genes and determine gene and protein function. Several smaller informatics companies, such as DoubleTwist, an applications service provider, are creating "research portals" to make libraries and databases accessible to individual researchers and small and midsized companies via the Internet.[19,20] Bioinformatics will accelerate the identification of gene function and the determination of genetic tests' clinical utility for specific populations.

## COMMERCIAL DISAPPOINTMENTS

Although genetic profiling has become fundamental to contemporary drug development, commercial predictive genetic tests are lacking. The market absence of this technology is profound when placed in the context of industry expectations in the mid-1990s. According to a 1996 industry survey, nearly 150 biotech companies (about a third of the respondents) were offering or developing genetic tests.[21] Few companies actually have commercialized this technology beyond newborn screening programs or with genetic-based treatments. Genzyme, the largest genetic testing company in the United States and perhaps the world, has dominated these markets. Most of the other companies that have attempted to market predictive genetic testing technology have struggled with disappointments and changed to a drug research and development emphasis. In 1999, for example, OncorMed was purchased by Gene Logic, and Medical Science Systems streamlined its focus and operations and recast itself as Interlueken Genetics.

The first broad effort to commercialize predictive genetic testing for a common adult-onset disorder involved BRCA1-based tests to assess susceptibility to some hereditary forms of breast cancer. In 1996 and 1997, three small biotech companies (OncorMed, Genetics & IVF Institute, Myriad Genetic Laboratories) introduced these tests onto the market. At least one of the companies offered the general public direct access; another engaged in aggressive direct-to-consumer marketing and estimated tremendous market demand despite the limited clinical utility of its test.[22] These companies did not experience the immediate, broad market demand they anticipated. Rather, they (1) drew tremendous public and medical community criticism and scrutiny, (2) highlighted the absence of regulation of predictive genetic testing services, (3) triggered anxiety about the possible consequences (most notably discrimination by employers and insurers) of generating information through predictive genetic tests, and (4) helped to enact and even inspired many federal and state legislative and regulatory initiatives. This body of state legislation is directed at a range of entities that includes employers, disability insurers, health insurers, and life insurers.[23] Box 17-1 lists actions frequently prohibited under this legislation and some common exceptions. On the federal level, President Clinton recently issued an executive order to prohibit discrimination in federal employment based on genetic information.[24]

> ## BOX 17-1 STATE GENETICS LEGISLATION: PROHIBITED ACTIONS AND EXCEPTIONS
>
> **Frequently Prohibited Actions**
>
> - Use of genetic testing in general
> - Requiring or requesting a genetic test or information
> - Disclosing the results of a genetic test to third parties without prior informed consent
> - Discharging, refusing to hire, or refusing to promote by employers on the basis of the results of genetic tests
> - Affecting terms, conditions, or disbursements of benefits based on the results of genetic tests
> - Refusing to consider an application, or refusing to issue or renew an existing policy
> - Classifying information derived from a genetic test as a preexisting condition
> - Charging higher rates or premiums
> - Discriminating charges in brokerage fees or commissions
>
> **Common Exceptions**
>
> - To preempt the statute when a court proceeding is involved, such as forensic or paternity testing by court order
> - To preempt the statute from interfering with research

Modified from Mulholland WF, Jaeger AS: *Jurimetrics* 39:317, 1999.

## REGULATORY UNCERTAINTY, MARKET REJECTION, AND THE NEED FOR CHANGE

When a company sells a predictive genetic test for another to perform, whether a hospital, physician, or other health care provider, that product is regulated by the U.S. Food and Drug Administration (FDA) as a medical device under the Medical Device Amendments to the Food, Drug, and Cosmetic Act[25] and under the Safe Medical Devices Act of 1990.[26] However, companies can commercialize predictive genetic tests without FDA regulation by performing their tests themselves as clinical services and selling access.[27] Users or their health care providers simply send samples to the company, and the company performs the testing and returns results. Under these circumstances, companies even may use ingredients in their tests that are not produced with FDA-assured manufacturing quality control.[9,22] Tests offered in this manner often are referred to as "home brews."

The direct federal regulation of predictive genetic testing services is limited to standard regulation of laboratories performing testing services on human samples for clinical use, known as the Clinical Laboratory Improvement Amendments (CLIA) (Box 17-2).[28-30] However, CLIA regulate testing proficiency, meaning accuracy, not clinical utility.[21] As long as a company providing a predictive genetic testing service achieves the mandated level of accuracy in determining the presence or absence of the particular endpoint (genetic characteristic) tested for, CLIA are satisfied. The company's claims about what test results mean to an individual's health are not regulated under CLIA.

In the foreseeable future, it is unlikely that the FDA will voluntarily assert jurisdiction over predictive genetic tests offered by commercial entities as clinical services. First, the

## BOX 17-2 CLINICAL LABORATORY IMPROVEMENT AMENDMENTS (CLIA): STANDARDS, REQUIREMENTS, AND OBLIGATIONS

**Basic Obligations of Certified Laboratories**

Maintain a quality assurance/quality control program adequate to ensure the validity and reliability of the tests performed.

Meet requirements concerning proper collection, transportation, and storage of specimens and reporting of test results.

Maintain the records, equipment, and facilities necessary for the laboratory's effective operation.

Employ only personnel who meet the qualifications established by the Department of Health and Human Services (HHS)

Qualify under a proficiency-testing program that meets HHS standards.

**Personnel Requirements**

Laboratories performing moderately complex tests must satisfy specific personnel requirements prescribed by CLIA.

CLIA define mandatory qualifications and functions for the laboratory director, technical consultant, and testing personnel.

CLIA hold laboratory directors responsible for the overall administration of laboratories.

**Patient Test Management**

Laboratories performing moderately complex and complex procedures must implement systems to ensure optimum patient specimen integrity and positive identification throughout the pretesting, testing, and posttesting processes.

**Proficiency Testing (PT)**

All laboratories performing moderately complex and complex procedures must participate in an approved PT program for each specialty and subspecialty in which they conduct tests.

Certified laboratories must be evaluated quarterly in every procedure and in every category of testing covered by their certification.

Laboratories are required to make PT results reasonably available to any person on request.

Failure to meet these requirements constitutes a "condition level" violation of CLIA, which may trigger suspension, limitation, or revocation of certification or alternative sanctions, including on-site monitoring, termination of Medicaid/Medicare approval for any specialty not subjected to PT, and civil money penalties.

**Quality Control (QC) and Assurance**

Although CLIA do not mandate a demonstration of clinical validity, laboratories must demonstrate analytical validity and test accuracy.

CLIA set forth general QC requirements and additional requirements for specialties.

CLIA regulations establish a process for FDA review of the QC features of both existing and new medical devices, including instruments, kits, and test systems that are classified as moderately complex.

FDA has undergone significant reforms under the Food and Drug Administration Modernization Act of 1997. The FDA now is digesting tremendous internal change and under pressure to be "transparent" and responsive to innovative technologies that may significantly improve human health. These pressures make the voluntary assumption of additional regulatory responsibilities unlikely.

> *FDA also has not had positive experience taking strong regulatory positions in the testing area. Its last few attempts to protect the public from too much self-knowledge proved to be an institutional bellyache. In the late 1980s the FDA adopted a complete ban on HIV home testing kits, which came under considerable derision. Accusations of paternalism were leveled and public health experts argued that without encouraging testing of populations not apparently at-risk, efforts to control spread of the disease would not be effective. FDA retreated from its position in 1995. Similar efforts to block the distribution of drug-testing kits drew comparable attacks.[9]*

Nevertheless, there are viable proposals for and ongoing initiatives to introduce federal regulation of predictive genetic testing services. In 1997 a task force of the National Institutes of Health and Department of Energy Working Group on Ethical, Legal, and Social Implications (ELSI) of the HGP issued a report on genetic testing (Box 17-3).[21,30] The task force's recommendations included modifying CLIA to address issues associated with predictive genetic testing and establishing an advisory committee on how to regulate this technology.[21] In 1999, HHS Secretary Donna Shalala assembled an Advisory Committee on Genetic Testing, whose recommendations are forthcoming. Also in 1999, a Genetic Testing Working Group to the Clinical Laboratory Improvement Advisory Committee (CLIAC) at the Centers for Disease Control and Prevention (CDC) issued recommendations for quality assurance programs for laboratory molecular genetic tests.[31]

Besides the absence of any reliable regulatory assurance of efficacy (clinical utility) for predictive genetic testing, even FDA-approved medical products often have difficulty gaining acceptance. In contrast with the standard market entry of innovative new medical products, most notably the nearly 100 biotech-based drugs introduced into commerce in the mid-to-late 1990s, the aggressive attempts to commercialize BRCA1 testing directly to consumers without any regulatory assurance have raised widespread criticism about predictive genetic testing and market rejection of these tests and others. Some of this BRCA testing was broadly marketed despite having grossly limited clinical utility for the general population. Test results were subject to misinterpretation and overreliance because of the vulnerable target patient population and limited clinical data, inviting criticism and suspicion. Consequently, commercial predictive genetic testing has been met with skepticism from the health care community. Similarly, the public has been educated about predictive genetic testing largely through highly publicized criticism about the alleged premature and overly aggressive commercialization of this particular testing technology.

Renewed public attention is focusing on the in-house predictive genetic testing services that escape quality assurance through FDA regulation, including FDA assurance of manufacturing quality control over the ingredients used in these tests.[10] In 1999, for example, the national media reported on a woman who underwent surgeries to remove her ovaries after receiving a false-positive BRCA1 test result from OncorMed.[32,33]

Predictive genetic tests are becoming less expensive, more automated, and increasingly relevant to common disorders. While the prevalence of clinically useful predictive genetic tests is still generally limited, both the medical community and the public should be-

## BOX 17-3  TASK FORCE ON GENETIC TESTING: KEY PRINCIPLES AND RECOMMENDATIONS

### Validity and Utility of Genetic Tests

Data establishing clinical benefits and risks, from both positive and negative test results, must be a prerequisite for clinical practice.

When subject identifiers are retained and tests are intended for clinical use, an institutional review board (IRB) must review and approve protocols for development of predictive genetic tests.

### Laboratory Quality and Certification

A national accreditation program should be established for laboratories performing genetic tests.

The College of American Pathologists and American College of Medical Genetics should administer a national accreditation program for laboratories performing genetic tests and periodically publish lists of the laboratories in compliance.

Reimbursement for genetic tests should be limited to those tests performed by laboratories included on these lists.

### Informed Consent, Confidentiality, and Discrimination

Whenever a specimen can be linked to a subject, informed consent must be obtained for validation studies.

Predictive genetic testing must be voluntary; informed consent must be obtained; and the decision whether to undergo testing must not jeopardize care.

Except in extreme circumstances, test results must be released only to individuals for whom the test subject has given consent.

Individuals must not be subjected to discrimination based on test results.

### HHS Advisory Committee

The HHS secretary should create an advisory committee to address implementation of the task force's recommendations.

### Human Subject Guidelines

The Office of Protection of Research Subjects from Research Risks (OPRR) should develop IRB guidelines for reviewing protocols for predictive genetic testing.

### Provider Competence

The task force endorsed establishment of the National Coalition for Health Professional Education in Genetics (NCHPREG) by the American Medical Association, the American Nurses Association, and the National Human Genome Research Institute.

Genetics curricula should be developed, recognizing inherited risk factors and issues associated with genetic tests and testing services.

---

come accustomed to using this technology to prevent, screen, and predict common disorders and better evaluate the course of treatment. Only through incremental, positive experience using predictive genetic tests will the medical community and public achieve the education necessary to reap the potential health care benefits this technology offers. Efforts by industry sponsors and government supporters to educate directly are no substitute, as demonstrated by the inability of the U.S. government, World Trade Organization, and companies such as Monsanto to contain mistrust of genetically modified food.[34]

In the absence of significant change, the disconnection between predictive genetic testing and the medical community will keep this technology generally removed from delivery of care, and tests that carry clinical utility will become more prevalent for increasingly expansive population groups. Given the challenges of interpreting and delivering information derived from predictive genetic testing, the worst-case scenario for mainstreaming this technology in primary care may be to disregard instances of clinical utility, hinder emerging testing capabilities, and then impose predictive genetic testing on the medical community and the public through concerns about liability.

This scenario is becoming more probable in light of recent judicial decisions. In addition to state legislation that codifies causes of action such as wrongful birth and wrongful life, wrongful conception and related tort causes of action affect predictive genetic testing.[35] Courts are becoming increasingly receptive to health care providers under duties to warn both patients and family members of genetic susceptibilities.[36-38] Too often, innovative medical technologies forced into use through legal liability are seriously questioned later. The most noted recent example is the use of autologous bone marrow transplants in women with breast cancer, an extraordinarily dangerous, painful, and costly treatment given to thousands of women in the 1990s.[39,40] The study supporting efficacy of the treatment and relied on for more than a decade while contrary data were slowly compiled now has been discredited, with allegations of scientific misconduct and research fraud.[39]

## A PROPOSAL FOR CHANGE

To make predictive genetic testing commercially viable and available, this technology must be treated similar to other new medical technologies. Predictive genetic testing must enter the marketplace through a regulatory process that offers assurance of safety, efficacy and clinical utility, and market responsibility. Given the likely emergence of a broad spectrum of such tests, the proposed regulatory framework is necessary to distinguish and endorse the use of the technology that carries clinical utility.

The most obvious options are to (1) introduce meaningful FDA review, (2) modify CLIA regulations to address the issue of clinical utility, or (3) formalize a compliance process conducted by relevant professional societies, particularly those that already are authorized to issue CLIA accreditation, most notably the College of American Pathologists. Although many industry representatives support variations of the professional society approach, this may be too little, too late, in light of the present stigma surrounding predictive genetic testing and resulting disconnection between this technology and the medical community. The same is true regarding CLIA. Although modifying CLIA may prove a meaningful supplemental measure to improve the credibility of predictive genetic testing, the medical community also is aware of the limitations of CLIA. More than 150,000 CLIA-certified laboratories are in need of oversight,[9] and CLIA is marred by a history of reporting deficiencies and insufficient laboratory inspections.[21] CLIA alone is unreliable as a laboratory quality assurance measure.

The most viable option to introduce the needed regulatory framework is to regulate predictive genetic testing through the FDA pursuant to an amendment to the Medical De-

> ## BOX 17-4   CRITERIA FOR HUMANITARIAN DEVICE CLASSIFICATION
>
> - Designed to benefit a target disease population of not more than 4000 individuals in the United States
> - Will not be available otherwise
> - Has no alternative available to treat or diagnose the disease or condition
> - Will not expose patients to unreasonable or significant risk of illness or injury
> - Provides health benefits that outweigh associated risks

vices Act (MDA). The FDA is familiar with regulating medical devices and similar technologies, and FDA regulation would carry assurances of compliance with manufacturing standards and responsible advertising and marketing. The latter is crucial to alleviate concerns raised with direct-to-consumer overselling of BRCA testing.

In addition, pursuant to the *Medtronic* line of cases,[41] compliance with FDA oversight could reduce exposure to liabilities while accelerating establishment of standard care practices. A provision in the MDA prohibits states from creating requirements for manufacturers in addition to what the MDA already mandates, and many courts have interpreted this provision to mean MDA preemption of common law product liability claims brought by individuals against manufacturers. According to a recent federal district court decision, although MDA preemption is limited, the FDA may preempt state product liability claims by imposing specific requirements on manufacturers.[42]

Moreover, if predictive genetic testing services were regulated similar to medical devices, companies would be more likely to sell them as testing kits rather than assume the hassles associated with running commercial CLIA laboratories, especially if CLIA were implemented in a more reliable manner. If sold as kits and directly regulated by the FDA as medical devices, the technology might even qualify for some regulatory benefits, including those associated with classification as a humanitarian device for use in target subpopulations (Box 17-4). These devices, which would not be economically feasible to manufacture for the slated uses and populations without the benefits, may be granted an FDA exemption from the effectiveness requirements of sections 514 (performance standards) and 515 (premarket approval) of the Federal Food, Drug, and Cosmetic Act.[43]

## SUMMARY

Predictive genetic testing must enter the marketplace of routine medical care as do other new medical products: through a regulatory framework that carries assurances of safety, efficacy, and market responsibility. An incremental, controlled introduction into health care of predictive genetic testing technology with defined clinical utility will build provider and public acceptance and help ensure proper use.

Although public and provider education has been promoted as a predecessor or even a substitute for regulation and related legislation, the most meaningful education is through responsible use. Such an approach is essential for predictive genetic testing because aggressive attempts to commercialize have stigmatized the technology by highlighting the absence of reliable regulatory assurance of clinical utility and market responsibility. The health care community may be more familiar with complications associated with providing this technology, such as misinterpretation of results, patient overreliance, and susceptibility to discrimination, than with the technology itself.

In the absence of the government intervention proposed in this chapter, predictive genetic testing technology is likely to remain stigmatized and discredited, distinguished from other health care products, and disconnected from primary care even after development of myriad testing capabilities for common disorders with defined clinical utility. The resulting lost opportunities to improve preventive health care and treatment are unacceptable, and forced integration of the technology into health care en masse through imposition of liability is equally unacceptable because of the complicated nature of the technology.

Predictive genetic testing capabilities will expand exponentially over the next several years through the coupling of genetic research and information technology and the importance placed on genetic profiling, pharmacogenomics, and pharmacogenetics in drug development. This technology will be fundamental in delivering tomorrow's quality health care. Instances of testing with clinical utility must be embraced by practitioners as opportunities to improve the quality of health care today and in the future.

## REFERENCES

1. Collins FS et al: New goals for the U.S. Human Genome Project: 1998-2003, *Science* 282:682-683, 1998.
2. Agres T: It holds key for making sense of biology, *Drug Discov Dev,* January/February 2000, pp 11-12.
3. Hood L, Rowen L: Genes, genomes, and society. In Rothstein MA, editor: *Genetic secrets,* New Haven, Conn, 1997, Yale University Press.
4. Watson MS: The regulation of genetic testing. In Long C, editor: *Genetic testing and the use of information,* Washington, DC, 1999, American Enterprise Institute.
5. Pettipher R, Holford R: Pharmacogenetics paves the way, *Drug Discov Dev,* January/February 2000, pp 53-54.
6. Silver LM: The meaning of genes and "genetic rights," *Jurimetrics* 40:9, 1999.
7. Bazell R: *Her-2: the making of Herceptin, a revolutionary treatment for breast cancer,* New York, 1998, Random House.
8. Johns Hopkins University Human Genome Initiative genome database, www.gdb. org.
9. Huang A: FDA regulation of genetic testing: institutional reluctance and public guardianship, *Food Drug* 53:555, 1998.
10. Rothstein M, Hoffman S: Genetic testing, genetic medicine, and managed care, *Wake Forest Law Review* 34:854, 1999.
11. Andrews L, Fullarton J, Holtzman N, Motulsky G, editors: *Assessing genetic risks: implications for health and social policy,* Washington, DC, 1994, National Academy Press.
12. Cancer screening saves lives of Jewish women, *Cancer Res Week,* Feb 15, 1999.
13. Long C: Introduction. In Long C, editor: *Genetic testing and the use of information,* Washington, DC, 1999, American Enterprise Institute.
14. Shaywitz DA, Ausiello DA: Can drug giants survive the biomedical revolution? *Wall Street Journal,* Feb 8, 2000.
15. Garet G: What's it worth, *Drug Discov Dev,* September 1999, p 67.
16. Branca MA: SNPs surge ahead, *Drug Discov Dev,* September 1999, p 77.
17. Gillis C: Code cracking, *Cyber Esq,* Winter 1999.
18. Moore SD: Orchid Biocomputers Internet service to spot drug side effects using DNA, *Wall Steet Journal,* Oct 19, 1999.

19. Thayer AM: BioInformatics for the masses, *C&EN,* Feb 7, 2000.

20. Fisher LM: Surfing the human genome: data bases of genetic code are moving to the web, *New York Times,* Sept 20, 1999.

21. Task Force on Genetic Testing: *Promoting safe and effective genetic testing in the United States,* Baltimore, 1998, Johns Hopkins University Press.

22. Malinowski MJ, Blatt RJR: Commercialization of genetic testing services: the FDA, market forces, and biological tarot cards, *Tulane Law Review* 71:1211, 1997.

23. Mulholland WF, Jaeger AS: Genetic privacy and discrimination: a survey of state legislation, *Jurimetrics* 39:317, 1999.

24. Executive Order to prohibit discrimination in federal employment based on genetic information, *Federal Register* 65:6877, 2000.

25. Public Law 94-295, 90 Stat 539 (codified at 15 USC § 55 [1994] and sections of 21 USC).

26. Public Law 101-629, 104 Stat 4511 (codified in 21 USC §§ 301-383 note, 42 USC §§ 263b-263n).

27. Medical devices, classification/reclassification; restricted devices; analyte specific reagents, *Federal Register* 61:10,484 (1996) (to be codified at 21 CFR pts 809 & 864).

28. Public Law 100-578, 102 Stat 2903 (codified at 42 USC §§ 201 note, 263a, 263a note).

29. Health Care Financing Administration: Clinical laboratory improvement amendments, www.hcfa.gov/medicare/hsqb/clia.htm.

30. Malinowski MJ: *Biotechnology: law, business, and regulation,* New York, 1999, Aspen.

31. Williams LO, Cole EC: *General recommendations for quality assurance programs for laboratory molecular genetic tests,* Atlanta, 1999, Centers for Disease Control and Prevention.

32. Peres J: Genetic testing can save lives—but errors leave scars, *Chicago Tribune,* Sept 26, 1999.

33. Weiss R: Genetic testing's human toll: in unregulated field, errors can upend lives and mean unneeded surgery, *Washington Post,* July 21, 1999.

34. Caution needed: a protocol on trade in GMOs, *Economist,* Feb 5, 2000.

35. *McAllister v HA,* 347 NC 638, 496 SE2d 577 (1998).

36. Severin MJ: Genetic susceptibility for specific cancers: medical liability of the clinician, *Cancer* 86(suppl 11):2564-2569, 1999.

37. *Safer v Estate of Pack,* 677 A2d 1188 (NJ Super 1996), *cert denied,* 683 A2d 1163 (NJ 1996).

38. *Pate v Threlkel,* 661 So 2d 278 (Fla 1995).

39. Kolata G, Eichenwald D: Insurer drops a therapy for breast cancer, *New York Times,* Feb 16, 2000.

40. Cancer study shuns bone marrow therapy, *New York Times,* March 4, 2000.

41. *Medtronic v Lohr,* 518 US 470 (1996).

42. *Haidak v Collagen Corporation,* No 98-30056-FHF (D Ma Oct 8, 1999).

43. US Food and Drug Administration: Requirements of laws and regulations, www.fda.gov/opacom/morechoices/smallbusiness/blubook.htm.

# CHAPTER 18

# Primary Care Genetics in an Unregulated Managed Market

*John D. Lantos*
*Timothy J. Aspinwall*

As new genetic discoveries diffuse from the research laboratory to the clinic, they create problems for primary care physicians. The practicing physician is in the familiar but increasingly untenable position of having to understand enough about new and understudied technology to know how to use it wisely and cost-effectively for patients with varying needs, expectations, and problems.

Primary care in America at the beginning of the twenty-first century is often thought to represent everything that is both good and lacking in American health care—cost-effectiveness, continuity of care, and an understanding of the whole patient. These values are largely theoretical, however, and primary care physicians and their patients face real dilemmas. It is not clear who really is a primary care physician or how physicians should collaborate with their specialist and paraprofessional colleagues to deliver high-quality, cost-effective, psychologically responsive care.[1] There is no consensus about professional identity, education, expertise, or accountability. It is not clear exactly what primary care physicians can do or should do, how they should be trained, how their training should be financed, or what these questions mean to academic medical centers.[2-5] Can primary care physicians provide as well as others with more training or provide better than those with less training? Should they become more like specialists, more like advanced practice nurses or physician assistants, or more like somebody else?

It is also not clear to whom today's primary care physicians are accountable or for whom they are working. They are expected to be patient advocates and also gatekeepers, to follow practice guidelines and exercise professional judgment, to respect patient autonomy and fulfill fiduciary obligations, and to meet productivity goals and ensure that patients are satisfied. Primary care physicians have not traditionally had a central teaching role, but academic medical centers are being asked to train more of them in ambulatory care settings. This new teaching responsibility will place an additional strain on today's primary care physicians. Furthermore, as more and more screening tests become available, physicians will have more tasks to accomplish in an ever-shortening office visit.[6]

Genetic testing represents an important area for examining ways in which primary care physicians can forge new identities and new professional roles. New genetic discoveries will offer great information and promise. For the foreseeable future, however, the Human Genome Project (HGP) will generate complex probabilistic information that is of uncertain value to any individual patient. In most cases, genetic tests do not provide definitive diagnostic information but rather more refined estimations of risk. Many of the tests will be costly, and no simple interventions will be available for many of the diseases.[7]

Furthermore, primary care physicians work within large, integrated health delivery systems. These systems operate within fixed budgets, rewarding physicians who streamline care and limit costs and penalizing those who exceed budget limits.[8] At the same time, legal and bioethical doctrines demand that patients be informed of available treatment options and be encouraged to participate in the testing or treatment decisions. These realities create unique challenges for primary care physicians, who work at the interface between the macrocosm of economic and sociocultural forces and the microcosm of a particular physician-patient relationship. This chapter discusses how primary care physicians should respond to these challenges.

## GENETICS AND REGULATION OF MEDICAL INNOVATION

Although much of the speculation about the impact and implications of the HGP has been theoretical and general, the impact of new genetic tests has varied in different clinical situations. The dilemmas in cystic fibrosis screening are different than those surrounding screening for Huntington disease or Tay-Sachs disease.[9-11] In each situation the type of testing is different, so there are important differences in the sensitivity, specificity, cost, and complexity of the tests; in the sociodemographic characteristics of the affected populations; and in the implications of a positive test. As a result, general speculation about the implications of the HGP probably will not be useful.

Common themes still exist, however, including the ambiguities of technology development, deployment, and assessment in the United States. The conditions under which a new medical technology "becomes available" to practicing physicians are ambiguous and ever changing. Federal regulations govern the licensing of new drugs or devices, regulations are inherent in the process of funding and publishing scientific studies, and various rules and regulations define the tort liability system. Most of these regulations are convoluted, vary from state to state, and constantly change. They also perennially lag behind the activities they try to regulate.

New drugs and devices must be approved by the U.S. Food and Drug Administration (FDA) before they can be marketed in the United States.[12] The FDA drug approval process is more time-consuming and expensive than in most other countries.[13] Fewer drugs and devices are approved or marketed in the United States than in most European countries, but the U.S. regulation system has little postapproval regulation. Once a drug or device is approved for any indication, it may be used for other indications without rigorous testing. Thus a genetic test may be approved for a specific indication in a specific population and then used for less specific indications that have never been rigorously evaluated.

It is uncertain what regulatory process will govern diagnostic genetic testing. When a diagnostic testing kit is used by someone other than the manufacturer, it must be approved by the FDA, but not all tests will require such kits. In many cases, similar techniques for testing will be useful for diagnosing mutations in many different genes. Commercial laboratories are regulated, but that process is different from FDA approval.[14] As a result of this combination of technology and regulatory oversight, it is unclear whether new genetic tests will need to be officially approved in any form.

The ambiguous status of a new genetic test will be similar to that of a new surgical procedure such as embolization of cerebral arteriovenous malformations, a diagnostic device such as positron emission tomography, or a biological therapeutics such as cord blood stem cells. Such tests will be marketed long before they have been rigorously evaluated. Given the pace of scientific advances, regulatory processes must make a trade-off between protecting the public from inadequately tested innovations and facilitating access to potentially beneficial medical innovations. A process of loose oversight and half-regulated markets seems inevitable and perhaps desirable.[15] In the resulting zone of ambiguity, however, physicians cannot rely on the government and must think and act for themselves. Practice guidelines, statements from professional organizations, insurance reimbursement policies, and malpractice litigation may determine what tests should be offered.

## A "PREGENETIC" PARABLE

Prenatal screening with a blood test for alpha fetoprotein (AFP) began to be used in the 1970s.[16] Although largely experimental with little evidence of benefit, demand for the tests began to grow. In 1982 the American College of Obstetricians and Gynecologists (ACOG) stated that "routine [AFP] screening of all gravida is of uncertain value."[16]

In 1983 the FDA approved commercial kits for the radioimmunoassay of AFP. Although the clinical implications were unclear and target population was undefined, approval moved the test from the research laboratory to the commercial clinical laboratory, improving access dramatically. No new data were reported, but by 1985 the ACOG had changed its position, now stating that "it is imperative that every prenatal patient *be advised of the availability* of this test" (italics added).[16] The position change resulted from a legal assessment of the likelihood of a malpractice suit, which became a self-fulfilling prophecy. By 1990, courts were awarding plaintiffs damages because their physicians failed to offer prenatal AFP screening. Commercial availability of the test led a professional society's lawyers to recommend a change in physician practice patterns, which quickly became the standard of care (SOC).

AFP screening was widely used before data showed its efficacy as a population-based screening test. For physicians, testing seemed better than not testing. If they did not test and the infant was born with a neural tube defect (NTD), they could be sued. If a false-positive test led to further maternal anxiety or even an amniocentesis-induced miscarriage, those were known and accepted risks. Furthermore, in those halcyon days before capitation rates and covered lives, such testing made money for the physicians. It seemed to be win-win for physician and patient and lose-lose for payors and plaintiff's lawyers.

Emerging data on the efficacy of AFP screening were ambiguous. The initial results of the test in selected populations were better than those in general populations. False-positive and false-negative results led to further testing. AFP by itself was a poor test for trisomies, but in conjunction with human chorionic gonadotropin and estradiol, sensitivity and specificity increased.[18] This triple screen was evaluated as a test to guide the use of prenatal ultrasound or amniocentesis. Prenatal ultrasound had become virtually routine, however, despite the lack of evidence on its efficacy.[19] With genetic tests entering the mix of potential fetal diagnostics, and with the increased potential of prenatal testing, greater confusion may result rather than greater clarity.

This history suggests that the diffusion of technology follows a complex interplay of legal, political, scientific, and economic forces. A diagnostic test was discovered that seemed to have some usefulness in a limited population of patients. Based on this, some physicians began advocating routine testing, and a medical device company developed a commercial kit for inexpensive testing that was approved by the FDA. FDA approval led the lawyers at a professional obstetrics organization to recommend that the test be offered to all patients as a form of defensive medicine. Physicians soon echoed that sentiment. The defensive medicine strategy became the SOC. The existence of the test created the need and financial support for the infrastructure of other facilities necessary for follow-up of positive tests.

The brief history of prenatal serum AFP testing does not address the question of whether making AFP screening available to all pregnant women was beneficial. The availability of such testing has been temporally associated with a dramatic decrease in the number of children born with NTDs. The decrease seems partly attributable to detection of fetuses with NTDs in the second trimester and to late second-trimester abortions, which suggests that screening programs work. However, a decline in the rates of spina bifida and other NTDs in the United States began before the widespread use of prenatal diagnostic services, which indicates that environmental factors may have contributed significantly to defects. The increased use of folic acid during pregnancy dramatically lowers the incidence of NTDs, thus changing the characteristics of the test, since sensitivity and specificity depend on the underlying prevalence of the condition in the population.[20] Even if testing was appropriate in 1980, it may not be appropriate today.

This AFP scenario illustrates the kinds of dilemmas that primary care physicians will face with every new test or combination of tests that becomes available.

## STANDARD OF CARE, NONDIRECTIVE COUNSELING, AND ENTITLEMENTS

Will a SOC evolve that includes a set of recommendations for genetic screening tests, or will the SOC demand only a nondirective discussion of treatment options? To the extent that the SOC requires provision of certain services, those services will likely become entitlements. To the extent that the SOC requires only a discussion of possibilities, the interventions could be treated more easily as luxury items. Currently, for example, a mammogram every year for women over age 50 might be the SOC, with reimbursement from most insurance companies. Testing for younger women or at more frequent intervals might be discussed with patients, who may then choose to purchase earlier or more frequent mammograms with their own money.[21]

The status of a particular test may have other economic implications. As genetic screening develops, insurance companies may require testing as a precondition for application and may exclude certain conditions from coverage based on unacceptable susceptibility.[22] Further, insurance companies may choose to cover only certain treatment options, putting patients in the difficult position of accepting the covered treatment plan or fending for themselves. For example, genetic testing may reveal a nonlethal fetal abnormality that would require very expensive medical treatment after birth. If an insurance company has anticipated this in its policy drafting, it might choose to cover only an abortion and not the treatment.

Professional SOCs and financing mechanisms may force patients to undergo some tests, limit access to others, and encourage still others. Given the current national infatuation with market solutions to social and political problems, more market-driven allocation policies will probably drive the distribution of medical resources. If so, new tests and treatments will increasingly exist in a health policy "twilight zone," just outside the entitlement to health care but within the SOC. As with AFP, physicians will be encouraged or required to advise people of a test's availability, but the patient will have to pay for it. Genetic screening then may be treated similar to infertility treatments, orthodontics, or long-term psychotherapy, rather than newborn metabolic screening, immunizations, or other "core" interventions.

Primary care physicians must seek a balance among three opposing pairs of tensions: (1) medical judgment and legal considerations, (2) paternalism and autonomy, and (3) physician as the patient's fiduciary and physician as steward of societal resources.

## MEDICAL JUDGMENT AND LEGAL CONSIDERATIONS IN TREATMENT DECISIONS

Physicians are often accused of practicing "defensive medicine," or recommending a test or treatment they believe is unnecessary because a judge or a jury might determine that it was necessary. However, courts usually define the SOC according to what physicians do or what expert physicians say they should do.[23] Thus, if no other physician thinks a test is necessary, no expert would testify that it was the SOC, and a court would probably not find a failure to order the test or treatment to be malpractice.

More often, defensive medicine refers to situations involving disagreement *within* the profession about whether a test or treatment is appropriate. Experts could be found whose opinion is that a failure to order a test or treatment would be considered malpractice. Interestingly, such situations create a social pressure to adopt treatments before they are proved effective. The cautious physician is penalized for delaying the introduction of an inadequately studied intervention. The penalty can be an actual malpractice case or more often the fear of a malpractice case.[24] From a societal perspective this seems an inappropriate way to introduce new therapies, but from the practitioner's standpoint it is a rational choice. A new test or procedure may not be effective and may cost money, but it does not cost the practitioner money. This will change if the structure for reimbursement changes. Increasingly, physicians are at risk for expenditures. Such arrangements create a personal incentive not to use excessive treatments.

Institutional or public policies, such as tort liability laws and reimbursement rules, will always influence medical treatments. Some encourage excessive treatment; others lead to the withholding of potentially beneficial treatments. There is no value-neutral position. Any guidelines or policies will influence decisions one way or the other. Given this inevitability, primary care physicians must be more clear in the future about whom they are working for and how particular systems of care may distort their primary responsibility to their patients. Not all conflicts of interest are harmful, but unrecognized or unacknowledged conflicts can be dangerous if they secretly distort individual decisions and institutional policies. Such situations require a more complex analysis of patient autonomy.

## AUTONOMY AND PATERNALISM IN SITUATIONS OF UNCERTAINTY

Tensions between patient autonomy and physician paternalism have been resolved in recent years by the general presumption in favor of autonomy. Patients are given information and options. Then, if no convincing evidence suggests that the patient is decisionally incompetent, the ethical and legal consensus is that the patient must be permitted to choose between the medical options, even and especially in the fact of outcome uncertainty. Another shift seems to be occurring, however, that is more a matter of fact than of consensus. This shift is away from either physician paternalism or patient autonomy and toward decision-making mechanisms that are institutional rather than individual. Increasingly, the authority of physicians or patients in choosing among diagnostic or therapeutic interventions is being challenged by administrators and policymakers whose authority derives from perceived economic imperatives. In this environment, new treatment options may be presented to patients, who may be given the theoretical option to choose them by purchasing them.

Theories of patient autonomy and physician paternalism have developed around the idea that there is adequate information from which to choose and a capacity to implement choices. When information is insufficient to make decisions, and when the decision maker cannot implement a choice, autonomy and paternalism fade in significance. In genetic screening and treatment, some indications will be ambiguous and some treatment options economically unavailable. In these cases, autonomy and paternalism will become less significant in the physician-patient relationship.

The traditional physician-patient relationship includes providing both information and treatment. For the benefits of the information-laden technology of genetic screening and treatment to be fully realized, this autonomy-based paradigm needs to be maintained. With the many options and many psychological, social, and medical consequences, predetermined option packages cannot be dispensed to patients without discussing the issues, such as mental depression, privacy interests (insurance, employment), and family concerns about inherited diseases. Also, certain treatment options may be inappropriately included as a form of marketing strategy.

It is crucial that primary care physicians have sufficient resources to ensure that patients can obtain counseling about treatment options. This will help prevent informed consent from becoming a charade.

## SUMMARY

Physicians have always worked within the tension between their status as caregivers to individual patients and their role as symbolic agents of social morality. Even the typical tasks of allocating time among various patients or between patient care and other demands require a value judgment about the importance of a particular patient's needs or desires. The concerns about new genetic tests do not reflect a new type of conflict for physicians. Instead, they reflect that the decisions physicians must make are becoming more frequent and more complex, with less consensus about the moral values that should inform such decisions.

# REFERENCES

1. Rosenblatt RA, Hart LG, Gamliel S, et al: Identifying primary care disciplines by analyzing the diagnostic content of ambulatory care, *J Am Board Fam Pract* 8:34-45, 1995.
2. Grumbach K, Becker SH, Osborn EH, Bindman AB: The challenge of defining and counting generalist physicians: an analysis of Physician Masterfile data, *Am J Public Health* 85:1402-1407, 1995.
3. Christakis NA, Jacobs JA, Messikomer CM: Change in self-definition from specialist to generalist in a national sample of physicians, *Ann Intern Med* 121:669-675, 1994.
4. Markson LE, Cosler LE, Turner BJ: Implications of generalists' slow adoption of zidovudine in clinical practice, *Arch Intern Med* 154:497-504, 1994.
5. Crowder VB: Defining emergency medicine: are we generalists or specialists? *Ann Emerg Med* 23:869-872, 1994.
6. Wilson M: Pediatric generalist training: graduate medical education at a crossroads, *Curr Opin Pediatr* 6:513-518, 1994.
7. Savill J: Science, medicine, and the future: prospecting for gold in the human genome, *BMJ* 314(7073):43-45, 1997.
8. Hillman AL: HMO managers' views on financial incentives and quality, *Health Affairs,* Winter 1991, pp 207, 210-211.
9. Newborn screening for cystic fibrosis: a paradigm for public health genetics policy development, *MMWR* 4(RR-16):1-24, 1997.
10. Hayes CV: Genetic testing for Huntington's disease—a family issue, *N Engl J Med* 327(20):1449-1451, 1992.
11. Kaplan F: Tay-Sachs disease carrier screening: a model for prevention of genetic disease, *Genet Test* 2(4):271-292, 1998.
12. 51 USC Section 55.
13. Andersson F: The drug lag issue: the debate seen from an international perspective, *Int J Health Serv* 22(1):53-72, 1992.
14. 42 USC Section 201.
15. Altman SH, Rodwin MA: Halfway competitive markets and ineffective regulation: the American health care system, *J Health Polit Policy Law* 13(2):323-329, 1988.
16. Annas GJ: Is a genetic screening test ready when the lawyers say it is? *Hastings Center Report* 15(6):16-18, 1985.
17. Mennuti MT: Prenatal genetic diagnosis: current status, *N Engl J Med* 297:1004-1006, 1997.
18. Haddow JE, Palomaki GE, Knight GJ, et al: Prenatal screening for Down's syndrome with use of maternal serum markers, *N Engl J Med* 327(27):588-593, 1992.
19. Ecker JL, Frigoletto FD: Routine ultrasound screening in low-risk pregnancies: imperatives for further study, *Obstet Gynecol* 93:607-610, 1999.
20. Rosano A et al: Time trends in neural tube defect prevalence in relation to preventive strategies: an international study, *J Epidemiol Community Health* 53:630-635, 1999.
21. Morrison EH: Controversies in women's health maintenance, *Am Fam Physician* 55:1283-1290, 1995.
22. Ostrer H et al: Insurance and genetic testing: where are we now? *Am J Hum Genet* 52:565-577, 1993.
23. Meadow WL, Lantos J, Tanz RR, et al: Ought standard care be the standard of care? A study of the time to administration of antibiotics in children with meningitis, *Am J Dis Child* 147:40-44, 1993.
24. Lawthers AG et al: Physicians' perceptions of the risk of being sued, *J Health Polit Policy Law* 17:463, 468-469, 1992.

# CHAPTER 19

# Insurance and Employment Issues in Primary Care Genetics

*Timothy J. Aspinwall*

The predictive capacity of genetic testing creates two competing imperatives. On the one hand there is the social need for accessible, quality health care and the desire to maximize genetic medicine's benefits. On the other there are insurance companies and employers who control medical losses by limiting coverage of persons with costly genetic disorders. Clearly, there is much to gain or lose, depending on how genetic diagnostic and prognostic factors are used. The full potential of medical genetics can be approached only if people have access to testing and therapy without fear that their options for health care coverage or employment will be limited because of a medical diagnosis.

Insurers and employers will increasingly use genetic information as a determining factor to exclude people who may present a higher risk. People who fear such exclusion will choose to forego genetic testing or other beneficial medical care. Given present law and financial incentives, an insurer will use genetic information to limit potential liabilities by denying, limiting, or increasing the price of health coverage for persons who may present a higher than normal risk. The information needed for optimal medical care and family planning may also limit a person's opportunities to obtain health care and employment. Unless meaningful steps are taken to ensure access to health care, the benefits of medical genetics may be significantly compromised.

Individual scholars and working groups have addressed the fairness and practical consequences of employers and insurers using genetic information to make decisions regarding health coverage and employment. The American Society of Human Genetics (ASHG) appointed an ad hoc committee in 1995, and the National Institutes of Health/Department of Energy (NIH/DOE) Working Group created a task force in 1993.[2] Both groups recognize universal access to health care as the best remedy to genetic discrimination. Effective genetic counseling and informed consent in genetic testing are also important as effective intermediate measures or as part of a more comprehensive solution.

This chapter discusses how genetic discrimination is likely to reduce accessibility of health care for those who need it most and examines the implications for patients and primary caregivers. Principles of risk-based underwriting and legislation to protect against genetic discrimination are reviewed. Genetic discrimination among insurers and employers is likely to continue, regardless of current and pending legislation, as long as risk-based underwriting is the standard in health insurance. This makes it particularly important for primary caregivers to make sure that informed consent for genetic testing includes a careful discussion of the possible social and economic consequences.

## POTENTIAL FOR GENETIC DISCRIMINATION

Genetic discrimination can be defined as discrimination directed against an individual, family, or race of people based on an actual or perceived genetic variation from the "normal" human genotype.[3] The potential for discrimination against persons with genetic illness or those at increased risk presents significant social and clinical issues relating to the availability of health care and the optimal use of genetic medicine.

A major period of genetic discrimination in the United States involved screening for sickle cell anemia among African-Americans during the 1970s. Both unaffected carriers and affected individuals were subject to discrimination. The U.S. Air Force and major commercial airlines excluded sickle cell carriers from service as pilots on the false grounds that carriers are at risk for high-altitude attacks.[4,5] A basic misunderstanding or indifference about the clinical distinction existed between an asymptomatic carrier and a person affected by the disease. Two aspects of this discrimination are of particular concern. First, the close association between sickle cell disease and race indicates a willingness to use genetics in ways that compound historical inequalities. Second, government and private industry demonstrated their readiness to adopt discriminatory policies without a full understanding of the disease or its manifestations.

Anecdotal evidence suggests that employers and insurers continue to practice genetic discrimination. In a 1996 study of 332 members of genetic support groups, 22% reported that they or a family member had been denied health insurance on the basis of a genetic condition in the family.[6] Although the respondents' impressions about the reasons for denial were highly subjective, 83% of those who had been asked about genetic diseases on their application were denied health insurance. In a 1992 study, 29 mailed responses described 41 instances of possible genetic discrimination; all except two involved insurance or employment.[3]

Although such anecdotal reports do not indicate the extent of genetic discrimination, insurers and employers have an economic incentive to use genetic information to project medical costs. At present, insurers do not use genetic testing, in part because it is not cost-effective.[5] There may be a ready market, however, if the cost of testing decreases.

## ACTUARIAL PRINCIPLES OF INSURANCE UNDERWRITING

The essential purpose of insurance is to provide a means by which individuals and organizations can limit uncertainty about potential losses by shifting risks to an insurance company in exchange for a certain sum of money. Health insurance companies rate individuals and groups according to their actuarially calculated level of risk in order to set premiums according to predicted loss. Three methods that insurers use for risk rating are as follows[7]:

1. Individual underwriting, in which individual applicants are rated according to their own risk characteristics
2. Experience underwriting, in which small or moderately sized groups of people are rated according to past experienced losses
3. Community rating, in which rates are set according to expected losses within a geographic area

The operating principle in this process is *equity;* the insurer is responsible to charge like premiums for like risks. This is distinct from a principle of *equality,* under which individuals or groups might be charged the same or similar premiums, regardless of risk. According to this principle of equity, an unfair cross-subsidy results if a policyholder is required to pay more or permitted to pay less than indicated by the calculated risk.

This concept of equity is mandated by the Unfair Trade Practices Act (UTPA), which prohibits insurers from (1) setting different premium levels for persons or groups who present the same level of risk or (2) charging the same premium for persons or groups who present different levels of risk.[8] This requirement preserves the financial solvency of insurance companies by assuring that risk liabilities do not exceed financial reserves. Also, if premiums do not reflect the level of risk, persons who present a lower risk will leave the risk pool, causing a rate increase for the remaining membership, which will cause another exodus, and so on. This concern is particularly relevant in a competitive insurance market, where one company's survival against the competition depends substantially on its ability to segment risks and set premiums accordingly.

### Criticism of Actuarial Equity

A forceful critique of the principle of equity as practiced in the insurance industry is that it fails to acknowledge significant differences between actuarial fairness and moral fairness.[9] The principle of equity may be a useful accounting tool, but some independent moral justification is necessary to give it any normative weight. One normative claim enlisted to support a system of actuarial fairness is that justice requires each person or voluntarily formed group to pay according to the risk they present. On this principle, like risks should be treated similarly, and there should be no forced cross-subsidies between groups or individuals with different levels of risk. Persons must be free to use or trade any of their own traits or abilities for their own advantage, regardless of any other social imperatives.[10] A powerful counter to this argument is that it fails to consider that initial inequalities, for which there may be no moral justification, can cause substantial inequalities in outcome.[11]

In the context of health insurance, actuarial equity has the practical effect of compounding or exacerbating inequalities. Although actuarial fairness requires that a person at high risk be charged a correspondingly higher premium, the person who is or may become seriously ill as a result of a genetic disorder is precisely the person who needs affordable health insurance. In the world of private health insurance, however, this person is likely to have the least access to affordable health care. This may be problematic depending on whether health insurance is viewed primarily as a business or as an instrument of social policy.[5] To the extent that the purpose of health insurance is to facilitate access to health care at an affordable and predictable cost, present applications of actuarial fairness should be reconsidered.

Life and disability insurance involve similar tensions between the social interest in maintaining generally accessible insurance coverage and the business interest in risk-based underwriting. Distinctions between disability and life insurance on the one hand and health insurance on the other shift the equities, however, such that the difference between actuarial fairness and moral fairness may not be as pronounced in the contexts of life and disability insurance.[12] A practical distinction is that the purchaser of life or disability insurance has substantial discretion to choose the value of the policy in terms of the lump sum to be paid in the event of death or the size and duration of disability payments. Thus a person at high risk for a disabling or fatal disease may opt to purchase insurance coverage far in excess of what he or she would otherwise choose, without sharing this risk information with the insurer. This may also be true with health insurance. The difference is that the payout on a health insurance policy is limited by the cost of treatment, which in most cases is substantially less than the value of the more expensive life or disability insurance policies. Thus the possibility of this type of market behavior by insurance consumers gives insurance companies a greater interest in knowing the health risks of individuals who apply to purchase life or disability insurance.

Another significant distinction is that the primary purpose of both life and disability insurance is to help ensure some financial support for oneself or one's family, whereas the purpose of health insurance is to help maximize and protect physical health. Health and money have qualitatively different values.[13] Money is an instrumental good that can only serve other ends; physical health is an intrinsic good with an independent value of its own. People think differently about their health than they do about their money. Losing one's health is not the same as losing money, and having one's health restored is not the same as a financial windfall. This distinction is apparent to health care providers, who often feel squeezed between their desire to deliver optimal health care and corporate pressures to optimize profits. These qualitative distinctions between money and health do not mean that one should always have priority over the other. In many situations, principles of distributive justice are likely to require reasonable trade-offs between the two.[13]

If formal qualitative distinctions do not fix a priority between health and money, an understanding of the practical implications may suggest an ordering of imperatives in this instance.[14] Life insurance and disability insurance are essentially part of a personal financial plan. Although access to a basic level of purchasing power is important to personal well-being, to the extent that reasonable financial alternatives exist to achieve this, the applicant for life or disability insurance has a less compelling claim to accessible insurance coverage than does the applicant for health insurance, to which few alternatives exist. However, some individuals may be able to invest enough in a medical savings account to cover any illness or injury. Such persons have no greater interest in health insurance than in life or disability insurance; their own financial means are sufficient. Conversely, individuals with little or no financial means have a strong interest in access to a means of continuing financial support and to health care. For the vast majority of the U.S. population, life insurance and disability insurance are desirable options. Most people would agree there is less imperative to advance individual discretionary financial goals by limiting risk-based underwriting than there is to protect access to affordable health care.

One reasonable alternative to risk-based underwriting in health insurance would be to require community rating. This would have the virtue of making health insurance equally accessible to members of a given community, while at the same time allowing insurers to adjust premiums according to risk. The difference is that insurers would be applying actuarial principles to a geographically defined community rather than to individuals or a self-selected group (see later discussion).

## EMPLOYER-SPONSORED HEALTH INSURANCE

More than 151 million people in the United States obtain their health coverage through their employer.[15,16] This makes employers the largest source of health coverage. Employers can offer health coverage through traditional means, purchasing coverage from an insurance company on behalf of their employees, or can self-insure by collecting premiums and paying medical costs through their own pool of funds or through stop-loss coverage purchased from a third-party insurer.

Most employers who purchase health coverage through an insurance company pay a premium that is set on the basis of *experience rating*.[2] That is, the risk of medical losses are calculated from a running average of claims submitted. This gives the employers an indirect but significant incentive to minimize potential medical expenses. Employers who self-insure have a more direct incentive to control medical losses because their own funds are at stake.

Self-insurance is increasingly the choice among employers. Approximately 65% of employers self-insure for medical expenses, and more than 80% of employers with more than 5000 employees are self-insured.[12] Two developments have contributed to the rise in self-insurance. First, increased accuracy in experience rating permits employers to predict their medical costs more precisely. Second, the Employee Retirement Income Security Act of 1974 (ERISA) frees self-insured employers from state insurance laws mandating certain coverages.[17,18] Thus the self-insured employer has sole authority to determine what type of coverage is offered and at what price. This includes the authority to exclude certain disorders from coverage and to charge higher prices to insure individuals at greater risk in order to make up for the increased cost of insuring those individuals. The only legal limitation on employer discretion is that changes in and pricing of coverage must be actuarially justified; employers are not permitted to be arbitrary.[8]

## CURRENT LEGISLATION

Public concern about the potential for employers and insurers to discriminate against persons with genetic disorders has led to state and federal legislation. Many states have enacted or have pending legislation to protect genetic privacy or restrict the use of genetic information.[19] The various state statutes offer different levels of protection, ranging from very comprehensive to disease specific. Because of the exemptions provided by ERISA, however, none of the state statutes can reach self-insured employers. Therefore any meaningful legislation regarding insurance or employer discrimination in health care will be at the federal level (Table 19-1).

## TABLE 19-1

# Federal Protections Against Genetic Discrimination

| | Symptomatic (e.g., Sickle Cell) | Susceptible (e.g., BRCA1) | Presymptomatic (e.g., Huntington) | Autosomal Dominant Carrier (e.g., Neuro-fibromatosis) |
|---|---|---|---|---|
| **AMERICANS WITH DISABILITIES ACT** | | | | |
| Insurance | Limited protection; allows actuarial distinctions | Limited protection; allows actuarial distinctions | Limited protection; allows actuarial distinctions | Limited protection; allows actuarial distinctions |
| Employment | Significant protection | Possible protection | Significant protection | Protection unlikely |
| **HEALTH INSURANCE PORTABILITY AND ACCOUNTABILITY ACT** | | | | |
| Insurance | Protects continuity of individual policy | Protects continuity of individual policy | Protects continuity of individual policy | Protects continuity of individual policy |
| Employment | Allows portability between group policies | Allows portability between group policies | Allows portability between group policies | Allows portability between group policies |
| **GENETIC NONDISCRIMINATION IN HEALTH INSURANCE AND EMPLOYMENT ACT** | | | | |
| Insurance | Limited protections; Allows distinctions based on physical examination | Significant protection (symptoms not evident) | Significant protection (symptoms not evident) | Significant protection (symptoms not evident) |
| Employment | Allows distinctions based on physical examination | Significant protection (symptoms not evident) | Significant protection (symptoms not evident) | Significant protection (symptoms not evident) |
| **GENETIC INFORMATION NONDISCRIMINATION IN HEALTH INSURANCE ACT** | | | | |
| Insurance | Limited protections; Allows distinctions based on physical examination | Significant protection (symptoms not evident) | Significant protection (symptoms not evident) | Significant protection (symptoms not evident) |
| Employment | No protection | No protection | No protection | No protection |

## Americans with Disabilities Act

The Americans with Disabilities Act (ADA) appears to forbid employers and insurers from discriminating against individuals on the basis of a physical or mental disability.[20] In the context of health insurance, however, substantial gaps exist in the protections afforded to individuals. The ADA prohibits insurers and self-insured employers from arbitrarily discriminating against individuals in the formulation and implementation of a health care plan. It does *not* prohibit actuarially based differentiation based on a risk analysis, which may take into account disability or susceptibility to disease. Therefore an insurer or employer may not be arbitrary in distinctions between individuals, but actuarially justified differences are permitted. The result is that an insurer or self-insured employer may set a higher premium for persons with a genetic disorder.

In the context of an employer's hiring and promotion decisions, the ADA is likely but not certain to provide protection for employees. The ambiguity here relates to whether the particular genetic disorder qualifies as a disability under the ADA. The ADA defines disability in an individual as any of the following[20]:

1.  A physical or mental impairment that substantially limits one or more major life activities
2.  A record of such impairment
3.  Being regarded as having such an impairment

Individuals who are presymptomatic for a disease that will inevitably become symptomatic, such as Huntington disease, or who are asymptomatic but genetically susceptible, such as with BRCA1 or BRCA2, are likely to be protected under the ADA. The statute is vague on this point, but a recent U.S. Supreme Court ruling and the Equal Employment Opportunity Commission's (EEOC's) *Compliance Manual* provide some guidance. The Supreme Court ruled that an asymptomatic woman who was positive for human immunodeficiency virus (HIV) was disabled because she had chosen not to bear children and therefore was limited in a major life activity.[21] Therefore the ADA would probably protect a person with a genetic disorder who is limited in a major life activity. Similarly, the EEOC's opinion, which is not binding on the courts, is that individuals who are either presymptomatic or susceptible to genetic disease and suffer discrimination are disabled under the third part of the ADA definition: they are regarded as having an impairment. However, neither the Supreme Court nor the EEOC has addressed whether the ADA protects an asymptomatic carrier, such as a person with neurofibromatosis.[22,23] Such a person would probably be protected under the first or third part of the ADA definition, if the person had limited a major life activity or suffered discrimination.

Given the likely interpretation of the ADA, an employer or insurer interested in controlling health care costs will be able to do so through traditional risk-based underwriting but will not be legally free to limit their risks through discriminatory hiring practices.

## Health Insurance Portability and Accountability Act of 1996

The Health Insurance Portability and Accountability Act (HIPAA), also known as the Kennedy-Kassenbaum Act, is intended to (1) provide continuity in group health insurance coverage when an employee changes jobs and (2) help persons with individual nongroup health insurance keep their policies in force.[24] The HIPAA has been partially successful.

The HIPAA prohibits an employer health plan from discriminating against a new employee or family member on the basis of health and strictly limits preexisting condition exclusions. A preexisting condition is defined as a condition "for which medical advice, diagnosis, care, or treatment was recommended or received within the six month period ending on the enrollment date [in the new health plan]."[24] Such an exclusion may last a maximum of 1 year, but this maximum period must be reduced by the amount of time that the employee or family member was covered under their previous health plan.

In the case of individual nongroup health insurance, the HIPAA does not offer portability (if a person moves to a new service area), but it does limit the conditions under which an insurer can cancel or refuse to renew. A health insurance policy will remain in force at the insured's option unless the following occur[8]:

1. The insured fails to pay the premiums.
2. The insured commits fraud (e.g., intentionally gives a false answer on the insurance application).
3. The insurer stops offering coverage in the relevant market.
4. The insured moves out of the service area.
5. The individual ceases to be a member in the association that offered the insurance.

With respect to group health plans, the HIPAA forbids insurers from treating a genetic condition as a preexisting condition unless there has been a diagnosis. Group health plans may not discriminate against individuals who are presymptomatic, disease susceptible, or asymptomatic carriers as having a preexisting condition.[8] In the context of individual nongroup health insurance, the HIPAA provides no preexisting condition limitations.

Although the HIPAA offers substantial protections, individual and group insurers remain free to use risk-based underwriting to determine premiums and what types of coverage to offer. Policyholders may have the legal option to join a new group plan or to keep an individual policy in force, but the cost of exercising such an option may effectively preclude it.

## Pending Legislation and Policy Proposals

Public concern about the limitations of the ADA and HIPAA has led Democrats and Republicans to introduce separate bills in the Senate and the House of Representatives. The stated purpose of each bill is to provide more comprehensive protection against genetic discrimination. The Democratic bill would provide protection against both insurance and employment discrimination, and the Republican bill would cover only insurance. Neither bill, however, would give complete protection in either category.

The *Genetic Nondiscrimination in Health Insurance and Employment Act*, sponsored by Democrats in the House of Representatives and the Senate, would prohibit insurers and employers from discriminating on the basis of "predictive genetic information."[25] The insurance provisions would make it unlawful for an insurer to discriminate against members of a group plan or an individual policyholder by denying coverage or adjusting premiums based on "predictive genetic information." The section on employment would prohibit employers from discriminating against individuals in decisions to hire, promote, discharge, or otherwise classify employees on the basis of genetic information.

A significant limitation of this bill is that "predictive genetic information" refers primarily to the results of DNA tests and specifically excludes information obtained by physical examination. This limitation is significant because many genetic disorders can be accurately diagnosed by physical examination.

Federal employees and applicants for federal employment are now similarly protected against employment discrimination. Under the terms of an executive order issued by President Clinton in 2000, federal employers are prohibited from discriminating against persons based on "protected genetic information."[26] The protections provided by this order are also limited in that the definition of "protected genetic information" excludes information obtained by physical examination.

The *Genetic Information Nondiscrimination in Health Insurance Act,* sponsored by Senate Republicans, would provide protection to individuals and groups against insurance discrimination by health insurers.[27] The protections and limitations set forth in the Republican bill are very similar to those in the Democratic bill. Again, the restrictive definition of "predictive genetic information" allows health insurers to discriminate on the basis of information derived through family history and physical examination.

A strong argument can be made for more comprehensive protections, but some criticize antidiscrimination legislation as being unfair to insurers and employers.[28] A central concern is that individuals at high risk will take advantage of private information to purchase in greater amounts than they would otherwise and at prices that do not reflect their unusually high level of risk. This is possible only when there is a basic asymmetry of essential information or a prohibition against risk taking. This poses a threat to insurers because they are denied the ability to price their policies according to projected risk. Not only is this unfair, they claim, but it jeopardizes their financial stability. In the most extreme case the private health insurance market could dissolve. These claims are highly empirical, and little evidence suggests that the effects of privacy and antidiscrimination legislation would be so severe. However, these concerns should be taken seriously.

## COMMUNITY RATING

One way to reduce the problem of discrimination without causing a potential threat to health insurers is to require community rating in health insurance. Under a system of community rating, information about a given individual's health is irrelevant to the insurer. The insurer is concerned with the aggregate risk of a community, and individuals are charged premiums that reflect the community risk. This method of rating is actuarially sound, and it protects individual access to affordable health care.

The limitation of community rating is that it cannot be sustained in a market that also offers individual and experience rating. Individuals and associations at lower risk will leave the community-rated pool to obtain lower premiums. An example of such an exodus can be seen in the experiences of the early nonprofit Blue Cross/Blue Shield plans, which have historically used community rating. Beginning in the 1940s, employers and unions, which tend to have relatively healthy risk pools, began to move out of community-rated plans into risk-rated plans.[29] This migration of the lower risk groups has continued to pressure the Blue Cross/Blue Shield plans, which are now increasingly abandoning their nonprofit status and adopting individual risk and experience rating.[2] The market has made it necessary for them to do so.

Given the unsustainability of community-rated plans in a market that includes competing risk-rated plans, several states, including New York and Massachusetts, have enacted legislation requiring community rating in health insurance.[30] Under community rating, persons who would be classified as a high risk by insurance underwriters will be eligible for more affordable health coverage. The necessary and anticipated implication is that the healthy population will subsidize the less healthy population within a given community of insured persons. A less anticipated implication is that poor and underserved persons will be forced to subsidize the health care of more wealthy persons within an economically diverse community. This result reflects the higher price of health care in more affluent areas; also, with any standard benefits plan, high-income groups will spend more on health care than low-income groups.[31,32]

Community rating is not a perfect solution, but it does offer affordable access and could substantially eliminate genetic discrimination in health care.

## GENETIC COUNSELING AND INFORMED CONSENT

With the continuing possibility of genetic discrimination, primary care providers must help patients considering genetic testing to make a clearly informed decision. Because of the medical complexity and the range of social and economic consequences, substantial counseling is usually a prerequisite for a well-informed decision. Patients not only must understand highly probabilistic information, but also must decide whether the benefits of such information exceed the possible adverse consequences relating to insurance and employment (not to mention social and psychological implications). Patients should be informed that if an insurer pays for a test, that same company will probably obtain the results. They should also be reminded that providing false answers on an insurance application constitutes fraud, and this is a basis for policy cancellation. Patients should also understand that the physician in charge may be legally required to make reasonable efforts to notify any of the patient's relatives who the test shows to be at risk and who may benefit from early diagnosis and treatment.[33,34] Additionally, patients need to consider that when one of their relatives applies for insurance, the insurer may ask whether the applicant knows of any relatives with particular genetic conditions. Although individuals may benefit from knowledge about their relative's genetic conditions, this information can make them vulnerable to genetic discrimination. Thus patients must consider their relative's circumstances as well as their own.

Few patients will be able to understand such information and make a well-considered decision in one meeting. A consensus group on informed consent and genetic testing recommends that informed consent be treated as a process rather than an event.[35] Under this model, patients should be offered genetic counseling to help them explore their values and concerns. This should be done through a series of discussions rather than a single encounter. Also, patients should be given explicit freedom to change their mind at any stage. The informed consent process should help the patient reach a decision that is "intentional, substantially noncontrolled, and based upon substantial understanding."[35,36]

## SUMMARY

Patients who may benefit from genetic testing face a dilemma. Their decision reflects some of the same tensions that society has been unable to resolve. The desire to maximize the benefits of genetic medicine and maintain access to health care conflicts with the cost-saving measures used by insurers and employers. As long as risk-based underwriting remains common practice in health insurance, patients will have to make difficult choices. Most often a series of competing considerations will need to be balanced against each other. In this process the primary care provider's participation is essential to help the patient make the best choices possible in an imperfect context.

# REFERENCES

1. The Ad Hoc Committee on Genetic Testing/Insurance Issues: Genetic testing and insurance, *Am J Hum Genet* 56:327-331, 1995.
2. NIH/DOE Working Group on Ethical, Legal, and Social Implications of Human Genome Research: *Genetic information and health insurance,* 93-3686, Bethesda, Md, 1993, Task Force on Genetic Information and Insurance.
3. Billings P et al: Discrimination as a consequence of genetic testing, *Am J Hum Genet* 50:476, 1992.
4. Lombardo P: Genetic confidentiality: what's the big secret? *University of Chicago Law School Roundtable* 3:589, 1996.
5. Gostin L: Genetic discrimination: the use of genetically based diagnostic tests by employers and insurers, *Am J Law Med* 17:109, 1991.
6. Lapham E, Kozma C, Weiss J: Genetic discrimination: perspectives of consumers, *Science* 274:621-624, 1996.
7. Ostrer H et al: Insurance and genetic testing: where are we now? *Am J Human Genet* 52:565-577, 1993.
8. Holmes E: Solving the insurance/genetic fair/unfair discrimination dilemma in light of the Human Genome Project, *Kentucky Law J* 85:503, 1996-97.
9. Daniels N: Insurability and the HIV epidemic: ethical issues in underwriting, *Milbank Q* 68:497, 1990.
10. Nozick R: *Anarchy, state, and utopia,* New York, 1974, Basic Books.
11. Rawls J: *A theory of justice,* Cambridge, Mass, 1971, Belknap.
12. Rothstein M: Genetics, insurance, and the ethics of genetic counseling, *Mol Genet Med* 3:159-177, 1993.
13. Sunstein C: *Free markets and social justice,* New York, 1997, Oxford University Press.
14. Jonsen A, Toulmin S: *The abuse of casuistry: a history of moral reasoning,* Berkeley, Calif, 1988, University of California Press.
15. Kuttner R: The American health care system: employer-sponsored health coverage, *N Engl J Med* 340:248, 1999.
16. Fronstin P: Sources of health insurance and characteristics of the uninsured: analysis of the March 1998 current population survey, Washington, DC, 1998, Employee Benefit Research Institute.
17. 29 USC Section 1001.
18. Greely H: Health insurance, employment discrimination, and the genetics revolution. In Kelves D, Hood L, editors: *The code of codes: scientific and social issues in the Human Genome Project,* Cambridge, Mass, 1992, Harvard University Press.
19. Davis H, Mitrus J: Genetic privacy and discrimination: a survey of state legislation, *Jurimetrics* 39:317, 1999.
20. 42 USC Section 12101.
21. *Bragdon v Abbott,* 118 S Ct 2196 (1998).
22. Bornstein R: Genetic discrimination, insurability and legislation: a closing of the legal loopholes, *J Law Public Policy* 4:551, 1996.

23. Andrews L: Genetic Fallout: New Technologies Are Changing the Legal Landscape, *Trial,* December 1995, pp 20, 25.

24. 29 USC Section 1181.

25. HR 2457, S 1322, 106th Congress (1999). (To be reintroduced under new bill number in 107th Congress.)

26. Executive Order 13145, *Federal Register* 65:6877, 2000.

27. S 543, 106th Congress (1999). (To be reintroduced under new bill number in 107th Congress.)

28. Epstein R: The legal regulation of genetic discrimination: old responses to new technology, *Boston University Law Review* 74: 1-23, 1997.

29. Light D: The ethics of corporate health insurance, *Business Professional Ethics J* 10: 49, 1997.

30. 501 McKinney's (NY) Section 323(a) (1992); Mass Ann Laws Ch 495.

31. Goldman D: Redistributional consequences of community rating: *Health Serv Res* 32:71, 1997.

32. Newhouse J: *Free for all: lessons learned from the RAND health insurance experiment,* Cambridge, 1993, Harvard University Press.

33. The American Society of Human Genetics Social Issues Subcommittee on Familial Disclosure: Professional disclosure of familial genetic information, *Am J Hum Genet* 62:474, 1998.

34. *Safer v Estate of Pack,* 291 NJ Super 619, 677 A2d 1188 (1996).

35. Geller G et al: Genetic testing for susceptibility to adult-onset cancer: the process and content of informed consent, *JAMA* 277: 1467, 1997.

36. Appelbaum P, Lidz C, Meisel A: *Informed consent: legal theory and clinical practice,* New York, 1987, Oxford University Press.

# APPENDIX

## FINDINGS AND RECOMMENDATIONS OF THE INSTITUTE OF MEDICINE COMMITTEE ON ASSESSING GENETIC RISKS

## OVERALL PRINCIPLES

**The committee recommends that vigorous protection be given to autonomy, privacy, confidentiality, and equity.** These principles should be breached only in rare instances and only when the following conditions are met: (1) the action must be aimed at an important goal—such as the protection of others from serious harm—that outweighs the value of autonomy, privacy, confidentiality, or equity in the particular instance; (2) it must have a high probability of realizing that goal; (3) there must be no acceptable alternatives that can also realize the goal without breach of these principles; and (4) the degree of infringement of the principle must be the minimum necessary to realize the goal.

**The committee recommends that regardless of the institutional structure of the entity offering genetic testing or other genetics services, there be a mechanism for advance review of the new genetic testing or other genetics services not only to assess scientific merit and efficacy, but also to ensure that adequate protections are in place for autonomy, privacy, confidentiality, and equity.** The usual standards for review of research should be applied no matter what the setting. In particular, an institutional review board (IRB) should review the scientific and ethical issues related to new tests and services in academic research centers, state public health departments, and commercial enterprises. These reviews should include any proposed investigational use of genetic tests, as well as more extensive pilot studies. In all instances the review body should include people from inside and outside the institution, including community representatives, preferably consumers of genetic services. In the clinical practice setting, professional societies should be encouraged to review studies and issue guidelines, thereby supplementing the guidance provided by IRBs.

**The committee also recommends that the National Institutes of Health (NIH) Office of Protection from Research Risks provide guidance and training on how review bodies should scrutinize the risks to human subjects of genetic testing.** IRBs may also need technical advice from a local advisory group on genetics. To the extent that a National Advisory Committee on Genetic Testing and its Working Group on Genetic Testing are established, these bodies should be consulted by IRBs and the NIH Office of Protection from Research Risks.

From Institute of Medicine Committee on Assessing Genetic Risks: *Implications for health and social policy,* Washington, DC, 1994, National Academy Press.

All laboratories offering genetic testing are included under the Clinical Laboratory Improvement Amendments of 1988 (CLIA88), and the committee recommends that the Health Care Financing Administration expand its existing lists of covered laboratory tests to include the full range of genetic tests now in use.

New tests, not validated elsewhere, that are added to the battery of tests should be considered investigational if they are used to make a clinical decision. The committee recommends that IRB approval be obtained in universities, commercial concerns, and other settings where new tests for additional disorders are being undertaken, even if the tests rely on existing technologies. IRB approval should be obtained before new tests are added to newborn screening.

## AUTONOMY

### Informed Consent

The committee recommends that for a proper informed consent to be obtained from a person who is considering whether to undergo genetic testing, the person should be given information about the risks, benefits, efficacy, and alternatives to the testing; information about the severity, potential variability, and treatability of the disorder being tested for; and information about the subsequent decisions that will be likely if the test is positive (e.g., whether the person will have to make a decision about abortion). Information should also be disclosed about any potential conflicts of interest of the person or institution offering the test (e.g., equity holdings or ownership of the laboratory performing the test, dependence on test reimbursement to cover the costs of counseling, patents). The difficulty in applying the traditional mechanisms for achieving informed consent should not be considered an excuse for failing to respect a patient's autonomy and need for information.

The committee recommends that research be undertaken to determine what patients want to know in order to make a decision about whether or not to undergo a genetic test. People may have less interest in information about the label for the disorder and its mechanisms of action than they have in information about how certainly the test predicts the disorder, what effects the disorder has on physical and mental functioning, and how intrusive, difficult, or effective any existing treatment protocol would be. Research is also necessary to determine the advantages and disadvantages of various means of conveying that information (e.g., through specialized genetic counselors, primary care providers, single-disorder counselors, brochures, videos, audiotapes, and computer programs). People also need to know about potential losses of insurability or employability or social consequences that may result from knowledge about the disorder for which testing is being discussed.

### Multiplex Testing

Performing multiple genetic tests on a single sample of genetic material—often using techniques of automation—has been called *multiplex testing*. **The committee recommends that informed consent be gained in advance of such multiplex testing.** New means (such as interactive or other types of computer programs, videotapes, and brochures) should be developed to provide people—in advance of testing—with the information described in the previous recommendations, such as descriptions of the nature of tests that are included in multiplex testing and the nature of the disorders being tested for. A health care provider or counselor should also provide information about each of the tests, or if that is not possible because of the number of tests being grouped together, the provider or counselor should supply information about the categories of disorders so that the person will be able to make an informed decision about whether to undergo the testing.

**The committee identified the area of multiplex testing as one in which more research is needed to develop ways to ensure that patient autonomy is recognized.** The more general research the committee has advocated on determining what information should be conveyed and how it should be conveyed should be supplemented with additional research dealing with the unique case of multiplex testing where many disorders could be tested for at once, and those disorders may have differing characteristics. **In multiplexing, tests should be grouped so that tests requiring similar demands for informed consent and education and counseling may be offered together.** Only certain types of tests should be multiplexed; some tests should only be offered individually, especially tests for untreatable fatal disorders (e.g., Huntington disease).

**The committee also recommends that research be undertaken to make decisions about which tests to group together in multiplex testing, based on the type of information the tests provide.** The committee believes strongly that tests for untreatable disorders should not be multiplexed with tests for disorders that can be cured or prevented by treatment or by avoidance of particular environmental stimuli.

# VOLUNTARINESS

**The committee reaffirms that voluntariness should be the cornerstone of any genetic testing program.** The committee found no justification for a state-sponsored mandatory public health program involving genetic testing of adults, or for unconsented-to genetic testing of patients in the clinical setting.

### Screening and Testing of Children

**The committee recommends that newborn screening programs be voluntary. The decision to make screening mandatory should require evidence that—without mandatory screening—newborns will not be screened for treatable illnesses in time to institute effective treatment (e.g., in PKU or congenital hypothyroidism).** The committee bases its recommendation and preference for voluntariness on evidence from studies of existing mandated and voluntary programs that demonstrate that the best interests of the child can be served without abrogating the principle of voluntariness. Voluntary programs have delivered services as well or better than mandated programs. There is no evidence that a serious harm will result if autonomy is recognized, just as there is no evidence that mandating newborn screening is necessary to ensure that the vast majority of newborns are screened.

**The committee recommends that newborn screening should not be undertaken in state programs unless there is a clear, immediate benefit to the particular infant being**

**screened.** In particular, screening should not be undertaken if presymptomatic identification of the infant and early intervention make no difference, if necessary and effective treatment is not available, or if the disorder is untreatable and screening is being done to provide information merely to aid the parents' (or the infant's) future reproductive plans. **The committee recommends that states that screen newborns have an obligation to ensure treatment of those detected with the disorder under state programs, without regard to ability to pay for treatment.**

**The committee recommends that in the clinical setting, children generally be tested only for disorders for which a curative or preventive treatment exists and should be instituted at that early stage.** Childhood screening is not appropriate for carrier status, untreatable childhood diseases, and late-onset diseases that cannot be prevented or forestalled by early treatment. Because only certain types of genetic testing are appropriate for children, tests specifically directed to obtaining information about carrier status, untreatable childhood diseases, or late-onset diseases should not be included in the multiplex tests offered to children. Research should be undertaken to determine the appropriate age for testing and screening for genetic disorders in order to maximize the benefits of therapeutic intervention and to avoid the possibility that genetic information will be generated about a child when there is no likely benefit to the child in the immediate future.

**The majority of the committee recommends that carrier status of newborns and other children be reported to parents only after the parents have been informed of the potential benefits and harms of knowing the carrier status of their children.** Because of the risk of stigma for the newborn, such pretest information should be provided to parents when they are informed about newborn screening. Provision should be made for answering any questions the parents may have; these questions are best answered in the context of genetic counseling. The decisions of the parents about whether to receive such information should always be respected. **Where such information is not disclosed after parents are given the option to get such information and then knowingly refuse the information, the courts should take this policy analysis and the recommendation of this committee into consideration and not find liability if parents sue because the carrier status of their child was not disclosed and they subsequently give birth to an affected child.** Research is needed on the consequences of revealing carrier status in newborns to identify both harms and benefits from disclosing such information in the future.

### Subsequent Uses

**The committee recommends that before genetic information is obtained from individuals (or before a sample is obtained for genetic testing), they (or, in the case of minors, their parents) be told what specific uses will be made of the information or sample; how—and for how long—the information or sample will be stored; whether personal identifiers will be stored; and who will have access to the information or sample, and under what conditions.** They should also be informed of future anticipated uses for the sample, asked permission for those uses, and told what procedures will be followed if the possibility for currently unanticipated uses develops. The individuals should have a right to consent or to object to particular uses of the sample or information.

**Subsequent anonymous use of samples for research is permissible, including in state newborn screening programs.** Except for such anonymous use, the newborn specimen should not be used for additional tests without informed consent of the parents or guardian.

If genetic test samples are collected for family linkage studies or clinical purposes, they should not be used for law enforcement purposes (except for body identification). If samples are collected for law enforcement purposes, they should not be accessible for other nonclinical uses such as testing for health insurance purposes.

## CONFIDENTIALITY

### Disclosure to Spouses and Relatives

**As a matter of general principle, the committee believes that patients should be encouraged and aided in sharing appropriate genetic information with spouses.** Mechanisms should be developed to aid a tested individual in informing his or her spouse and relatives about the individual's genetic status and informing relatives about genetic risks. These mechanisms would include the use of written materials, referrals for counseling, and so forth.

**On balance, the committee recommends that health care providers not reveal genetic information about a patient's carrier status to the patient's spouse without the patient's permission. Furthermore, information about misattributed paternity should be revealed to the mother but should not be volunteered to the woman's partner.** Although confidentiality may be breached to prevent harm to third parties, the harm envisioned by the cases generally has been substantial and imminent. The spouse's claim of future harm due to the possibility of later conceiving a child with a genetic disorder would not be a sufficient reason to breach confidentiality. The committee found no evidence of a trend on the part of people to mislead their spouses about their carrier status. Moreover, since most people *do* tell their spouses about genetic risks, breaching of confidentiality would be needed only rarely.

**The committee believes that patients should share genetic information with their relatives so that the relatives may avert risks or seek treatment.** Health care providers should discuss with patients the benefit of sharing information with relatives about genetic conditions that are treatable or preventable or that involve important reproductive decision making. **The committee believes that the disadvantages of informing relatives over the patient's refusal generally outweigh the advantages, except in the rare instances described above.**

**The committee recommends that confidentiality be breached and relatives informed about genetic risks only when attempts to elicit voluntary disclosure fail, there is a high probability of irreversible or fatal harm to the relative, the disclosure of the information will prevent harm, the disclosure is limited to the information necessary for diagnosis or treatment of the relative, and there is no other reasonable way to avert the harm.** When disclosure is to be attempted over the patient's refusal, the burden should be on the person who wishes to disclose to justify to the patient, to an ethics committee, and perhaps in court that the disclosure was necessary and met the committee's test.

If there are any circumstances in which the geneticist or other health care professional could breach confidentiality and disclose information to a spouse, relative, or other third party—for example, to an employer—those circumstances should be explained in advance of testing; and, if the patient wishes, the patient should be given the opportunity to be referred to a health care provider who will protect confidentiality.

**On a broader scale, the committee recommends that:**

• **all forms of genetic information be considered confidential and not be disclosed without the individual's consent** (except as required by law), including genetic information that is obtained through specific genetic testing of a person as well as genetic information about a person that is obtained in other ways (e.g., physical examination, knowledge of past treatment, or knowledge of a relative's genetic status);

• **confidentiality of genetic information should be protected no matter who obtains or maintains that information,** including genetic information collected or maintained by health care professionals, health care institutions, researchers, employers, insurance companies, laboratory personnel, and law enforcement officials; and

• **to the extent that current statutes do not ensure such confidentiality, they should be amended so that disclosure of genetic information is not required.**

**The committee recommends that codes of ethics of those professionals providing genetics services (such as those of the National Society of Genetic Counselors [NSGC], or of geneticists, physicians, and nurses) contain specific provisions to protect autonomy, privacy, and confidentiality.** The committee endorses the NSGC statement of a guiding principle on confidentiality of test results:

> *The NSGC support individual confidentiality regarding results of genetic testing. It is the right and responsibility of the individual to determine who shall have access to medical information, particularly results of testing for genetic conditions.*

The committee also endorses the principles on DNA banking and DNA data banking contained in the 1990 ASHG statement.

**To further protect confidentiality, the committee recommends that:**

• **patients' consent be obtained before the patient's name is provided to a genetic disease registry and that consent be obtained before information is redisclosed;**

• **each entity that receives or maintains genetic information or samples have procedures in place to protect confidentiality,** including procedures limiting access on a need-to-know basis, identifying an individual who has responsibility for overseeing security procedures and safeguards, providing written information to each employee or agent regarding the need to maintain confidentiality, and taking no punitive action against employees for bringing evidence of confidentiality breaches to light;

• **any entity that releases genetic information about an individual to someone other than that individual ensure that the recipient of the genetic information has procedures in place to protect the confidentiality of the information:**

• **any entity that collects or maintains genetic information or samples separate them from personal identifiers** and instead link the information or sample to the individual's name through some form of anonymous surrogate identifiers;

• **the person have control over what parts of his or her medical record are available to which people;** if an optical memory card is used, this could be accomplished through a partitioning-off of data on the card; and

• **any individual be allowed access to his or her genetic information in the context of appropriate education and counseling,** except in the early research phases during the development of genetic testing when an overall decision has been made that results based on the experimental procedure will not be released and the subjects of the research have been informed of that restriction prior to participation.

### Discrimination in Insurance and Employment

**In general, the committee recommends that principles of autonomy, privacy, confidentiality, and equity be maintained, and the disclosure of genetic information and the taking of genetic tests should not be mandated.** Such a position, however, is in conflict with some current practices in insurance and employment.

Although more than half the U.S. population (approximately 156 million people) is covered by some kind of insurance, the use of genetic information in medical underwriting decisions about life insurance appears to raise different and somewhat lesser concerns than the use of genetic information in health insurance underwriting. More of life insurance has historically been medically underwritten. Complaints of genetic discrimination in life insurance have been made. Apparently, fewer Americans believe that life insurance is a basic right. In contrast. the Canadian Privacy Commission believes that life insurance is a basic right, and recommends that Canadians be permitted to purchase up to $100,000 in basic life insurance without genetic or other restrictions; underwriting for larger amounts of life insurance could be subject to a variety of life-style and health restrictions, including the use of genetic information. **Most of the committee agrees with the spirit of the Canadian commission's recommendation that a** *limited* **amount of life insurance be available to everyone without regard to health or genetic status. However, health insurance was considered a much more pressing ethical, legal, and social issue.**

**The committee recommends that legislation be adopted so that medical risks, including genetic risks, not be taken into account in decisions on whether to issue or how to price health care insurance.** Because health insurance differs significantly from other types of insurance in that it regulates access to health care, an important social good, risk-based health insurance should be eliminated. A means of access to health care should be available to every American without regard to the individual's present health status or condition, including genetic makeup. Any health insurance reform proposals need to be evaluated to determine their effect on genetic testing and the use of genetic information in health insurance.

**The committee recommends that the unfair practices highlighted by the** *McGann* **case be prevented.**\* Such situations could be eliminated by Congress in three ways. First, the antidiscrimination provision of the Employee Retirement Income Security Act (ERISA), section 510, could be amended to prohibit various types of employer conduct. For example, the legislation could prohibit: (1) the alteration of benefits or the alteration of benefits without a certain notice period; (2) the reduction of coverage for only a single medical condition; (3) the reduction of benefits after a claim for benefits already had been submitted, and so forth. At the very least, the committee recommends that an amendment be adopted making those practices illegal.

A second way of legislatively preventing *McGann*-type situations would be to amend the ERISA preemption provision, section 514. By amending this section to limit the preemptive effect of ERISA (e.g., that permits ERISA provisions to override state insurance

---

\*A case involving employer changes in health coverage to cut "losses" on an employee with AIDS.

regulation) or to eliminate ERISA preemption entirely, the result would be to allow the states to regulate self-insured employer benefits in the same way that state insurance commissions regulate commercial health insurance benefits. Although state regulation may be preferable to no regulation, it could lead to the burdensome multiplicity of state regulations that ERISA was intended to eliminate. For this reason, the committee believes that federal prohibition of the type of conduct in the *McGann* case would be preferable.

A third way to eliminate discrimination in employee health benefits by self-insured employers would be to amend section 501 of the Americans with Disabilities Act (ADA). The ADA is essentially neutral on the issue of health benefits; clauses on preexisting conditions, medical underwriting, and other actuarially based practices, to the extent permitted by state law, do not violate the ADA. Thus, the ADA could be amended to prohibit differences in health benefits that result in discrimination against individuals with disabilities. Amending the ADA in this manner would, in effect, mandate uniform coverage (although it is not clear what conditions would be covered) at community rates for employees. If Congress wanted to mandate that all employers offer a package of health benefits, a good argument could be made that it ought to do so separately and not via amendments to the ADA.

**The committee recommends that legislation be adopted so that genetic information cannot be collected on prospective or current employees unless it is clearly job related.** Sometimes employers will have employees submit to medical examinations to see if they are capable of performing particular job tasks. The committee recommends that if an individual consents to the release of genetic information to an employer or potential employer, the releasing entity should not release specific information, but instead answer only yes or no regarding whether the individual was fit to perform the job at issue.

**The committee recommends that the Equal Employment Opportunity Commission recognize that the language of the ADA provides protection for presymptomatic people with a genetic profile for late-onset disorders, unaffected carriers of disorders that might affect their children, and people with genetic profiles indicating the possibility of increased risk of a multifactorial disorder.** The committee also recommends that state legislatures adopt laws to protect people from genetic discrimination in employment. In addition, the committee recommends an amendment to the ADA (and adoption of similar state statutes) limiting the type of medical testing employers can request or the medical information they can collect to that which is job related.

**Ultimately, new laws on a variety of other topics may also be necessary to protect autonomy, privacy, and confidentiality in the genetics field, and to protect people from inappropriate decisions based on their genotypes.** The ability of genetics to predict health risks for asymptomatic individuals and their potential offspring presents challenges in the ethical and social spheres. **The committee recommends that careful consideration be given to the development of policies for the implementation of genetic testing and the handling of genetic test results.**

# GLOSSARY

**adenine (A)** Nitrogenous base, one member of the base pair AT (adenine and thymine).

**allele** Alternative form of a genetic locus; a single allele for each locus is inherited separately from each parent (e.g., at a locus for eye color the allele might result in blue or brown eyes).

**amino acid** Any of a class of 20 molecules that are combined to form proteins in living things. The sequence of amino acids in a protein and thus protein function are determined by the genetic code.

**amplification** Increase in the number of copies of a specific DNA fragment; can be in vivo or in vitro. *See also* cloning, polymerase chain reaction.

**arrayed library** Individual primary recombinant clones (hosted in phage, cosmid, yeast artificial chromosome, or other vector) that are placed in two-dimensional arrays in microtiter dishes. Each primary clone can be identified by the identity of the plate and the clone location (row and column) on that plate. Arrayed libraries of clones can be used for many applications, including screening for a specific gene or genomic region of interest and physical mapping. Information gathered on individual clones from various genetic linkage and physical map analyses is entered into a relational database and used to construct physical and genetic linkage maps simultaneously; clone identifiers serve to interrelate the multilevel maps. *See also* genomic library, library.

**autoradiography** Technique that uses x-ray film to visualize radioactively labeled molecules or fragments of molecules; used in analyzing length and number of DNA fragments after they are separated by gel electrophoresis.

**autosome** Chromosome not involved in sex determination. The diploid human genome consists of 46 chromosomes, 22 pairs of autosomes, and one pair of sex chromosomes (the X and Y chromosomes).

**bacterial artificial chromosome (BAC)** Vector used to clone DNA fragments (100- to 300-kb insert size; average, 150 kb) in *Escherichia coli* cells. Based on naturally occurring F-factor plasmid found in the bacterium *E. coli*. *See also* cloning vector.

**bacteriophage** *See* phage.

**base pair (bp)** Two nitrogenous bases (adenine and thymine or guanine and cytosine) held together by weak bonds. Two strands of DNA are held together in the shape of a double helix by the bonds between base pairs.

**base sequence** Order of nucleotide bases in a DNA molecule.

**base sequence analysis** Method, sometimes automated, for determining the base sequence.

**biotechnology** Set of biological techniques developed through basic research and now applied to research and product development. In particular, industry's use of recombinant DNA, cell fusion, and new bioprocessing techniques.

**bp** *See* base pair.

---

From Human Genome Project Information website: www.ornl.gov/hgmis. Sponsored by the U.S. Department of Energy Human Genome Program.

**cDNA** *See* complementary DNA.

**centimorgan (cM)** Unit of measure of recombination frequency. One centimorgan is equal to a 1% chance that a marker at one genetic locus will be separated from a marker at a second locus due to crossing-over in a single generation. In humans, 1 cM is equivalent, on average, to 1 million base pairs.

**centromere** Specialized chromosome region to which spindle fibers attach during cell division.

**chromosome** Self-replicating genetic structure of cells containing the cellular DNA that bears the linear array of genes in its nucleotide sequence. In *prokaryotes,* chromosomal DNA is circular, and the entire genome is carried on one chromosome. *Eukaryotes* consist of a number of chromosomes whose DNA is associated with different types of proteins.

**clone** Exact copy made of biological material, such as a DNA segment (a gene or other region), a whole cell, or a complete organism.

**clone bank** *See* genomic library.

**cloning** Using specialized DNA technology to produce multiple, exact copies of a single gene or other segment of DNA to obtain enough material for further study. This process is used by researchers in the Human Genome Project and is referred to as *cloning DNA.* The resulting cloned (copied) collections of DNA molecules are called *clone libraries.* A second type of cloning exploits the natural process of cell division to make many copies of an entire cell. The genetic makeup of these cloned cells, called a *cell line,* is identical to the original cell. A third type of cloning produces complete, genetically identical animals, such as the famous Scottish sheep, Dolly.

**cloning vector** DNA molecule originating from a virus, a plasmid, or the cell of a higher organism, into which another DNA fragment of appropriate size can be integrated without loss of the vector's capacity for self-replication; vectors introduce foreign DNA into host cells, where it can be reproduced in large quantities. Examples are plasmids, cosmids, and yeast artificial chromosomes; vectors are often recombinant molecules containing DNA sequences from several sources.

**cM** *See* centimorgan.

**code** *See* genetic code.

**codon** *See* genetic code.

**complementary DNA (cDNA)** DNA that is synthesized from a messenger RNA template; the single-stranded form is often used as a probe in physical mapping.

**complementary sequence** Nucleic acid-base sequence that can form a double-stranded structure by matching base pairs with another sequence; the complementary sequence to GTAC is CATG.

**conserved sequence** Base sequence in a DNA molecule (or an amino acid sequence in a protein) that has remained essentially unchanged throughout evolution.

**contig** Group of cloned (copied) pieces of DNA representing overlapping regions of a particular chromosome.

**contig map** Map depicting the relative order of a linked library of small overlapping clones representing a complete chromosomal segment.

**cosmid** Artificially constructed cloning vector containing the *cos* gene of phage *lambda.* Cosmids can be packaged in *lambda* phage particles for infection into *E. coli;* this permits cloning of larger DNA fragments (up to 45 kb), which can be introduced into bacterial hosts in plasmid vectors.

**crossing-over** Breaking during meiosis of one maternal and one paternal chromosome, exchange of corresponding sections of DNA, and rejoining of the chromosomes. This process can result in an exchange of alleles between chromosomes. *See also* recombination.

**cytosine (C)** Nitrogenous base, one member of the base pair GC (guanine and cytosine).

**deletion map** Description of a specific chromosome that uses defined mutations (specific deleted areas in the genome) as "biochemical signposts," or markers for specific areas.

**deoxyribonucleotide** *See* nucleotide.

**diploid** Full set of genetic material consisting of paired chromosome, with one chromosome from each parental set. Most animal cells, except the gametes, have a diploid set of chromosomes. The diploid human genome has 46 chromosomes. *See also* haploid.

**DNA (deoxyribonucleic acid)** Molecule that encodes genetic information. DNA is a double-stranded molecule held together by weak bonds between base pairs of nucleotides. The four nucleotides in DNA contain the bases: adenine (A), guanine (G), cytosine (C), and thymine (T). In nature, base pairs form only between A and T and between G and C; thus the base sequence of each single strand can be deduced from that of its partner.

**DNA probe** *See* probe.

**DNA replication** Use of existing DNA as a template for the synthesis of new DNA strands. In humans and other eukaryotes, replication occurs in the cell nucleus.

**DNA sequence** Relative order of base pairs, whether in a fragment of DNA, a gene, a chromosome, or an entire genome. *See also* base sequence analysis.

**domain** Discrete portion of a protein with its own function. The combination of domains in a single protein determines it overall function.

**double helix** The shape that two linear strands of DNA assume when bonded together.

**electrophoresis** Method of separating large molecules (e.g., DNA fragments, proteins) from a mixture of similar molecules. An electric current is passed through a medium containing the mixture, and each kind of molecule travels through the medium at a different rate, depending on its electrical charge and size. Separation is based on these differences. Agarose and acrylamide gels are the media commonly used for electrophoresis of proteins and nucleic acids.

**endonuclease** Emzyme that cleaves its nucleic acid substrate at internal sites in the nucleotide sequence.

**enzyme** Protein that acts as a catalyst, speeding the rate at which a biochemical reaction proceeds but not altering the direction or nature of the reaction.

*Escherichia coli* Common bacterium that has been studied intensively by geneticists because of its small genome size, normal lack of pathogenicity, and ease of growth in the laboratory.

**EST** Expressed sequence tag. *See* sequence tagged site.

**eukaryote** Cell or organism with membrane-bound, structurally discrete nucleus and other well-developed subcellular compartments. Eukaryotes include all organisms except viruses, bacteria, and blue-green algae. *See also* chromosome, prokaryote.

**evolutionarily conserved** *See* conserved sequence.

**exogenous DNA** DNA originating outside an organism.

**exon** Protein-coding DNA sequence of a gene. *See also* intron.

**exonuclease** Enzyme that cleaves nucleotides sequentially from free ends of a linear nucleic acid substrate.

**expressed gene** *See* gene expression.

**flow cytometry** Analysis of biological material by detection of the light-absorbing or fluorescing properties of cells or subcellular fractions (i.e., chromosomes) passing in a narrow stream through a laser beam. An absorbance or fluorescence profile of the sample is produced. Automated sorting devices are used to fractionate samples and sort successive droplets of the analyzed stream into different fractions, depending on the fluorescence emitted by each droplet.

**flow karyotyping** Use of flow cytometry to analyze and separate chromosomes on the basis of their DNA content.

**fluorescence in situ hybridization (FISH)** Physical mapping approach that uses fluorescein tags to detect hybridization of probes with metaphase chromosomes and with less-condensed somatic interphase chromatin.

**gamete** Mature male or female reproductive cell (sperm or ovum) with a haploid set of chromosomes (23 for humans).

**gel electrophoresis** DNA separation technique important in DNA sequencing. Standard sequencing procedures involve cloning DNA fragments into special sequencing cloning vectors that carry tiny pieces of DNA. The next step is to determine the base sequence of the tiny fragments by a special procedure that generates a series of even tinier DNA fragments that differ in size by only one base. These nested fragments are separated by gel electrophoresis, in which the DNA pieces are added to a gelatinous solution, allowing the fragments to work their way down through the gel. Smaller pieces move faster and will reach the bottom first. Movement through the gel is hastened by applying an electrical field to the gel.

**gene** Fundamental physical and functional unit of heredity. A gene is an ordered sequence of nucleotides located in a particular position on a particular chromosome that encodes a specific functional product (i.e., protein or RNA molecule).

**gene expression** Process by which a gene's coded information is converted into the structures present and operating in the cell. Expressed genes include those that are transcribed into mRNA and then translated into protein and those that are transcribed into RNA but not translated into protein (e.g., transfer and ribosomal RNAs).

**gene family** Group of closely related genes that make similar products.

**gene library** *See* genomic library.

**gene mapping** Determination of the relative positions of genes on a DNA molecule (chromosome or plasmid) and of the distance, in linkage units or physical units, between them.

**gene product** Biochemical material, either RNA or protein, resulting from expression of a gene. The amount of gene product is used to measure a gene's activity; abnormal amounts can be correlated with disease-causing alleles.

**genetic code** Sequence of nucleotides, coded in triplets (codons) along the mRNA, that determines the sequence of amino acids in protein synthesis. The DNA sequence of a gene can be used to predict the mRNA sequence, and the genetic code can in turn be used to predict the amino acid sequence.

**genetic engineering technology** *See* recombinant DNA technology.

**genetic map** *See* linkage map.

**genetic material** *See* genome.

**genetics** Study of the patterns of inheritance of specific traits.

**genome** All the genetic material in the chromosomes of a particular organism; its size is generally given as its total number of base pairs.

**genome project** Research and technology development effort aimed at mapping and sequencing some or all of the genome of humans and other organisms.

**genomic library** Collection of clones made from a set of randomly generated overlapping DNA fragments representing the entire genome of an organism. *See also* arrayed library, library.

**genomic sequence** Order of the subunits, called *bases,* that make up a particular fragment of DNA in a genome. DNA is a long molecule made up of four different kinds of bases, which are abbreviated A, C, T, and G. DNA fragment that is 10 bases long might have a base sequence of, for example, ATCGTTCCTG. The particular sequence of bases encodes important information in an individual's genetic blueprint and is unique or each individual (except identical twins).

**guanine (G)** Nitrogenous base, one member of the base pair GC (guanine and cytosine).

**haploid** Single set of chromosomes (half the full set of genetic material) in the egg and sperm cells of animals and in the egg and pollen cells of plants. Humans have 23 chromosomes in their reproductive cells. *See also* diploid.

**heterozygosity** Presence of different alleles at one or more loci on homologous chromosomes.

**homeobox** Short stretch of nucleotides whose base sequence is virtually identical in all the genes that contain it. It has been found in many organisms, from fruit flies to humans. In the fruit fly a homeobox appears to determine when particular groups of genes are expressed during development.

**homologous chromosome** Chromosome containing the same linear gene sequences as another, each derived from one parent.

**homology** Similarity in DNA or protein sequences between individuals of the same species or among different species.

**human gene therapy** Insertion of normal DNA directly into cells to correct a genetic defect.

**Human Genome Initiative** Collective name for several projects begun in 1986 by the U.S. Department of Energy (DOE) to (1) create an ordered set of DNA segments from known chromosomal locations, (2) develop new computational methods to analyzing genetic map and DNA sequence data, and (3) develop new techniques and instruments for detecting and analyzing DNA. This DOE initiative is now known as the *Human Genome Program.* The national effort, led by DOE and the National Institutes of Health (NIH), is known as the *Human Genome Project.*

**hybridization**—Process of joining two complementary strands of DNA or one each of DNA and RNA to form a double-stranded molecule.

**in situ hybridization** Use of a DNA or RNA probe to detect the presence of the complementary DNA sequence in cloned bacterial or cultured eukaryotic cells.

**in vitro** Outside a living organism.

**informatics** Study of the application of computer and statistical techniques to the management of information. In genome projects, informatics includes the development of methods to search databases quickly, to analyze DNA sequence information, and to predict protein sequence and structure from DNA sequence data.

**interphase** Period in the cell cycle when DNA is replicated in the nucleus; followed by mitosis.

**intron** DNA base sequence interrupting the protein-coding sequence of a gene; this sequence is transcribed into RNA but is cut out of the message before it is translated into protein. *See also* exon.

**karyotype** Photomicrograph of an individual's chromosomes arranged in a standard format showing the number, size, and shape of each chromosome type; used in low-resolution physical mapping to correlate gross chromosomal abnormalities with the characteristics of specific diseases.

**kilobase (kb)** Unit of length for DNA fragments equal to 1000 nucleotides.

**library** Unordered collection of clones (i.e., cloned DNA from a particular organism), whose relationship to each other can be established by physical mapping. *See also* arrayed library, genomic library.

**linkage** Proximity of two or more markers (e.g., genes, RFLP markers) on a chromosome; the closer the markers, the lower the probability that they will be separated during DNA repair or replication processes (binary fission in prokaryotes, mitosis or meiosis in eukaryotes), and thus the greater the probability that they will be inherited together.

**linkage map** Map of the relative positions of genetic loci on a chromosome, determined on the basis of how often the loci are inherited together. Distance is measured in centimorgans (cM).

**localize** Determination of the original position (locus) of a gene or other marker on a chromosome.

**locus (*pl.* loci)** Position on a chromosome of a gene or other chromosome marker; also, the DNA at that position. The use of locus is sometimes restricted to mean regions of DNA that are expressed. *See also* gene expression.

**long-range restriction mapping** Restriction enzymes are proteins that cut DNA at precise locations. Restriction maps depict the positions on chromosomes of restriction enzyme cutting sites. These are used as biochemical "signposts," or markers of specific areas along the chromosomes. The map will detail the positions on the DNA molecule that are cut by particular restriction enzymes.

**macrorestriction map** Map depicting the order of and distance between sites at which restriction enzymes cleave chromosomes.

**mapping** *See* gene mapping, linkage map, physical map.

**marker** Identifiable physical location on a chromosome (e.g., restriction enzyme cutting site, gene) whose inheritance can be monitored. Markers can be expressed regions of DNA (genes) or some segment of DNA with no known coding function but whose pattern of inheritance can be determined. *See also* restriction fragment length polymorphism.

**megabase (Mb)** Unit of length for DNA fragments equal to 1 million nucleotides and about equal to 1 cM.

**meiosis** Process of two consecutive cell divisions in the diploid progenitors of sex cells. Meiosis results in four rather than two daughter cells, each with a haploid set of chromosomes.

**messenger RNA (mRNA)** RNA that serves as a template for protein synthesis. *See also* genetic code.

**metaphase** Stage in mitosis or meiosis during which the chromosomes are aligned along the equatorial plane of the cell.

**mitosis** Process of nuclear division in cells that produces daughter cells that are genetically identical to each other and to the parent cell.

**mRNA** *See* messenger RNA.

**multifactorial or multigenic disorder** *See* polygenic disorder.

**multiplexing** Sequencing approach that uses several pooled samples simultaneously, greatly increasing sequencing speed.

**mutation** Any heritable change in DNA sequence. *See also* polymorphism.

**nitrogenous base** Nitrogen-containing molecule having the chemical properties of a base.

**nucleic acid** Large molecule composed of nucleotide subunits.

**nucleotide** Subunit of DNA or RNA consisting of a nitrogenous base (adenine, guanine, thymine, or cytosine in DNA; adenine, guanine, uracil, or cytosine in RNA), a phosphate molecule, and a sugar molecule (deoxyribose in DNA, ribose in RNA). Thousands of nucleotides are linked to form a DNA or RNA molecule. *See also* base pair, DNA, RNA.

**nucleus** Cellular organelle in eukaryotes that contains the genetic material.

**oncogene** Gene with one or more forms associated with cancer. Many oncogenes are directly or indirectly involved in controlling the rate of cell growth.

**overlapping clones** *See* genomic library.

**P1-derived artificial chromosome (PAC)** Vector used to clone DNA fragments (100- to 300-kb insert size, average, 150 kb) in *Escherichia coli* cells. Based on bacteriophage (a virus) P1 genome. *See also* cloning vector.

**PAC** *See* P1-derived artificial chromosome.

**PCR** *See* polymerase chain reaction.

**phage** Virus for which the natural host is a bacterial cell.

**physical map** Map of the locations of identifiable landmarks on DNA (e.g., restriction enzyme cutting sites, genes), regardless of inheritance. Distance is measured in base pairs. For the human genome, the lowest resolution physical map is the banding patterns on the 24 different chromosomes; the highest resolution map would be the complete nucleotide sequence of the chromosomes.

**plasmid** Autonomously replicating, extrachromosomal circular DNA molecules, distinct from the normal bacterial genome and nonessential for cell survival under nonselective conditions. Some plasmids are capable of integrating into the host genome. A number of artificially constructed plasmids are used as cloning vectors.

**polygenic disorder** Genetic disorder resulting from the combined action of alleles of more than one gene (e.g., heart disease, diabetes, some cancers). Although such disorders are inherited, they depend on the simultaneous presence of several alleles; thus the hereditary patterns are usually more complex than those of single-gene disorders. *See also* single-gene disorders.

**polymerase (DNA or RNA)** Enzyme that catalyzes the synthesis of nucleic acids on pre-existing nucleic acid templates, assembling RNA from ribonucleotides or DNA from deoxyribonucleotides.

**polymerase chain reaction (PCR)** Method for amplifying a DNA base sequence using a heat-stable polymerase and two 20-base primers, one complementary to the (+) strand at one end of the sequence to be amplified and the other complementary to the (−) strand at the other end. Because the newly synthesized DNA strands can subsequently serve as additional templates for the same primer sequences, successive rounds of primer annealing, strand elongation, and dissociation produce rapid and highly specific amplification of the desired sequence. PCR also can be used to detect the existence of the defined sequence in a DNA sample.

**polymorphism** Difference in DNA sequence among individuals. Genetic variations occurring in more than 1% of a population would be considered useful polymorphisms for genetic linkage analysis. *See also* mutation.

**positional cloning** Technique used to identify genes, usually those associated with diseases, based on their location on a chromosome. This is in contrast to the older, "functional cloning" technique that relies on some knowledge of a gene's protein product. For most diseases, researchers have no such knowledge.

**primer** Short, preexisting polynucleotide chain to which new deoxyribonucleotides can be added by DNA polymerase.

**probe** Single-stranded DNA or RNA molecules of specific base sequence, labeled radioactively or immunologically, that are used to detect the complementary base sequence by hybridization.

**prokaryote** Cell or organism lacking a membrane-bound, structurally discrete nucleus and other subcellular compartments. Bacteria are prokaryotes. *See also* chromosome, eukaryote.

**promoter** Site on DNA to which RNA polymerase will bind and initiate transcription.

**protein** Large molecule composed of one or more chains of amino acids in a specific order; the order is determined by the base sequence of nucleotides in the gene coding for the protein. Proteins are required for the structure, function, and regulation of cells, tissues, and organs, and each protein has unique functions. Examples are hormones, enzymes, and antibodies.

**purine** Nitrogen-containing, double-ring, basic compound that occurs in nucleic acids. The purines in DNA and RNA are adenine and guanine.

**pyrimidine** Nitrogen-containing, single-ring, basic compound that occurs in nucleic acids. The pyrimidines in DNA are cytosine and thymine; in RNA, cytosine and uracil.

**random method** *See* shotgun method.

**rarecutter enzyme** *See* restriction enzyme cutting site.

**recombinant clone** Clone containing recombinant DNA molecules.

**recombinant DNA molecules** Combination of DNA molecules of different origin that are joined using recombinant DNA technologies.

**recombinant DNA technology** Procedure used to join DNA segments in a cell-free system (an environment outside a cell or organism). Under appropriate conditions, a recombinant DNA molecule can enter a cell and replicate there, either autonomously or after it has become integrated into a cellular chromosome.

**recombination** Process by which progeny derive a combination of genes different from that of either parent. In higher organisms, this can occur by crossing-over.

**regulatory region, regulatory sequence** DNA base sequence that controls gene expression.

**resolution** Degree of molecular detail on a physical map of DNA, ranging from low to high.

**restriction enzyme (endonuclease)** Protein that recognizes specific, short nucleotide sequences and cuts DNA at those sites. Bacteria contain more than 400 such enzymes that recognize and cut more than 100 different DNA sequences.

**restriction enzyme cutting site** Specific nucleotide sequence of DNA at which a particular restriction enzyme cuts the DNA. Some sites occur frequently in DNA (e.g., every several hundred base pairs), others much less frequently (rarecutter; e.g., every 10,000 base pairs).

**restriction fragment length polymorphism (RFLP)** Variation between individuals in DNA fragment sizes cut by specific restriction enzymes; polymorphic sequences that result in RFLPs are used as markers on both physical maps and genetic linkage maps. RFLPs are usually caused by mutation at a cutting site. *See also* marker.

**ribonucleic acid (RNA)** Chemical found in the nucleus and cytoplasm of cells; it is important in protein synthesis and other chemical activities of the cell. The structure of RNA is similar to that of DNA. There are several classes of RNA molecules, including messenger RNA, transfer RNA, ribosomal RNA, and other small RNAs, each serving a different purpose.

**ribonucleotide** *See* nucleotide.

**ribosomal RNA (rRNA)** Class of RNA found in the ribosomes of cells.

**ribosomes** Small cellular components of specialized ribosomal RNA and protein; site of protein synthesis. *See also* ribonucleic acid (RNA).

**RNA** *See* ribonucleic acid.

**sequence** *See* base sequence.

**sequence tagged site (STS)** Short (200- to 500-bp) DNA sequence that has a single occurrence in the human genome and a known location and base sequence. Detectable by polymerase chain reaction, STSs are useful for localizing and orienting the mapping and sequence data reported from many different laboratories and serve as landmarks on the developing physical map of the human genome. *Expressed sequence tags* (ESTs) are STSs derived from cDNAs.

**sequencing** Determination of the order of nucleotides (base sequences) in a DNA or RNA molecule or the order of amino acids in a protein.

**sex chromosome** X or Y chromosome in humans that determines the sex of an individual. Females have two X chromosomes in diploid cells; males have an X and a Y chromosome. The sex chromosomes are the twenty-third chromosome pair in a karyotype. *See also* autosome.

**shotgun method** Sequencing method that involves randomly sequencing tiny cloned pieces of the genome, with no knowledge of the piece's original location on a chromosome. This can be contrasted with *directed* strategies, in which pieces of DNA from adjacent stretches of a chromosome are sequenced. Directed strategies eliminate the need for complex reassembly techniques. Because there are advantages to both strategies, researchers use both random (or shotgun) and directed strategies in combination to sequence the human genome. *See also* genomic library, library.

**single-gene disorder** Hereditary disorder caused by a mutant allele of a single gene (e.g., Duchenne muscular dystrophy, retinoblastoma, sickle cell disease). *See also* polygenic disorders.

**somatic cell** Any cell in the body, except gametes and their precursors.

**Southern blotting** Transfer by absorption of DNA fragments separated in electrophoretic gels to membrane filters for detection of specific base sequences by radiolabeled complementary probes.

**STS** *See* sequence tagged site.

**tandom repeat sequences** Multiple copies of the same base sequence on a chromosome; used as a marker in physical mapping.

**technology transfer** Process of converting scientific findings from research laboratories into useful products by the commercial sector.

**telomere** Each end (extremity) of a chromosome. This specialized structure is involved in the replication and stability of linear DNA molecules. *See also* DNA replication.

**thymine (T)** Nitrogenous base, one member of the base pair AT (adenine and thymine).

**transcription** Synthesis of an RNA copy from a sequence of DNA (a gene); the first step in gene expression. *See also* translation.

**transfer RNA (tRNA)** Class of RNA having structures with triplet nucleotide sequences that are complementary to the triplet nucleotide coding sequences of mRNA. The role of tRNAs in protein synthesis is to bond with amino acids and transfer them to the ribosomes, where proteins are assembled according to the genetic code carried by mRNA.

**transformation** Process by which the genetic material carried by an individual cell is altered by incorporation of exogenous DNA into its genome.

**Translation** Process in which the genetic code carried by mRNA directs the synthesis of proteins from amino acids. *See also* transcription.

**tRNA** *See* transfer RNA.

**uracil** Nitrogenous base normally found in RNA but not DNA; uracil is capable of forming a base pair with adenine.

**vector** *See* cloning vector.

**virus** Noncellular biological entity that can reproduce only within a host cell. Viruses consist of nucleic acid covered by protein; some animal viruses are also surrounded by membrane. Inside the infected cell, the virus uses the synthetic capability of the host to produce progeny virus.

**VLSI** Very-large-scale integration, allowing more than 100,000 transistors on a chip.

**yeast artificial chromosome (YAC)** Vector used to clone DNA fragments (up to 400 kb); it is constructed from the telomeric, centromeric, and origin sequences needed for replication in yeast cells. *See also* cloning vector.

# BIBLIOGRAPHY

## Guide to Articles

## 1. Human Genome Project: Goals, Methods, Achievements, and Critics

Abuelo D: Medical genetics: past, present and future, *Med Health RI* 82:152-154, 1999.

Annas G, Sherman E: The Human Genome Project: social policy research priorities, *Polit Life Sci* 11:254-259, 1992.

Cohen M: 1994 ASHG Presidential Address: Who are we? Where are we going? Anticipating the 21st century, *Am J Hum Genet* 56:1-10, 1995.

Collins FS: Taking stock of the genome project, *Science* 262:20-22, 1993.

Collins FS: Medical and ethical consequences of the Human Genome Project, *J Clin Ethics* 2:260-267 1994.

Collins FS: Shattuck lecture: medical and societal consequences of the Human Genome Project, *N Engl J Med* 341:28-37, 1999.

Dickman S: We're not just readouts of our genes: Harvard professor criticizes Human Genome Project, *Ann Oncol* 5:669-670, 1994.

Fetters MD, Doukas DJ, Phan KL: Family physicians perspectives on genetics and Human Genome Project, *Clin Genet* 56:28-34, 1999.

Fost N: Ethical issues in genetics, *Pediatr Clin North Am* 39:79-89, 1992.

Greenberg DS: Exit Dr. Watson, the genome chief, *Lancet* 339:980-981, 1992.

High-level ethics committee needed to guide genetics policy, *Nature* 385:756, 1997.

Jordan E: The Human Genome Project: where did it come from, where it is going? *Am J Hum Genet* 51:1-6, 1992.

Knoppers BM, Hirtle M, Lormeau S: Ethical issues in international collaborative research on the human genome: the HGP and HGDP, *Genomics* 34:272-282, 1996.

Lessick M, Williams J: The Human Genome Project: implications for nursing, *Medsurg Nurs* 3:49-58, 1994.

Lyttle J: Issues concerning ethical conduct and genetic mapping raised at Montreal meeting, *CMAJ* 156:411-412, 1997.

McCabe ER: The new biology enters the generalist pediatrician's office: lessons from the Human Genome Project, *Pediatr Rev* 20:314-319, 1999.

McCrary SV, Allen B, Moseley R, et al: Ethical and practical implications of the human genome initiative for family medicine, *Arch Fam Med* 2:1158-1163, 1993.

McKusick V: Mapping and sequencing the human genome, *N Engl J Med* 320:910-915, 1989.

Murray TH, Livny E: The Human Genome Project: ethical and social implications, *Bull Med Libr Assoc* 83:14-21, 1995.

New goals for the U.S. Human Genome Project: 1998-2003, *Science* 282:682-689, 1998.

Rice E: The Human Genome Project and gene therapy: a genetic counselor's perspective, *J Perinat Neonatal Nurs* 12:16-25, 1998.

Stephenson J: Ethics group drafts guidelines for control of genetic material and information, *JAMA* 184:279, 1998.

Watson JD: The Human Genome Project: past, present and future, *Science* 248:44-48, 1990.

World Health Organization, Human Genetics Programme: Proposed International Guidelines on Ethical Issues in Medical Genetics and Genetic Services. Part II, *Law Hum Genome Rev* 9:239-251, 1998.

## 2. Scientific and Clinical Issues

### 2.1 Methods of Testing and Screening
#### 2.1a Preimplantation Diagnosis

Eighth International Working Group on Preimplantation Genetics, Ninth International Conference on Prenatal Diagnosis and Therapy, *J Assist Reprod Genet* 16:161-220, 1999.

Findlay I, Matthews P, Quirke P: Preimplantation genetic diagnosis using fluorescent polymerase chain reaction: results and future developments, *J Assist Reprod Genet* 16:199-206, 1999.

Grifo JA, Tang YX, Krey L: Update in preimplantation genetic diagnosis, *Acad NY Acad Sci* 828:162-165, 1997.

Handyside AH, Scriven PN, Ogilvie CM: The future of preimplantation genetic diagnosis, *Hum Reprod* 4:249-255, 1998.

International working Group on Preimplantation Genetics: Preimplantation diagnosis: an alternative to prenatal diagnosis of genetic and chromosomal disorders, *J Assist Reprod Genet* 16:161-164, 1999.

Pergament E, Fiddler M: The expression of genes in human preimplantation embryos, *Prenat Diagn* 18:1366-1373, 1998.

Rechitsky S, Strom C, Verlinsky O, et al: Accuracy of preimplantation diagnosis of single-gene disorders by polar body analysis of oocytes, *J Assist Reprod Genet* 16:192-198, 1999.

Second International Symposium on Preimplantation Genetics, *J Assist Reprod Genet* 14:423-485, 1997.

Verlinsky O, Rechitsky S, Cieslak, et al: Preimplantation diagnosis of single disorders, *Tsitol Genet* 32:14-22, 1998.

Wells D, Sherlock JK: Strategies for preimplantation genetic diagnosis of single gene disorders by DNA amplification, *Prenat Diagn* 18:1389-401, 1998.

### 2.1b  Prenatal Diagnosis

Bahado-Singh R, Oz U, Kovanci E: A high-sensitivity alternative to "routine" genetic amniocentesis: multiple urinary analytes, nuchal thickness, and age, *Am J Obstet Gynecol* 180:169-173, 1999.

Bianchi DW: Fetal cells in the maternal circulation: feasibility for prenatal diagnosis, *Br J Haematol* 105:574-583, 1999.

Bowman JE: Prenatal screening for hemoglobinopathies, *Am J Hum Genet* 48:433-438, 1991.

Drugan A, Johnson MP, Evans MI: Ultrasound screening for fetal chromosome anomalies, *Am J Med Genet* 90:98-107, 2000.

Eng CM, Schechter C, Robinowitz: Prenatal genetic carrier testing using triple disease screening, *JAMA* 278:1268-1272, 1997.

Heckerling PS, Verp MS: A cost-effectiveness analysis of amniocentesis and chorionic villus sampling for prenatal genetic testing, *Med Care* 32:863-880, 1994.

Kuppermann M, Goldberg JD, Nease RF, et al: Who should be offered prenatal diagnosis? The 35-year-old question, *Am J Public Health* 89:160-163, 1999.

Lamvu G, Kuller JA: Prenatal diagnosis using fetal cells from the maternal circulation, *Obstet Gynecol Surv* 52:433-437, 1997.

Macmillian C: Genetics and developmental delay, *Semin Pediatr Neurol* 5:39-44, 1998.

Van den Veyver IB, Roa BB: Applied molecular genetic techniques for prenatal diagnosis, *Curr Opin Gynecol* 10:97-103, 1998.

Willner JP: Reproductive genetics and today's patient options: prenatal diagnosis, *Mt Sinai J Med* 65:173-177, 1998.

Yang EY, Cass DL, Sylvester KG, et al: Fetal gene therapy: efficacy, toxicity, and immunologic effects of early gestation recombinant adenovirus, *J Pediatr Surg* 34:235-241, 1999.

### 2.2  Gene Therapy
### 2.2a  Somatic

Alton EW, Geddes DM: Gene therapy for cystic fibrosis: a clinical perspective, *Gene Ther* 2:88-95, 1995.

Choate KA, Khavari PA: Direct cutaneous gene delivery in a human genetic skin disease, *Hum Gene Ther* 8:1659-1665, 1997.

Eming SA, Morgan JR, Berger A: Gene therapy for tissue repair: approaches and prospects, *Br J Plast Surg* 50:491-500, 1997.

Hou Z, Nguyen Q, Frenkel B, et al: Osteoblast-specific gene expression after transplantation of marrow cells: implications for skeletal gene therapy, *Proc Natl Acad Sci USA* 96:7294-7299, 1999.

Schofiels JP, Caskey CT: Non-viral approaches to gene therapy, *Br Med Bull* 51:56-71, 1995.

Senut MC, Gage FH: Prenatal gene therapy: can the technical hurdles be overcome? *Mol Med Today* 5:152-156, 1999.

US Food and Drug Administration, Center for Biologics Evaluation and Research: Guidance for human somatic cell therapy and gene therapy, *Hum Gene Ther* 9:1513-1524, 1998.

VA Palo Alto Health Care System, Stanford University School of Medicine: High-efficiency gene transfer and pharmacologic selection of genetically engineered human keratinocytes, *Biotechniques* 25:274-280, 1998.

Ye X, Rivera VM, Zoltick P: Regulated delivery of therapeutic proteins after in vivo somatic cell gene transfer, *Science* 283:88-91, 1999.

### 2.2b Germline
Gordon JW: Micromanipulation of embryos and germ cells: an approach to gene therapy? *Am J Med Genet* 35:206-214, 1990.

## 3. Ethical, Legal, and Social Implications

### 3.1 Law and Policy
Annas G: The Human Genome Project as social policy: implications for clinical medicine, *Bull NY Acad Med* 68:126-134, 1992.

Annas G: Privacy Rules for DNA databanks, *JAMA* 270:2346-2350, 1993.

Bossart J, Pearson B: Commercialization of gene therapy—the evolution of licensing and rights issues, *Trends Biotechnol* 13:290-294, 1995.

Clayton EW: The dispersion of genetic testing: regulatory and liability issues, *Hastings Cent Rep* 25:568-597, 1995.

Cohen-Haguenauer O: Overview of regulation of gene therapy in Europe: a current statement including reference to US regulation, *Hum Gene Ther* 6:773-785, 1995.

Juengst ET: Human genome research and the public interest: progress notes from an American science policy experiment, *Am J Hum Genet* 54:121-128, 1994.

Wilfond BS, Nolan K: National policy development from the clinical application of genetic diagnostic technologies: lessons from cystic fibrosis, *JAMA* 270:2948-2954, 1993.

### 3.2 Laboratory Regulations and Standards
McGovern MM, Benach MO: Quality assurance in molecular genetic testing laboratories, *JAMA* 281:835-840, 1999.

Milunsky A: Commercialization of clinical genetic laboratory services: in whose best interest? *Obstet Gynecol* 81:627-629, 1993.

Schwartz MK: Genetic testing and the clinical laboratory improvement amendments of 1988: present and future, *Clin Chem* 45:739-745, 1999.

### 3.3 Access to Treatment and Economics
Lebacqz K: Fair shares: Is the genome project just? *CTNS Bull Center Theol Nat Sci* 13:1-16, 1993.

Vaillancourt-Rosenau P: Reflections on the cost consequences of the new gene technology for health policy, *Int J Technol Assess Health Care* 10:546-561, 1994.

### 3.4 Discrimination
#### 3.4a Employment
Andrews LB, Jaeger AS: Confidentiality of genetic information in the workplace, *Am J Law Med* 17:75-108, 1991.

Colby JA: An analysis of genetic discrimination legislation proposed by the 105th Congress, *Am J Law Med* 24:443-480, 1998.

Faden RR, Kass NE: Genetic screening technology: ethical issues in access to tests by employers and health insurance companies, *J Soc Sci* 49:75-88, 1993.

Hendriks A: Genetics, human rights and employment: American and European perspectives, *Med Law* 16:557-565, 1997.

Jacobs LA: At-risk for cancer: genetic discrimination in the workplace, *Oncol Nurs Forum* 25:475-480, 1998.

Lapham EV, Kozma C, Weiss JO: Genetic discrimination: perspectives of consumers, *Science* 274:621-624, 1996.

Lehrman S: Job discrimination based on genetics for California ban, *Nature* 393:611, 1998.

Wadman M: Law urged to check genetic discrimination, *Nature* 386:312, 1997.

#### 3.4b Insurance
Geller G, Bernhart BA, Doksum T, et al. Decision-making about breast cancer susceptibility testing: how similar are the attitudes of physicians, nurse practitioners, and at-risk women? *J Clin Oncol* 16:2868-2876, 1998.

Jecker NS: Genetic testing and the social responsibility of private health insurance companies, *J Law Med Ethics* 21:109-116, 1993.

Kapp MB: Medicolegal, employment and insurance issues in APOE genotyping and Alzheimer's disease, *Ann NY Acad Sci* 802:139-148, 1996.

McEwen JE, McCathy K, Reilly R: A survey of life insurance companies concerning use of genetic information, *Am J Hum Genet* 53:33-45, 1993.

Moseley R, Crandall L, Dewar M, et al: Ethical implications of a complete human gene map for insurance, *Business Professional Ethics J* 10:69-82, 1991.

Murray TH: Genetics and the moral mission of health insurance, *Hastings Cent Rep* 22:2-17, 1992.

O'Neil O: Genetic information and insurance: some ethical issues, *Philos Trans R Soc Lond Biol Sci* 352:1087-1093, 1997.

Ostrer H, Allen W, Candall LA, et al: Insurance and genetic testing: where are we now? *Am J Hum Genet* 52:565-577, 1993.

Rothstein MA: Genetics, insurance, and the ethics of genetic counseling, *Mol Genet Med* 3:159-177, 1993.

Sandburg P: Genetic information and life insurance: proposal for an ethical European policy, *Soc Sci Med* 40:1549-1559, 1995.

Slaughter LM: Genetic information must remain private to prevent discrimination, *Genet Test* 2:17-35, 1998.

Wadman M: Bill tightens law against genetic discrimination by health insurers, *Nature* 394:306, 1998.

Wellcome Trust, London: Genetics and insurance in Britain: why more than just the Atlantic divides the English-speaking nations, *Nat Genet* 20:119-121, 1998.

Wingrove KJ, Norris J, Barton PL, et al: Experiences and attitudes concerning genetic testing and insurance in a Colorado population: a survey of families diagnosed with fragile X syndrome, *Am J Med Genet* 64:378-381, 1996.

### 3.5 Genetic Testing and Screening
#### 3.5a Individual

Allan D: Ethical boundaries in genetic testing, *CMAJ* 154:241-244, 1996.

Biesecker LG, Collins FS, DeRenzo EG, et al: Case: responding to a request for genetic testing that is still in the lab, *Camb Q Healthc Ethics* 4:387-400, 1995.

Bove CM, Fry ST, MacDonald DJ: Presymptomatic and predisposition genetic testing: ethical and social considerations, *Semin Oncol Nurs* 13:135-140, 1997.

Brown ML, Kessler LG: The use of gene tests to detect hereditary predisposition to cancer: economic considerations, *J Natl Cancer Inst* 87:1131-1136, 1995.

Burnside JW: Ethical quandries in genetic testing, *Tex Med* 93:46-49, 1997.

Evans DG: Genetic testing for cancer predisposition: need and demand, *J Med Genet* 32:161, 1995.

Fitzpatrick JL, Hahn C, Costa T, et al: The duty to recontact: attitudes of genetics service providers, *Am J Hum Genet* 64:852-860, 1999.

Fost N: Ethical implications of screening asymptomatic individuals, *FASEB J* 6:2813-2817, 1992.

Grady C: Ethics and genetic testing, *Adv Intern Med* 44:389-411, 1999.

Holtzman NA: Medical and ethical issues in genetic screening—an academic view, *Environ Health Perpect* 104(suppl 5):987-990, 1996.

Jones SL, Krysa LW: Comfort care interventions in a preimplantation genetic testing program, *Holist Nurs Pract* 12:20-29, 1998.

Kadlec JV, McPherson RA: Ethical issues in screening and testing for genetic diseases, *Clin Lab Med* 15:989-999, 1995.

Kapp MB: Ethical and legal implications of advances in genetic testing technology, *Leg Med* 305, 1994.

Kelley WN: The impact of gene therapy on medicine and society, *Ann NY Acad Sci* 716:18-22, 1994.

Kimyai-Asadi A, Terry PB: Ethical considerations in pulmonary genetic testing and gene therapy, *Am J Respir Crit Care Med* 155:3-8, 1997.

Leonard DG: The future of molecular genetic testing, *Clin Chem* 54:726-731, 1999.

Marshall E: Gene therapy's growing pains, *Science* 268:1050-1055, 1995.

Wilke J: From a survivor: the emotional experience of genetic testing, *J Psychosoc Nurs Ment Health Serv* 33:28-37, 1995.

Williams JK: Genetic testing: implications for professional nursing, *J Prof Nurs* 14:184-188, 1998.

Whittaker L: Clinical applications of genetic testing: implications for the family physician, *Am Fam Physician* 53:2077-2084, 1996.

Young DS, Leonard DG: Issues in genetic testing, *Clin Chem* 45:915-926, 1999.

#### 3.5b Population

Baird PA: Identifying people's genes: ethical aspects of DNA sampling in populations, *Perspect Biol Med* 38:159-166, 1995.

Clarke A: Population screening for genetic susceptibility to disease, *BMJ* 311:35-38, 1995.

Jorde LB, Watkins WS, Kere J, et al: Gene mapping in isolated populations: new roles for old friends? *Hum Hered* 50:57-65, 2000.

Penticuff JH: Ethical dimensions in genetic screening: a look into the future, *J Obstet Gynecol Neonatal Nurs* 25:785-789, 1996.

University of Central Lancashire, Preston, UK: Genetic screening and ethics: European perspectives, *J Med Philos* 23:255-273, 1998.

### 3.5c Preimplantation Diagnosis

Draper H, Chadwick R: Beware! Preimplantation genetic diagnosis may solve some old problems but it also raises new ones, *J Med Ethics* 25:114-120, 1999.

Eisenberg VH, Schenker JG: Preembryo research: medical aspects and ethical considerations, *Obstet Gynecol Surv* 52:565-574, 1997.

Grifo JA, Tang YX, Krey L: Update in preimplantation genetic diagnosis: age, genetics and infertility, *Ann NY Acad Sci* 828:162-165, 1997.

Hadassah University Medical Center, Dept of OB/GYN, Jerusalem: Preimplantation genetic diagnosis: principles and ethics, *Hum Reprod* 13:2238-2245, 1998.

King DS: Preimplantation genetic diagnosis and the 'new' eugenics, *J Med Ethics* 25:176-182, 1999.

Persson I: Equality and selection for existence, *J Med Ethics* 25:130-136, 1999.

Raeburn JA: Commentary: preimplantation diagnosis raises a philosophical dilemma, *BMJ* 311:540, 1995.

Schulman JD, Edwards RG: Preimplantation diagnosis in disease control, not eugenics, *Hum Reprod* 11:463-464, 1996.

Verlinsky O, Rechitsky S, Cieslak J, et al: Preimplantation diagnosis of single disorders, *Tsitol Genet* 32:14-22, 1998.

### 3.5d Prenatal Diagnosis

American Academy of Pediatrics: Prenatal genetic diagnosis for pediatricians, *Pediatrics* 93:1010-1014, 1994.

Kaplan D: Prenatal screening and its impact on persons with disabilities, *Clin Obstet Gynecol* 36:605-612, 1993.

Kielstein R, Sass H: Right not to know or duty to know? **Prenatal** screening for polycystic renal disease, *J Med Philos* 17:395-405, 1992.

### 3.5e Newborn Screening

Bowman JE: Legal and ethical issues in newborn screening, *Pediatrics* 83:894-896, 1989.

Hiller EH, Landenburger G, Natowicz MR: Public participation in medical policy-making and the status of consumer autonomy: the example of newborn-screening programs in the United States, *Am J Public Health* 87:1280-1288, 1997.

Holtzman NA: What drives neonatal screening programs? *N Engl J Med* 325:802-804, 1991.

Mitchell JA, Petroski G: Evaluation of a statewide program in genetic diseases, *Am J Med Genet* 78:217-225, 1998.

Neonatal Intensive Care Unit, Winchester Medical Center, Winchester, VA: Expanding the newborn screen: terrific or troubling? *Am J Matern Child Nurs* 23:266-271, 1998.

Penticuff JH: Ethical dimensions in genetic screening: a look into the future, *J Obstet Gynecol Neonatal Nurs* 25:785-789, 1996.

Stoddard JJ, Farrell PM: State to state variations in newborn screening policies, *Arch Pediatr Adolesc Med* 151:561-564, 1997.

University of Central Lancashire, Preston, UK: Genetic screening and ethics: European perspectives, *J Med Philos* 23:255-273, 1998.

### 3.5f Pediatric Testing

Clayton EW: Removing the shadows of the law from the debate about genetic testing of children, *Am J Med Genet* 57:630-634, 1995.

Clayton EW: Genetic testing in children, *J Med Philos* 22:233-251, 1997.

Elger BS, Harding TW: Testing adolescents for a hereditary breast cancer gene (BRCA1): respecting their autonomy is in their best interest, *Arch Pediatr Adolesc Med* 154:113-119, 2000.

Fryer A: Genetic testing of children, *Arch Dis Child* 73:97-99, 1995.

Kodish ED: Testing children for cancer genes: the rule of earliest onset, *J Pediatr* 135:390-395, 1999.

Lessick M, Faux S: Implications of genetic testing of children and adolescents, *Holist Nurs Pract* 12:38-46, 1998.

Malkin D, Friend SH: Screening for cancer susceptibility in children, *Curr Opin Pediatr* 6:46-51, 1994.

Williams JK, Lessick M: Genome research: implications for children, *Pediatr Nurs* 22:40-46, 1996.

### 3.6 Gene Therapy
#### 3.6a Somatic

Fletcher JC, Richter G: Human fetal gene therapy: moral and ethical questions, *Hum Gene Ther* 7:1605-1614, 1996.

Kimyai-Asadi A, Terry PB: Ethical considerations in pulmonary genetic testing and gene therapy, *Am J Respir Crit Care Med* 155:3-8, 1997.

Lindemann A, Rosenthal FM, Hase S, et al: Guidelines for the design and implementation of clinical studies in somatic cell therapy and gene therapy, the German working group for gene therapy, *J Mol Med* 73:207-211, 1995.

McDonough PG: The ethics of somatic and germline gene therapy, *Ann NY Acad Sci* 816: 378-382, 1997.

Parens E: The goodness of fragility: on the prospect of human capacities, *Kennedy Inst Ethics J* 5:141-153, 1995.

#### 3.6b Germline

Berger EM, Gert BM: Genetic disorders and the ethical status of germ-line therapy, *J Med Philos* 16:667-683, 1991.

Billings PR, Hubbard R, Newman SA: Human germline gene modification: a dissent, *Lancet* 353:1873-1875, 1999.

Gordon JW: Genetic enhancement in humans, *Science* 283:2023-2024, 1999.

Gordon JW: Germline alteration by gene therapy: assessing and reducing the risks, *Mol Med Today* 4:468-470, 1999.

Jeungst E: Germ-line gene therapy: back to basics, *J Med Philos* 16:587-592, 1991.

Juengst ET: "Prevention" and goals of genetic medicine, *Hum Gene Ther* 6:1595-1605, 1995.

McCullough LB: The management of instability and incompleteness: clinical ethics and abstract expressionism, *J Med Philos* 22:1-10, 1997.

Peters T: Playing god and germline intervention, *J Med Philos* 20:365-386, 1995.

Philipps University, Marburg, Germany: Interventions in the human genome: some moral and ethical considerations, *J Med Philos* 23:303-317, 1998.

Wilson JM, Wivel NA: Potential risk of inadvertent germ-line gene transmission: statement from the American Society of Gene Therapy to the NIH Recombinant DNA Advisory Committee, March 12, 1999, *Hum Gene Ther* 10:1593-1595, 1999.

### 3.7 Privacy, Confidentiality, and Disclosure

Annas GJ: Genetic prophecy and genetic privacy—can we prevent the dream from becoming a nightmare? *Am J Public Health* 85:1196-1197, 1995.

Ault A: Drug industry hopes to moderate genetic privacy laws, *Nat Med* 4:6, 1998.

Berry RM: The genetic revolution and the physician's duty of confidentiality: the role of the old Hippocratic virtues in the regulation of the new genetic intimacy, *J Leg Med* 18:401-441, 1997.

Botkin JR, McMahon WM, Smith KR, et al: Privacy and confidentiality in the publication of pedigrees: a survey of investigators and biomedical journals, *JAMA* 279:1801-1812, 1998.

Chadwick R: The Icelandic database—do modern times need modern sagas? *BMJ* 319:441-444, 1999.

Deftos LJ: The evolving duty to disclose the presence of genetic disease to relatives, *Acad Med* 73:962-968, 1998.

Early CL, Strong LC: Certificates of confidentiality: a valuable tool for protecting genetic data, *Am J Hum Genet* 57:727-731, 1995.

Fuller BP, Kahn MJ, Barr PA, et al: Privacy in genetics research, *Science* 285:1359-1361, 1999.

Lebacqz K: Genetic privacy: no deal for the poor, *Dialog* 33:39-48, 1994.

McAbee GN, Sherman J, Davidoff-Feldman B: Physician's duty to warn third parties about the risk of genetic diseases, *Pediatrics* 102:140-142, 1998.

Motulsky AG: If I had a gene test, what would I have and who would I tell? *Lancet* 354:35-37, 1999.

Olick RS: Disclosing genetic information to family members: do old paradigms fit the new medicine? *NJ Med* 97:43-46, 2000.

Palca J: Keeping genetic information under wraps, *Hastings Cent Rep* 27:6, 1997.

Reilly PR, Boshar MF, Holtzman SH: Ethical issues in genetic research: disclosure and informed consent, *Nat Genet* 15:16-20, 1997.

Stephenson J: Ethics group drafts guidelines for control of genetic material and information, *JAMA* 279:184, 1998.

**3.8 Informed Consent**

Clayton EW, Steinberg KK, Khoury MJ: Informed consent for genetic research on stored tissue samples, *JAMA* 274:1786-1792, 1995.

Council on Ethical and Judicial Affairs, American Medical Association: Multiplex genetic testing, *Hastings Cent Rep* 28:15-21, 1998.

Enserink M: Iceland Oks private health databank, *Science* 283:13, 1999.

Geller G: Commentary: weighing burdens and benefits rather than competence, *BMJ* 318: 1065-1066, 1939.

Lyttle J: Is informed consent possible in the rapidly evolving world of DNA sampling? *CMAJ* 156:257-258, 1997.

Rieger PT, Pentz RD: Genetic testing and informed consent, *Semin Oncol Nurs* 15:104-115, 1999.

**3.8a Adults**

Annas GJ, Elias S: Confusing law and ethics: why the committee's report on informed consent should be reconsidered, *Womens Health Issues* 3:25-26, 1993.

Elias S, Annas GJ: Generic consent for genetic screening, *N Engl J Med* 330:1611-1613, 1994.

Goldworth A: Informed consent in the human genome enterprise. Special section. Designs of life: choice, control, and responsibility in genetic manipulation, *Camb Q Healthc Ethics* 4:296-303, 1995.

**3.8b Children and Adolescents**

Dickerson, DL: Can children and young people consent to be tested for adult onset genetic disorders? *BMJ* 318:1063-1065, 1999.

Lessick M, Faux S: Implications of genetic testing of children and adolescents, *Holist Nurs Pract* 12:38-46, 1998.

Weir RF, Horton JR: Genetic research, adolescents, and informed consent, *Theor Med* 16:347-373, 1995.

## 4. Genetic Education

American Society of Clinical Oncology: Resource document for curriculum development in cancer genetics education, *J Clin Oncol* 15:2157, 1997.

Banke MG, Gettig EA, Rittmeyer LJ, et al: What is a gene? *Pa Med* 100:24-25, 1997.

Collins FS, Bochm K: Avoiding casualties in the genetic revolution: the urgent need to educate physicians about genetics, *Acad Med* 74:48-49, 1999.

Hetteberg CG, Prows CA, Deets C, et al: National survey of genetics content in basic nursing preparatory programs in the United States, *Nurs Outlook* 47:168-180, 1999.

Holtzman NA: Primary care physicians as providers of frontline genetic services, *Fetal Diagn Ther* 18(suppl):213-219, 1993.

Jenkins J: Educational issues related to cancer genetics, *Semin Oncol Nurs* 13:141-144, 1997.

Johnson SM, Kurtz ME, et al: Teaching the process of obtaining informed consent to medical students, *Acad Med* 67:598-600, 1992.

Kolb SE, Aguilar MC, Dinenberg M, et al: Genetics education for primary care providers in community health settings, *J Community Health* 24:45-59, 1999.

Leavitt FJ: Educating nurses for their role in bioethics, *Nurs Ethics* 3:39-52, 1996.

McElhinney T, Lajkowicz C: The new genetics & nursing education, *Nurs Health Care* 15:10, 1994.

Monsen RB: Nursing takes leading role in genetics education: coalition formed to increase provider awareness on genetics technologies, *Am J Nurs* 28:11, 1996.

Olopade OI, Offit K, Garber JE: Genetic testing for susceptibility to cancer, Task Force on Cancer Genetics Education, *JAMA* 279:1612-1613, 1998.

Parker LS: Bioethics for human geneticists: models for reasoning and methods for teaching, *Am J Hum Genet* 54:137-147, 1991.

## 5. Public Health and Epidemiology

Bogardus ST Jr, Concato J, Feinstein AR: Clinical epidemiological quality in molecular genetic research: the need for methodological standards, *JAMA* 281:1919-1926, 1999.

Bondy M, Mastromarino C: Ethical issues of genetic testing and their implications in epidemiologic studies, *Ann Epidemiol* 7:363-366, 1997.

Clayton EW: What should be the role of public health in newborn screening and prenatal diagnosis? *Am J Prev Med* 16:111-115, 1999.

Coughlin SS: The intersection of genetics, public health, and preventative medicine, *Am J Prev Med* 16:89-90, 1999.

Ellsworth DL, Manolio TA: The emerging importance of genetics in epidemiologic research. I. Basic concepts in human genetics and laboratory technology, *Ann Epidemiol* 9:1-16, 1999.

Holtzman NA, Andrews LB: Ethical and legal issues in genetic epidemiology, *Epidemiol Rev* 19:163-174, 1997.

Khoury MJ: From genes to public health: the applications of genetic technology in disease prevention, *Am J Public Health* 86:1717-1722, 1996.

Kirby RS: Analytical resources for assessment of clinical genetics services in public health: current status and future prospects, *Teratology* 61:9-16, 2000.

Tang D, Warburton D, Tannenbaum SR, et al: Molecular and genetic damage from environmental tobacco smoke in young children, *Cancer Epidemiol Biomarkers Prev* 8:427-431, 1999.

## 6. Managed Care

Amonkar MM, Madhaven S, Rosenbluth SA, et al: Barriers and facilitators to providing common preventive screening services in managed care settings, *J Community Health* 24:229-247, 1999.

Gates EA: Reproductive health under managed care: expanding provider obligations, *Semin Perinatol* 22:233-240, 1998.

Mark HF, Prence E, Beauregard L, Greenstein R: The impact of managed care on genetic testing laboratories in the United States, *Cytobios* 88:43-52, 1996.

McCullough LB: Molecular medicine, managed care, and the moral responsibilities of patients and physicians, *J Med Philos* 23:3-9, 1998.

Ross JS: Molecular pathology and managed care: challenges and opportunities, *Diagn Mol Pathol* 7:189-191, 1998.

## 7. Genetic Counseling

Ad Hoc Committee on Genetic Counseling: Genetic counseling, *Am J Med Genet* 27:240-242, 1975.

Anderson G: Nondirectiveness in prenatal genetics: patients read between the lines, *Nurs Ethics* 6:126-136, 1999.

Bartels DM, LeRoy BS, McCarthy P, et al: Nondirectiveness in genetic counseling: a survey of practitioners, *Am J Med Genet* 72:172-179, 1997.

Berkenstadt M, Shiloh S, Barkai G, et al: Perceived personal control (PPC): a new concept in measuring outcome of genetic counseling, *Am J Med Genet* 82:53-59, 1999.

Botkin JR: Genetic counseling: making room for beneficence, *J Clin Ethics* 6:182-184, 1995.

Bowles, Biesecker B, Marteau TM: The future of genetic counseling: an international perspective, *Nat Genet* 22:133-137, 1999.

Cohn GM, Miller RC, Gould M, et al: Impact of genetic counseling on primary and preventative care in obstetrics and gynecology, *J Reprod Med* 44:7-10, 1999.

Kuska B: Group seeks approach to genetic counseling, *J Natl Cancer Inst* 87:485-486, 1995.

Lawler AM, Gearhart JD: Genetic counseling for patients who will be undergoing treatment with assisted reproductive technology, *Fertil Steril* 70:412-413, 1998.

Loescher LJ: The family history component of cancer genetic risk counseling, *Cancer Nurs* 22:96-102, 1999.

Mahowald MB, Verp MS, Anderson RR: Genetic counseling: clinical and ethical challenges, *Annu Rev Genet* 32:547-559, 1998.

Mehlman MJ, Kodish ED, Whitehouse P, et al: The need for anonymous genetic counseling and testing, *Am J Hum Genet* 58:393-397, 1996.

Milunsky JM, Milunsky A: Genetic counseling in perinatal medicine, *Obstet Gynecol Clin North Am* 24:1-17, 1997.

Patients' understanding of medical risks: implications for genetic counseling, *Obstet Gynecol* 93:910-914, 1999.

Rice E: The Human Genome Project and gene therapy: a genetic counselor's perspective, *J Perinat Neonatal Nurs* 12:16-25, 1998.

Sharpe NF: Psychological aspects of genetic counseling, *Am J Med Genet* 50:234-238, 1994.

Steiner-Grossman P, David KL: Involvement of rabbis in counseling and referral for genetic conditions: results of a survey, *Am J Hum Genet* 53:1359-1365, 1993.

Walsh A: Presymptomatic testing for Huntington's disease: the role of genetic counseling, *Med Health RI* 82:168-170, 1999.

Zare N, Sorenson JR, Heeren T: Sex of provider as a variable in effective genetic counseling, *Soc Sci Med* 19:671-675, 1984.

## 8.   Reproductive Decisions

Beck MN: Eugenic abortion: an ethical critique, *CMAJ* 143:181-186, 1990.

Clayton EW: Reproductive genetic testing: regulatory and liability issues, *Fetal Diagn Ther* 8:39-59, 1993.

Denayer L, Evers-Kiebooms G, De Boeck K, et al: Reproductive decision making of aunts and uncles of a child with cystic fibrosis: genetic risk perception and attitudes toward carrier identification and prenatal diagnosis, *Am J Med Genet* 44:104-111, 1992.

## 9.   Psychological Consequences

Black RB: Prenatal diagnosis and fetal loss: psychological consequences and professional responsibilities, *Am J Med Genet* 35:586-587, 1990.

## 10.   Cultural and Ethnic Differences

Brett KM, Schoendorf KC, Kiely JL: Differences between black and white women in the use of prenatal care technologies, *Am J Obstet Gynecol* 170:41-46, 1994.

Browner CH, Preloran M, Press NA: The effects of ethnicity, education and an informational video on pregnant women's knowledge and decisions about a prenatal diagnostic screening test, *Patient Educ Couns* 27:135-146, 1996.

Cavalli-Sforza LL: The Chinese Human Genome Diversity Project, *Proc Natl Sci USA* 95:11501-11503, 1998.

Dodson M, Williamson R: Indigenous peoples and the morality of the Human Genome Diversity Project, *J Med Ethics* 25:204-208, 1999.

Dyson SM: "Race," ethnicity and haemoglobin disorders, *Soc Sci Med* 47:121-131, 1998.

Garte S: The role of ethnicity in cancer susceptibility gene polymorphisms: the example of CYP1A1, *Carcinogenesis* 19:1329-1332, 1998.

Hughes C, Gomez-Caminero A, Benkendorf J, et al: Ethnic differences in knowledge and attitudes about BRCA1 testing in women at increased risk, *Patient Educ Couns* 32:51-62, 1997.

Kudzma EC: Culturally competent drug administration, *Am J Nurs* 99:46-51, 1999.

Lehrman S: Coalition to pursue ethnic concerns over gene research, *Nature* 392:428, 1998.

Lerman C, Hughes C, Benkendorf JL, et al: Racial differences in testing motivation and psychological distress following pretest education for BRCA1 gene testing, *Cancer Epidemiol Biomarkers Prev* 8:361-367, 1999.

McPherson EC: Ethical implications of the Human Genome Diversity Project, *Nurs Connect* 8:36-43, 1995.

Shriver MW, Smith MW, et al: Ethnic-affiliation estimation by use of population-specific DNA markers, *Am J Hum Genet* 60:957-964, 1997.

Smith MW, Mendoza RP: Ethnicity and pharmacogenetics, *Mt Sinai J Med* 63:285-290, 1996.

Stewart JA, Dundas R, Howard RS, et al: Ethnic differences in incidence of stroke: prospective study with stroke register, *BMJ* 318:967-971, 1999.

University of California, Los Angeles, Dept of Psychiatry and Biobehavioral Sciences: Characteristics of women who refuse an offer of prenatal diagnosis: data from the California maternal serum alpha fetoprotein blood test experience, *Am J Med Genet* 78:433-445, 1998.

Wallace RW: The Human Genome Diversity Project: medical benefits versus ethical concerns, *Mol Med Today* 4:59-62, 1998.

## 11. Gender Differences

### 11.1 Providers

Wertz DC: Provider biases and choices: the role of gender, *Clin Obstet Gynecol* 36:521-531, 1993.

Wertz DC: Providers gender and moral reasoning: a proposed agenda for research on providers and patients, *Fetal Diagn Ther* 8(suppl 1):81-89, 1993.

Wertz DC: Is there a "woman's ethic" in genetics: a 37-nation survey of providers, *J Am Med Womens Assoc* 52:33-38, 1997.

Wertz DC, Fletcher JC: Moral reasoning among medical geneticists in eighteen nations, *Theor Med* 10:123-138, 1989.

### 11.2 Patients

Aro AR, Hakonen A, Hietala M, et al: Acceptance of genetic testing in a general population: age, education and gender differences, *Patient Educ Couns* 32:41-49, 1997.

Bird CE, Reiker PP: Gender matters: an integrated model for understanding men's and women's health, *Soc Sci Med* 48:745-755, 1999.

Cassel CK: Policy implications of the Human Genome Project for women, *Womens Health Issues* 7:225-229, 1997.

Kehoe P, Krawczak M, Harper PS, et al: Age of onset in Huntington disease: sex specific influence of apolipoprotein E genotype and normal CAG repeat length, *J Med Genet* 36:108-111, 1999.

Mahowald MB: A feminist standpoint for genetics, *J Clin Ethics* 7:333-340, 1996.

Mahowald MB: Gender justice in genetics, *Womens Health Issues* 7:230-233, 1997.

Mahowald MB: The Human Genome Project and women, *Womens Health Issues* 7:204-205, 1997.

Mahowald MB: An overview of the Human Genome Project and its implications for women, *Womens Health Issues* 7:206-208, 1997.

Mahowald MB, Levinson D, Cassel C: The new genetics and women, *Milbank Q* 74:239-283, 1996.

## 12. Eugenics

Barondess JA: Medicine against society: lessons from the Third Reich, *JAMA* 276:1657-1661, 1996.

Barondess JA: The old eugenics and the new science, *Trans Am Clin Climatol Assoc* 109:174-180, 1998.

Beardsley T: China syndrome: China's eugenics law makes trouble for science and business, *Sci Am* 276:33-34, 1997.

Coutts MC, McCarrick PM: Eugenics, *Kennedy Inst Ethics J* 5:163-178, 1995.

Galton DJ, Galton CJ: Francis Galton: Eugenics today, *J Med Ethics* 24:99-105, 1998.

Garver KL, Gaver B: The Human Genome Project and eugenic concerns, *Am J Hum Genet* 54:148-158, 1994.

Hanauske-Abel HM: Not a slippery slope or sudden subversion: German medicine and national socialism in 1933, *BMJ* 313:1453-1463, 1996.

Henn W: Genetic screening with the DNA chip: a new Pandora's box? *J Med Ethics* 25:200-203, 1999.

Holtzman NA, Rothstein MA: Eugenics and genetic discrimination, *Am J Hum Genet* 50:457-459, 1992.

Kevles DJ: Eugenics and human rights, *BMJ* 319:435-438, 1999.

Koenig R: Watson urges "put Hitler behind us," *Science* 276:892, 1997.

Ledley FD: Distinguishing genetics and eugenics on the basis of fairness, *J Med Ethics* 20:157-164.

McGee G: Parenting in an era of genetics, *Hastings Cent Rep* 27:16-22, 1997.

Sher G, Feinmann MA: The day-to-day realities: commentary on the new eugenics and medicalized reproduction, *Camb Q Healthc Ethics* 4:313-315, 1995.

Testart J: The new eugenics and medicalized reproduction, *Camb Q Healthc Ethics* 4:304-312, 1995.

University of Central Lancashire, Preston, UK: Genetic screening and ethics: European perspectives, *J Med Philos* 23:255-273, 1998.

Wikler D: Can we learn from eugenics? *J Med Ethics* 25:183-194, 1999.

## 13. Sex Selection

Fletcher JC: Is sex selection ethical? *Prog Clin Biol Res* 128:333-348, 1983.

Hossain AM, Barik S, Rizk B, et al: Preconceptional sex selection: past, present, and future, *Arch Adrol* 40:3-14, 1998.

Kalaca C, Akin A: The issue of sex selection in Turkey, *Hum Reprod* 10:1631-1632, 1995.

Laland K, Kumm J, Feldman MW: Medical ethics and human reproduction: scientists predict unbalanced future with sex selection, *BMJ* 308:536, 1994.

Mao X, Wertz DC: China's genetic services providers' attitudes towards several ethical issues: a cross-cultural survey, *Clin Genet* 52:100-109, 1997.

Schulman JD: Ethical issues in gender selection by X/Y sperm separation, *Hum Reprod* 8:1541, 1993.

Sills ES, Kirman I, Thatcher SS III, et al: Sex selection of human spermatozoa: evolution of current techniques and applications, *Arch Gynecol Obstet* 261:109-115, 1998.

Simpson JL, Carson SA: The reproductive option of sex selection, *Hum Reprod* 14:870-872, 1999.

## 14.   Behavior Genetics

Alper JS, Beckwith J: Genetic fatalism and social policy: the implications of behavior genetics research, *Yale J Biol Med* 66:511-524, 1993.

Bouchard TJ Jr, Hur YM: Genetic and environmental influences on the continuous scales of the Myers-Briggs Type Indicator: an analysis based on twins reared apart, *J Pers* 66:135-149, 1998.

Hewitt JK: Behavior genetics and eating disorders, *Psychopharmacol Bull* 33:355-358, 1997.

Johnson AM, Vernon PA, McCarthy JM, et al: Nature vs nurture: are leaders born or made? A behavior genetic investigation of leadership style, *Twin Res* 1:216-223, 1998.

Sher L: Short note: behavioral genetic research: achievements and concerns, *Med Hypotheses* 50:265-266, 1998.

Thapar A, Holmes J, Poulton K, et al: Genetic basis of attention deficit and hyperactivity, *Br J Psychiatry* 174:105-111, 1999.

True WR, Xian H, Scherrer JF, et al: Common genetic vulnerability for nicotine and alcohol dependence in men, *Arch Gen Psychiatry* 56:655-661, 1999.

Wertz JS, Beckwith J: Genetic fatalism and social policy: the implications of behavior genetics research, *Yale J Biol Med* 66:511-524, 1993.

Weyher HF: Contributions to the history of psychology. CXII. Intelligence, behavior genetics, and the Pioneer Fund, *Psychol Rep* 82:1347-1374, 1993.

## 15.   Religion and Theology

Baylor College of Medicine, Texas Medical Center, Houston: Genetics, religion and ethics project, *Hum Gene Ther* 3:525-527, 1992.

Bell M, Stonemann Z: Reactions to prenatal testing: reflection of religiosity and attitudes toward abortion and people with disabilities, *Am J Ment Retard* 105:1-13, 2000.

Eisenberg VH, Schnenker JG: The ethical, legal and religious aspects of preembryo research, *Eur J Obstet Gynecol Reprod Biol* 75:11-24, 1997.

Eisenberg VH, Schnenker JG: Genetic engineering: moral aspects and control of practice, *J Assist Reprod Genet* 14:297-316, 1997.

Evans MI, Drugan A: Attitudes on the ethics of abortion, sex selection, and selective pregnancy termination among health care professionals, ethicists, and clergy likely to encounter such situations, *Am J Obstet Gynecol* 164:1092-1099, 1991.

Gustafson JM: A Christian perspective on genetic engineering, *Hum Gene Ther* 5:747-754, 1994.

Ismail MS: Serour GI: Assisted reproductive medicine: current Islamic bioethical rules, *Eur J Contracept Reprod Health Care* 2:161-165, 1997.

Lysaught MT: From clinic to congregation: religious communities and genetic medicine, *Christian Scholar's Review* 23:329-348, 1994.

Perlin E: Jewish bioethics and medical genetics, *J Religion Health* 33:333-340, 1994.

Peters T: "Playing God" and germline intervention, *J Med Philos* 20:365-386, 1995.

Stone R: Religious leaders oppose patenting genes and animals, *Science* 268:1126, 1995.

## 16. Conceptual Issues

### 16.1 Health and Disease

Boyle PJ: Genetic grammar: 'Health, Illness' and the Human Genome Project, *Hastings Cent Rep* 22(4):S1, 1992.

Hubbard R: Transparent women, visible genes, and new conceptions of disease, *Camb Q Healthc Ethics* 4:291-295, 1995.

Lippman A: Twice told tales: stories about genetic disorders, *Am J Hum Genet* 151:936-937, 1992.

### 16.2 Normalcy and Disability

Silvers A: Damaged goods: does disability disqualify people from just health care? *Mt Sinai J Med* 62:102-111, 1995.

Silvers A: Reconciling equality to difference: caring or justice for people with disabilities, *Hypatia* 10:30-55, 1995.

Strudler A: The social construction of genetic abnormality: ethical implications for managerial decisions in the workplace, *J Business Ethics* 13:839-848, 1994.

### 16.3 Species

Anderson WF: Genetic engineering and our humanness, *Hum Gene Ther* 5:755-760, 1994.

Hamilton MP: Genetic engineering and humanness: a revolutionary prospect, *Hum Gene Ther* 5:745-746, 1994.

### 16.4 Identity

Brock DW: The non-identity problem and genetic harm: the case of wrongful handicaps, *Bioethics* 9:269-275, 1995.

Elliot R: Identity and the ethics of gene therapy, *Bioethics* 7:27-40, 1993.

Levin M: A formal treatment of gene identity, genetic causation, and related notions, *Behav Philos* 22:49-58, 1994.

## 17. Diseases and Disorders

### 17.1 Huntington Disease

Almqvist EW, Bloch M, Brinkman R, et al: A worldwide assessment of the frequency of suicide, suicide attempts, or psychiatric hospitalization after predictive testing for Huntington disease, *Am J Hum Genet* 64:1293-1304, 1999.

Burgess MM, Adam S, Bloch M, et al: Dilemmas of anonymous predictive testing for Huntington disease: privacy vs. optimal care, *Am J Med Genet* 71:197-201, 1997.

Campodonico JR, Aylward E, Codori AM, et al: When does Huntington's disease begin? *J Int Neuropsychol Soc* 4:467-473, 1998.

Hayes CV: Genetic testing for Huntington's disease: a family issue, *N Engl J Med* 327:1449-1451, 1992.

Jankovic I, Beach J, Ashizawa T: Emotional and functional impact of DNA testing on patients with symptoms of Huntington's disease, *J Med Genet* 32:516-518, 1995.

Kirkwood SC, Siemers E, Stout JC, et al: Longitudinal cognitive and motor changes among presymptomatic Huntington disease gene carriers, *Arch Neurol* 56:563-568, 1999.

Klimek ML, Rohs G, Young L, et al: Multidisciplinary approach to management of a hereditary neurodegenerative disorder: Huntington disease, *Axone* 19:34-38, 1997.

Marder K, Zhao H, Myers RH, et al: Rate of functional decline in Huntington's disease, Huntington study group, *Neurology* 54:452-458, 2000.

Reddy PH, Williams M, Tagle DA: Recent advances in understanding the pathogenesis of Huntington disease, *Trends Neurosci* 22:248-255, 1999.

Rohs G, Klimek ML: Ethical, social and legal issues in Huntington disease: the nurse's role, *Axone* 17:55-59, 1996.

Sharpe NF: Presymptomatic testing for Huntington disease: is there a duty to test those under the age of eighteen years? *Am J Med Genet* 46:250-253, 1993.

Sharpe NF: Informed consent and Huntington disease: a model for communication, *Am J Med Genet* 50:239-246, 1994.

Walsh A: Presymptomatic testing for Huntington's disease: the role of genetic counseling, *Med Health RI* 82:168-170, 1999.

Wexler N: Genetics session: the human genome. Prognostications and predispositions, *Ann NY Acad Sci* 882:22-31, 1999.

Williams JK, Schutte DL, Evers CA, et al: *Image J Nurs Sch* 31:109-114, 1999.

**17.2 Breast Cancer**

Blackwood MA, Weber BL: BRCA1 and BRCA2: from molecular genetics to clinical medicine, *J Clin Oncol* 16:1969-1977, 1998.

Cassel CK: Breast cancer screening in older women: ethical issues, *J Gerontol* 47:126-130, 1992.

Coughlin SS, Khourly MJ, Steinberg KK: BRCA1 and BRCA2 gene mutations and risk of breast cancer: health perspectives, *Am J Prev Med* 16:91-98, 1999.

Fodor FH, Weston A, Bleiweiss IJ, et al: Frequency and carrier risk associated with common BRCA1 and BRCA2 mutations in Ashkenazi Jewish breast cancer patients, *Am J Hum Genet* 63:45-51, 1998.

Geller G, Bernhardt BA, Doksum T, et al: Decision-making about breast cancer susceptibility testing: how similar are the attitudes of physicians, nurse practitioners, and at-risk women, *J Clin Oncol* 16:2868-2876, 1998.

Geller G, Doksum T, Bernhardt BA, et al: Participation in breast cancer susceptibility testing protocols: influence of recruitment source, altruism, and family involvement on women's decisions, *Cancer Epidemiol Biomarkers Prev* 8:377-383, 1999.

Grann VR, Whang W, Jacobson JS, et al: Benefits and costs of screening Ashkenazi Jewish women for BRCA1 and BRCA2, *J Clin Oncol* 17:494-500, 1999.

Johns Hopkins School of Hygiene and Public Health: Epidemiology, prevention, and early detection of breast cancer, *Curr Opin Oncol* 10:492-497, 1998.

Kutner SE: Breast cancer genetics and managed care: the Kaiser Permanente experience, *Cancer* 86(suppl 1):2570-2574, 1999.

Lerman C, Hughes C, Lemon SJ, et al: What you don't know can hurt you: adverse psychologic effects in members of BRCA1-linked and BRCA2-linked families who decline genetic testing, *J Clin Oncol* 16:1640-1644, 1998.

Lerner BH: Great expectations: historical perspectives on genetic breast cancer testing, *Am J Public Health* 89:938-944, 1999.

Lessick M, Wickham R, Rewaldt M: Breast and ovarian cancer: genetic update and implications for nursing, *Medsurg Nurs* 6:341-349, 1997.

Mogilner A, Otten M, Cunningham JD, et al: Awareness and attitudes concerning BRCA gene testing, *Ann Surg Oncol* 5:607-612, 1998.

Rowley PT, Loader S: Attitudes of obstetrician-gynecologists toward DNA testing for a genetic susceptibility to breast cancer, *Obstet Gynecol* 88:611-615, 1996.

Wilcox-Honnold PM: Breast cancer and gene testing: risk, rationale, and responsibilities of primary care providers, *Prim Care Pract* 2:271-283, 1998.

**17.3 Down Syndrome**

Bromley B, Shipp T, Benacerraf BR: Genetic sonogram scoring index: accuracy and clinical utility, *J Ultrasound Med* 18:523-528, 1999.

Cole LA, Shahabi S, Oz UA, et al: Urinary screening tests for fetal Down syndrome. II. Hyperglycosylated hCG, *Prenat Diagn* 19:351-359, 1999.

Glover NM, Clover SJ: Ethical and legal issues regarding selective abortion of fetuses with Down syndrome, *Ment Retard* 14:207-214, 1996.

Spong CY, Ghidini A, Stanley-Christian H, et al: Risk of abnormal triple screen for Down syndrome is significantly higher in patients with female fetuses, *Prenat Diagn* 19:337-339, 1999.

University of Leeds, UK: Same day diagnosis of Down's syndrome and sex in single cells using multiplex fluorescent PCR, *Mol Pathol* 51:164-167, 1998.

Verma L, Macdonald F, Leedham P, et al: Rapid and simple prenatal DNA diagnosis of Down's syndrome, *Lancet* 352:9-12, 1998.

Wald NJ, Watt HC, Hackshaw AK: Integrated screening for Down's syndrome on the basis of tests performed during the first and second trimesters, *N Engl J Med* 341:461-467, 1999.

**17.4 Alzheimer Disease**

Antuono P, Beyer J: The burden of dementia: a medical and research perspective, *Theor Med Bioeth* 20:3-13, 1999.

Burgess MM: Ethical issues in genetic testing for Alzheimer disease: lessons from Huntington's disease, *Alzheimer Dis Assoc Disord* 8:71-78, 1994.

Cassel CK: Genetic testing and Alzheimer disease: ethical issues for providers and families, *Alzheimer Dis Assoc Disord* 12(suppl 3):S16-S20, 1998.

Coon DW, Davies H, McKibben C, Gallagher-Thompson D: The psychological impact of genetic testing for Alzheimer disease, *Genet Test* 3:121-131, 1999.

Daw EW, Heath SC, Wijsman EM: Multipoint oligogenic analysis of age-at-onset data with applications to Alzheimer disease, *Am J Hum Genet* 64:839-851, 1999.

Emilien G, Maloteaux J, Beyreuther K, et al: Alzheimer disease: mouse models pave the way for therapeutic opportunities, *Arch Neurol* 57:176-181, 2000.

Koenig BA, Silvererg HL: Understanding probabilistic risk in predisposition genetic testing for Alzheimer disease, *Genet Test* 3:55-63, 1999.

McConnell LM, Goldstein MK: The application of medical decision analysis to genetic testing: an introduction, *Genet Test* 3:65-70, 1999.

McConnell LM, Koenig BA, Greely HT, et al: Genetic testing and Alzheimer disease: has the time come? Alzheimer Disease Working Group of the Stanford Program in Genomics, Ethics & Society, *Nat Med* 4:757-759, 1998.

McConnell LM, Sanders GD, Owens DK: Evaluation of genetic test: APOE genotyping for the diagnosis of Alzheimer disease, *Genet Test* 3:47-53, 1999.

Rogaeva E, Premkumar S, Song Y, et al: Evidence for an Alzheimer disease susceptibility locus on chromosome 12 and for further locus heterogeneity, *JAMA* 280:614-618, 1998.

Samuels SC, Davis KL: Experimental approaches to cognitive disturbance in Alzheimer's disease, *Harv Rev Psychiatry* 6:11-22, 1998.

Schuttle DL: Genetic testing in Alzheimer's disease: benefits, risks and public policy, *J Gerontol Nurs* 24:17-23, 1998.

St George-Hyslop PH: Molecular genetics of Alzheimer's disease, *Biol Psychiatry* 47:183-199, 2000.

Tobin SL, Chun N, Powell TM, et al: The genetics of Alzheimer disease and the application of molecular tests, *Genet Test* 3:37-45, 1999.

Vladeck BC: Genetic testing for Alzheimer disease: a view from Washington, *Alzheimer Dis Assoc Disorder* 12(suppl 3):S29-S32, 1998.

Wu Z, Kinslow C, Pettigrew KD, et al: Role of familial factors in late-onset Alzheimer disease as a function of age, *Alzheimer Dis Assoc Disord* 12:190-197, 1998.

## 17.5 Vascular and Arterial Disease

Chang MW, Leiden JM: Gene therapy for vascular proliferative disorders, *Semin Interv Cardiol* 1:185-193, 1996.

Dominiczak AF, Negrin DC, Clark JS, et al: Genes and hypertension: from gene mapping in experimental models to vascular gene transfer strategies, *Hypertension* 35:164-172, 2000.

Duckers HJ, Nabel EG: Gene therapy for coronary artery disease: the University of Michigan program *Semin Interv Cardiol* 3:201-204, 1998.

Isner JM, Feldman LJ: Gene therapy for arterial disease, *Lancet* 344:1653-1654, 1994.

Isner JM, Walsh K, Symes J, et al: Arterial gene therapy for therapeutic angiogenesis in patients with peripheral artery disease, *Circulation* 91:2687-2692, 1995.

Kibbe M, Billar T, Tzeng E: Gene therapy and vascular disease, *Adv Pharmacol* 46:85-150, 1999.

Kullo IJ, Simari RD, Schwartz RS: Vascular gene transfer: from bench to bedside, *Arterioscler Thromb Vasc Biol* 19:196-207, 1999.

Losordo DW, Vale PR, Isner JM: Gene therapy for myocardial angiogenesis, *Am Heart J* 138:132-141, 1999.

Matsumura JS, Kim R, Shively VP: Characterization of vascular gene transfer using a novel cationic lipid, *J Surg Res* 85:339-345, 1999.

Meyerson SL, Schwartz LB: Gene therapy as a therapeutic intervention for vascular disease, *J Cardiovasc Nurs* 13:91-109, 1999.

Nabel EG: Gene therapy for cardiovascular disease, *Circulation* 91:541-548, 1995.

Rabbani R, Topol EJ: Strategies to achieve coronary arterial plaque stabilization, *Cardiovasc Res* 41:402-417, 1999.

Rosengart TK, Lee YL, Patel SR, et al: Angiogenesis gene therapy: phase I assessment of direct intramyocardial administration of an adenovirus vector expressing VEGF121 cDNA to individuals with clinically significant severe coronary artery disease, *Circulation* 100:468-474, 1999.

Rowland RT, Cleveland JC Jr, Meng X, et al: Potential gene therapy strategies in the treatment of cardiovascular disease, *Ann Thorac Surg* 60:721-728, 1995.

Svensson EC, Schwartz LB: Gene therapy for vascular disease, *Curr Opin Cardiol* 13:369-374, 1998.

Tio RA, Isner JM, Walsh K: Gene therapy to prevent restenosis, the Boston experience, *Semin Interv Cardiol* 3:205-210, 1998.

**17.6 Neurofibromatosis**

Bance M, Ramsden RT: Management of neurofibromatosis type 2, *Ear Nose Throat J* 78:91-94, 1999.

Brewer VR, Moore BD, Hiscock M: Learning disability subtypes in children with neurofibromatosis, *J Learn Disabil* 30:521-533, 1997.

Davis RE: Diagnosing neurofibromatosis type I in children, *Nurse Pract* 22:73-76, 1997.

Evans DG: Neurofibromatosis type 2: genetic and clinical features, *Ear Nose Throat J* 78:97-100, 1999.

Gabriel KR: Neurofibromatosis, *Curr Opin Pediatr* 9:89-93, 1997.

Johnson NS, Saal HM, Lovell AM, et al: Social and emotional problems in children with neurofibromatosis type 1: evidence and proposed interventions, *J Pediatr* 134:767-772, 1999.

Kulkantrakorn K, Geller TJ: Seizures in neurofibromatosis, *Pediatr Neurol* 19:347-350, 1998.

Mayo Clinic, Department of Medical Genetics; Neurofibromatosis: a common neurocutaneous disorder, *Mayo Clin Proc* 73:1071-1076, 1998.

Zvulunov A, Weitz R, Metzker A: Neurofibromatosis type 1 in childhood: evaluation of clinical and epidemiologic features as predictive factors for severity, *Clin Pediatr (Phila)* 37:295-299, 1998.

**17.7 Psychiatric Disorders**

Barondes SH: An agenda for psychiatric genetics, *Arch Gen Psychiatry* 56:549-552, 1999.

DeLisi LE, Crow TJ: Chromosome workshops 1998: current state of psychiatric linkage, *Am J Med Genet* 88:215-218, 1999.

Ginns EI, St Jean P, Philibert RA, et al: A genome-wide search for chromosomal loci linked to mental health wellness in relative at high risk for bipolar affective disorder among the Old Order Amish, *Proc Natl Acad Sci USA* 95:15531-15536, 1998.

Madrid A, Marachi JP: Medical assessment: its role in comprehensive psychiatric evaluation, *Child Adolesc Psychiatr Clin N Am* 8:257-270, 1999.

Owen MJ, Cardno AG: Psychiatric genetics: progress, problems, and potential, *Lancet* 354(suppl 1):SI11-SI14, 1999.

Pulver AE: Search for schizophrenia susceptibility genes, *Biol Psychiatry* 47:221-230, 2000.

Rutter M Silberg J, O'Connor T, Simonoff E: Genetics and child psychiatry. I. Advances in quantitative and molecular genetics, *J Child Psychol Psychiatry* 40:3-18, 1999.

**17.8 Phenylketonuria**

Chang TM, Prakash S: Therapeutic uses of microencapsulated genetically engineered cells, *Mol Med Today* 4:221-227, 1998.

Koch R, Moseley K, Ning J, et al: Long-term beneficial effects of the phenylalanine-restricted diet in late-diagnosed individuals with phenylketonuria, *Mol Genet Metab* 67:148-155, 1999.

Sarkissian CN, Shao Z, Blain F: A different approach to treatment of phenylketonuria degradation with recombinant phenylalanine ammonia lyase, *Proc Natl Acad Sci USA* 96:2339-2344, 1999.

Waisbren SE, Hamilton BD, St. James PJ, et al: Psychological factors in maternal phenylketonuria: women's adherence to medical recommendations, *Am J Public Health* 85:1636-1641, 1995.

Waisbren SE, Hanley W, Levy HL, et al: Outcome at age 4 years in offspring of women with maternal phenylketonuria: the Maternal PKU Collaborative Study, *JAMA* 283:756-762, 2000.

**17.9 Infectious Disease**

Bunnell BA, Morgan RA: Gene therapy for infectious diseases, *Clin Microbiol Rev* 11:42-56, 1998.

Colacino JM, Staschke KA: The identification and development of antiviral agents for the treatment of chronic hepatitis B virus infection, *Prog Drug Res* 50:259-322, 1998.

Curiel TJ, Piche A, Kasono K, et al: Gene therapy strategies for AIDS-related malignancies, *Gene Ther* 4:1284-1288, 1997.

Rondon IJ, Marasco WA: Intracellular antibodies (intrabodies) for gene therapy of infectious diseases, *Annu Rev Microbiol* 51:257-283, 1997.

Schraufnagel DE: Tuberculosis treatment for the beginning of the next century, *Int J Tuberc Lung Dis* 3:651-662, 1999.

**17.10 Thalassemia**

Dover GJ: Hemoglobin switching protocols in thalassemia: experience with sodium phenyl-butyrate and hydroxyurea, *Ann NY Acad Sci* 850:80-86, 1998.

Kuliev A, Rechitsky S, Verlinsky O, et al: Preimplantation diagnosis of thalassemias, *J Assist Reprod Genet* 15:219-225, 1998.

Trent RJ, Le H, Yu B: Prenatal diagnosis for thalassaemia in a multicultural society, *Prenat Diagn* 18:591-598, 1998.

Weatherall DJ: Thalassemia in the next millennium: keynote address, *Ann NY Acad Sci* 850:1-9, 1998.

**17.11 Cystic Fibrosis**

Glavac D, Ravnik-Glavak M, Potocnik U, et al: Screening methods for cystic fibrosis transmembrane conductance regulator (CFTR) gene mutations in non-human primates, *Pfluger Arch* 439(suppl 3):R12-R13, 2000.

Grubb BR, Boucher RC: Pathophysiology of gene-targeted mouse models for cystic fibrosis, *Physiol Rev* 79(suppl 1):S193-S214, 1999.

Hull J, Thomas AH: Contribution of genetic factors other than CFTR to disease severity in cystic fibrosis, *Thorax* 53:1018-1021, 1998.

Johns Hopkins Hospital, Dept of Pediatrics: Therapies directed at the basic defect in cystic fibrosis, *Clin Chest Med* 19:515-525, 1998.

Levenkron JC, Loader S, Rowley PT: Carrier screening for cystic fibrosis: test acceptance and one year follow-up, *Am J Med Genet* 73:378-386, 1997.

Lieu TA, Watson SE, Washington AE: The cost-effectiveness of prenatal carrier screening for cystic fibrosis, *Obstet Gynecol* 84:903-912, 1994.

Loader S, Caldwell P, Kozyra A, et al: Cystic fibrosis carrier population screening in the primary care setting, *Am J Hum Genet* 59:234-247, 1996.

Mennie ME, Compton ME, Filfillan A, et al: Prenatal screening for cystic fibrosis: psychological effects on carriers and their partners, *J Med Genet* 30:543-548, 1993.

Mennuti MT, Thomson E, Press N: Screening for cystic fibrosis carrier state, *Obstet Gynecol* 93:456-461, 1999.

Mischler EH, Wilfond BS, Fost N, et al: Cystic fibrosis newborn screening: impact on reproductive behavior and implications for genetic counseling, *Pediatrics* 102:44-52, 1998.

Proceedings of a 1997 Workshop: Newborn screening for cystic fibrosis: a paradigm for public health genetics policy development, *MMWR* 46:1-24, 1997.

Resnikoff JR, Conrad DJ: Recent advances in the understanding and treatment of cystic fibrosis, *Curr Opin Pulm Med* 4:130-134, 1998.

University of Rochester School of Medicine: Prenatal screening for cystic fibrosis carriers: an economic evaluation, *Am J Hum Genet* 63:1160-1174, 1998.

Vintzileos AM, Ananth CV: A cost-effectiveness analysis of prenatal carrier screening for cystic fibrosis, *Obstet Gynecol* 91:529-534, 1998.

**17.12 Sickle Cell Disease**

Ballas SK: Complications of sickle cell anemia in adults: guidelines for effective management, *Cleve Clin J Med* 66:48-58, 1999.

Beyer JE, Platt AF, Kinney TR, et al: Practice guidelines for the assessment of children with sickle cell pain, *J Soc Pediatr Nurs* 4:61-73, 1999.

Blouin MJ, Beauchemin H, Wright A, et al: Genetic correction of sickle cell disease: insights using transgenic mouse models, *Nat Med* 6:177-182, 2000.

Noonan SS: Sickle cell patients find a brand New World, *NJ Med* 96:23-25, 1999.

Olney RS: Preventing morbidity and mortality from sickle cell disease: a public health perspective, *Am J Prev Med* 16:116-121, 1999.

Overturf GD: Infections and immunizations of children with sickle cell disease, *Adv Pediatr Infect Dis* 14:191-218, 1999.

Silbergleit R, Jancis MO, McNamara RM: Management of sickle cell pain crisis in the emergency department at teaching hospitals, *J Emerg Med* 17:625-630, 1999.

Wang WC, Langston JW, Steen RG, et al: Abnormalities of the central nervous system in very young children with sickle cell anemia, *J Pediatr* 132:994-998, 1998.

Watkins KE, Hewes DK, Connelly A, et al: Cognitive deficits associated with frontal-lobe infarction in children with sickle cell disease, *Dev Med Child Neurol* 40:536-543, 1998.

Wilson Schaeffer JJ, Gil KM, Burchinal M, et al: Depression, disease severity, and sickle cell disease, *J Behav Med* 22:115-126, 1999.

### 17.13 Tay-Sachs Disease

Akerman BR, Natowicz MR, Kaback MM, et al: Novel mutations and DNA-based screening in non-Jewish carriers of Tay-Sachs disease, *Am J Hum Genet* 60:1099-1106, 1997.

Broide E, Zeigler M, Eckstein J, et al: Screening for carriers of Tay-Sachs disease in the ultraorthodox Ashkenazi Jewish community in Israel, *Am J Med Genet* 47:213-215, 1993.

Kaplan F: Tay-Sachs disease carrier screening: a model for prevention of genetic disease, *Genet Test* 2:271-292, 1998.

Levin M: Screening Jews and genes: a consideration of the ethics of genetic screening within the Jewish community: challenges and responses, *Genet Test* 3:207-213, 1999.

Prenatal genetic carrier testing using triple disease screening, *JAMA* 278:1268-1272, 1997.

## Books and Special Journal Issues

Andrews LB, Fullarton JE, Holtzman NA, et al: *Assessing genetic risks: implications for health and social policy,* Washington, DC, 1994, National Academy Press.

Baker D, Schuette J, Uhlmann W, editors: *A guide to genetic counseling,* New York, 1999, Wiley & Sons.

Bayerz K: *GenEthics: technological intervention in human reproduction as a philosophical problem,* 1994, Cambridge, UK, Cambridge University Press.

Bennett R: *The practical guide to the genetic family history,* New York, 1999, Wiley & Sons.

Bishop JE, Waldholz M: *Genome: the story of the most astonishing scientific adventure of our time,* New York, 1990, Simon & Schuster.

Bosk CL: *All God's mistakes: genetic counseling in a pediatric hospital,* Chicago, 1992, University of Chicago Press.

Bowman JE, Murray RF Jr: *genetic variation and disorders in peoples of African origin,* Baltimore, 1990, Johns Hopkins University Press.

Briggs T, Chandler AM, editors: *Biochemistry (Oklahoma notes),* New York, 1995, Springer-Verlag.

Buyse ML, editor: *Birth defects encyclopedia: the comprehensive, systematic, illustrated reference source for the diagnosis, delineation, etiology, biodynamics, occurrence, prevention, and treatment of human anomalies of clinical relevance,* Cambridge, Mass, 1990, Blackwell.

Chadwick D, Bock G, Whelan J, editors: *Human genetic information: science, law and ethics,* Chichester, UK, 1990, Wiley & Sons.

Chadwick RF, Shickle D, Henk AM, et al, editors: *The ethics of genetic screening,* Norwell, Mass, 1999, Kluwer.

Chirban JT, editor: *Health and faith: medical, psychological and religious dimensions,* Lanhan, Md, 1991, University Press of America.

Fisher NL: *Multicultural awareness in genetic counseling: a guide for genetics professionals,* Baltimore, 1995, Johns Hopkins University Press.

Fisher NL, editor: *Cultural and ethnic diversity,* Baltimore, 1996, Johns Hopkins University Press.

Fortun M, Mendelsohn E, editors: *The practices of human genetics,* New York, 1999, Kluwer.

Frankel MS, Reich A, editors: *The genetic frontier: ethics, law and policy,* Washington, DC, 1994, American Association for the Advancement of Science.

Gelehrter TD, Collins FS, Ginsburg D: *Principles of medical genetics,* Baltimore, 1998, Williams & Wilkins.

Gert B, Berger EM, Cahill EF, et al: *Morality and the new genetics: a guide for students and health care providers,* Sudbury, Mass, 1998, Jones & Bartlett.

Gould LG: *Cancer and genetics: answering your patients' questions,* 1997, PRR, Inc, American Cancer Society.

Griffins AJ: *An introduction to genetic analysis,* New York, 1993, Freeman.

Holtzman NA: *Proceed with caution: predicting genetic risks in the recombinant DNA era,* Baltimore, 1989, Johns Hopkins University Press.

Holtzman NA, Watson MS, editors: *Promoting safe and effective genetic testing in the United States,* Baltimore, 1998, Johns Hopkins University Press.

Hubbard R, Wald E: *Exploding the gene myth: how genetic information is produced and manipulated by scientists, physicians, employers, insurance companies, educators, and law enforcers,* Boston, 1993, Beacon Press.

Jorde LB: *Medical genetics,* St Louis, 1997, Mosby.

Kevles D: *In the name of eugenics: genetics and the uses of human heredity,* New York, 1985, Knopf.

Kevles DJ, Hood L, editors: *The Code of codes: scientific and social issues in the Human Genome Project,* Boston, 1992, Harvard University Press.

Lea DH, Jenkins JF, Francomano CA: *Genetics in clinical practice,* Boston, 1988, Jones & Bartlett.

Lyon J, Gorner P: *Altered fates: gene therapy and the retooling of human life,* New York, 1996, Norton.

Mahowald M: *Genes, women, equality,* New York, 2000, Oxford University Press.

Mange EJ: *Basic human genetics,* Sunderland, Mass, 1994, Sinauer Associates.

McKusick VA: *Mendelian inheritance in man: a catalogue of human genes and genetic disorders,* Baltimore, 1994, Johns Hopkins University Press.

Mehlman MJ, Botkin JR: *Access to the genome: the challenge to equality,* Washington, DC, 1998, Georgetown University Press.

Nelkin D, Lindee MS: *The DNA mystique: the gene as a cultural icon,* New York, 1995, Freeman.

Parens E, editor: *Enhancing human traits: ethical and social implications,* Washington, DC, 1998, Georgetown University Press.

Peters T: *Genetic issues of social justice,* Cleveland, 1998, Pilgrim Press.

Rothblatt M: *Unzipped genes: taking charge of baby-making in the new millennium,* Philadelphia, 1997, Temple University Press.

Rothenberg KH, Thomson EJ, editors: *Women and prenatal testing: facing the challenges of genetic technology,* Columbus, 1994, Ohio State University Press.

Rothstein MA, editors: *Genetic secrets: protecting privacy and confidentiality in the genetic era,* New Haven, Conn, 1997, Yale University Press.

Seashore MR, Wappner RS: *Genetics in primary care & clinical medicine,* Stamford, Conn, 1996, Appleton & Lange.

Smith DW: *Smith's recognizable patterns of human malformation,* Philadelphia, 1988, Saunders.

Special Issue: Development biology: frontiers for clinical genetics, *Clin Genet* 57, 2000.

Symposium: Genetics and the law: the ethical, legal and social implications of genetic technology and biomedical ethics, *University of Chicago Law School Roundtable* 3(2), 1996.

Symposium: Respecting genetic privacy, *Jurimetrics* 40(1), 1999.

Thompson L: *Correcting the code: inventing the genetic cure for the human body,* New York, 1994, Simon & Schuster.

Touchette N, Holtzman NA, Davis JG, et al: *Toward the 21st century: incorporating genetics into primary health care,* Plainview, NY, 1997, Cold Spring Harbor Laboratory Press.

US Department of Health and Human Services (USDHHS), National Institutes of Health, National Center for Human Genome Research: *Review of Ethical, Legal and Social Implications Program 1990-95,* Washington, DC, 1996, USDHHS.

Vogel F, Motulsky AG: *Human genetics: problems and approaches,* New York, 1997, Springer.

Weatherall DJ: *The new genetics and clinical practice,* New York, 1991, Oxford University Press.

Wertz D, Fletcher J, editors: *Ethics and human genetics: a cross-cultural perspective,* New York, 1989, Springer-Verlag.

## Policy Statements

American Society of Human Genetics: Maternal serum alpha-fetoprotein screening programs and quality control for laboratories performing maternal serum and amniotic fluid alpha-fetoprotein assays, *Am J Hum Genet* 40:75-82, 1987.

Proposed American Society of Human Genetics Position: Mapping/sequencing the human genome, *Am J Hum Genet* 143:101-102, 1988.

Update on MSAFP Policy Statement from the American Society of Human Genetics, *Am J Hum Genet* 45:332-334, 1989.

American Society of Human Genetics: Statement on cystic fibrosis screening, *Am J Hum Genet* 46:339, 1990.

American Society of Human Genetics Social Issues Committee: Report on genetics and adoption: points to consider, *Am J Hum Genet* 48:1009-1010, 1991.

American Society of Human Genetics Committee Report: The Human Genome Project: implications for human genetics, *Am J Hum Genet* 49:687-691, 1991.

American Academy of Pediatrics: Issues in newborn screening, *Pediatrics* 89:345-348, 1992.

American Society of Human Genetics: Statement on clinical genetics and freedom of choice, *Am J Hum Genet* 48:1011, 1992.

Frederick PL et al: Recommendations on predictive testing for germ line mutations among cancer-prone individuals, *Natl Cancer Inst* 84:1156-1159, 1992.

American Society of Human Genetics: Cystic fibrosis carrier screening, *Am J Hum Genet* 51:1443-1444, 1992.

American Academy of Pediatrics: Prenatal genetic diagnosis for pediatricians, *Pediatrics* 93:1010-1015, 1994.

American Society of Human Genetics: Genetic testing for breast and ovarian cancer predisposition, *Am J Hum Genet* 55:i-iv, 1994.

Institute of Medicine Subcommittee: *Assessing genetic risks: implications for health and social policy,* Washington, DC, 1994, National Academy Press.

American Society of Human Genetics/American College of Medical Genetics Report: Points to consider: ethical, legal, and psychosocial implications of genetic testing in children and adolescents, *Am J Hum Genet* 57:1233-1241, 1995.

American Society of Human Genetics Ad Hoc Committee on Insurance Issues in Genetic Testing: Background statement: genetic testing and insurance, *Am J Hum Genet* 56:327-331, 1995.

American College of Obstetricians and Gynecologists Technical Bulletin: An educational aid to obstetricians-gynecologists, *Genet Technol* 208:10, 1995.

American Academy of Pediatrics: Newborn screening fact sheets, *Pediatrics* 98:467-472, 1996.

American Society of Clinical Oncology: Genetic testing for cancer susceptibility, *J Clin Oncol* 14:1730-1736, 1996.

American Society of Human Genetics Report: Statement on informed consent for genetic research, *Am J Hum Genet* 59:471-474, 1996.

Burke W, Dal M, Garber J, et al: Consensus statement: genetic recommendations for follow-up care of individuals with an inherited predisposition to cancer. II. BRCA1 and BRCA2, *JAMA* 277:1003, 1997.

American Academy of Pediatrics: General principles in the care of children and adolescents with genetic disorders and other chronic health conditions, *Pediatrics* 99:643-644, 1997.

American Society of Human Genetics, Social Issues Subcommittee on Familial Disclosure: Professional disclosure on familial genetic information, *Am J Hum Genet* 62:474-483, 1998.

American Society of Human Genetics/American College of Medical Genetics: Genetic testing in adoption, *Am J Hum Genet* 66:761-767, 2000.

## Electronic Resources

Many websites are devoted to individual genetic conditions. Because these sites often change, however, they are not listed here. They can be found by using any search engine. Websites should be critically reviewed because some, particularly personal sites, may contain outdated or erroneous information.

Human Genomic Epidemiology Network: http://www.cdc.gov/genetics/hugenet/ Provides review articles for various human genome topics; aimed at medical and public health professionals.

Ethical, Legal, and Social Implications Program (ELSI) home page: http://www.nhgri.nih.gov/ELSI/ Provides good information and links policy, legislation, and funding opportunities.

ELSI materials: http://www.ornl.gov/hgmis/resource/elsi.html Provides news and information regarding ethical, legal, and social implications regarding genetics research.

ELSI in science: http://www.lbl.gov/Education/ELSI/ELSI.html Contains teaching modules designed to stimulate discussion on the implications of scientific research.

Genetic and biological resources links: www.er.doe.gov/production/ober/bioinfo center.html Provides links regarding the Human Genome Project.

Genetics glossary: http://www.kumc.edu/gec/glossnew.html Provides a list of genetics glossaries.

Gene tests: www.genetests.org Formerly "Helix"; provides a database of laboratories doing various genetic tests for diagnostics or only for research.

Gene Clinics: www.geneclinics.org Contains a collection of review and summary articles about genetic diseases; aimed at primary care physicians.

Gene therapy: http://www.mc.vanderbilt.edu/gcrc/gene/ index.html Provides a web course covering the basics of gene therapy with related links.

National Institutes of Health Office of Biotechnology Activities: http://www.nih.gov/od/oba/ Includes the former DNA Recombinant Advisory Committee (gene transfer, gene therapy) and the secretary's advisory committees on genetic testing and xenotransplantation.

National Human Genome Research Institute: www.nhgri.nih.gov Provides a wide variety of information, including genetic research, grant information, conferences, and news.

Primer on molecular genetics: www.ornl.gov/hgmis/publicat/primer/intro.html http://www.ornl.gov/hgmis/TRCAL.HTML Includes a calendar of training courses and workshops.

Human Genome Project publications: http://www.ornl.gov/hgmis/pulicat/publications. html

To Know Ourselves: http://www.ornl.gov/hgmis/publicat/tko/index. html Provides a review of the U.S. Department of Energy's (DOE's) role, history, and achievements in the Human Genome Project.

Educational resources: www.ornl.gov/hgmis/resource/education.html Provides news, information, and teaching materials regarding the Human Genome Project.

National Bioethics Advisory Committee home page:
http://www.bioethics.gov
Offers advice to the National Science and Technology Council and others on bioethical issues related to human biology and behavior.

*Online Mendelian Inheritance in Man* (OMIM):
http://www.ncbi.nlm.nih.gov/Omim
Provides a comprehensive, authoritative, and up-to-date human gene and genetic disorder catalog that supports medical genetics and the Human Genome Project.

*Promoting Safe and Effective Genetic Testing in the United States* (1997):
http://www.med.jhu.edu/tfgtelsi
Provides principles and recommendations by a joint NIH-DOE Human Genome Project group that examined the development and provision of gene tests in the United States.

Users' guide to genetics:
www.nhgri.nih.gov/DIR/VIP/SI/schedule.html
Contains a series of expert lectures done at the Smithsonian Institution.

Human gene testing:
www4.nas.edu/beyond/discovery.nsf/web/gene
Independent article that discusses the history of gene discovery and issues of testing; colon cancer treated specifically; good internal links.

US Department of Energy Human Genome Project home page:
www.ornl.gov/TechResource/HumanGenome/home.html

Healthweb:
www.healthweb.org

# INDEX